ENVIRONMENTAL DATA HANDLING
Georege B. Heaslip

THE MEASUREMENT OF AIRBORNE PARTICLES
Richard D. Cadle

ANALYSIS OF AIR POLLUTANTS
Peter O. Warner

ENVIRONMENTAL INDICES
Herbert Inhaber

URBAN COSTS OF CLIMATE MODIFICATION
Terry A. Ferrar, Editor

CHEMICAL CONTROL OF INSECT BEHAVIOR: THEORY AND
APPLICATION
H. H. Shorey and John J. McKelvey, Jr.

MERCURY CONTAMINATION: A HUMAN TRAGEDY
Patricia A. D'Itri and Frank M. D'Itri

POLLUTANTS AND HIGH RISK GROUPS
Edward J. Calabrese

SULFUR IN THE ENVIRONMENT, Parts I and II
Jerome O. Nriagu

ENERGY UTILIZATION AND ENVIRONMENTAL HEALTH
Richard A. Wadden, Editor

METHODOLOGICAL APPROACHES TO DERIVING ENVIRONMENTAL
AND OCCUPATIONAL HEALTH STANDARDS
Edward J. Calabrese

FOOD, CLIMATE, AND MAN
Margaret R. Biswas and Asit K. Biswas, Editors

CHEMICAL CONCEPTS IN POLLUTANT BEHAVIOR
Ian J. Tinsley

RESOURCE RECOVERY AND RECYCLING
A. F. M. Barton

QUANTITATIVE TOXICOLOGY
V. A. Filov, A. A. Golubev, E. I. Liublina, and N. A. Tolokontsev

QUANTITATIVE TOXICOLOGY

QUANTITATIVE TOXICOLOGY

(*Kolichestvennaya Toksikologiya*)

Selected Topics

V. A. FILOV

Sc.D.(Biol.), Chief, Experimental Laboratory, N. N. Petrov Institute of Oncology, Leningrad

A. A. GOLUBEV, M.D. (deceased)

E. I. LIUBLINA

Sc.D.(Biol.), Senior Scientific Worker, Laboratory for Industrial Toxicology, Institute of Industrial Hygiene and Occupational Diseases, Leningrad

N. A. TOLOKONTSEV

M.D., Chief, Human Ecology Section, Institute for Socioeconomic Problems, Leningrad

A Revised and Enlarged text
based on the 1973 Russian Edition
Translated by V. E. Tatarchenko

A WILEY-INTERSCIENCE PUBLICATION
JOHN WILEY & SONS
New York · Chichester · Brisbane · Toronto

Library of Congress Cataloging in Publication Data

Main entry under title:
Quantitative toxicology.
   (Environmental science and technology)

   Translation of a rev. and enl. text based on the 1973 ed.
of Kolichestvennaya toksikologiya by V. A. Filov and others.
   "A Wiley-Interscience publication."
   Bibliography pp. 422–447
   Includes index.
   1. Industrial toxicology—Mathematical models.
I. Filov, Vladimir Aleksandrovich, and others. II. Kolichestvennaya
toksikologiya. III. Tible. [DNLM: 1. Industrial
medicine. 2. Poisons. 3. Poisoning.
WA465 Q15]

RA1229. Q3613   615.9′02   78-12530
ISBN 0-471-02109-1

Printed in the United States of America
10 9 8 7 6 5 4 3 2 1

To the Memory of our Teacher, Professor Nikolai V. Lazarev

SERIES PREFACE

Environmental Science and Technology

The Environmental Science and Technology Series of Monographs, Textbooks, and Advances is devoted to the study of the quality of the environment and to the technology of its conservation. Environmental science therefore relates to the chemical, physical, and biological changes in the environment through contamination or modification, to the physical nature and biological behavior of air, water, soil, food, and waste as they are affected by man's agricultural, industrial, and social activities, and to the application of science and technology to the control and improvement of environmental quality.

The deterioration of environmental quality, which began when man first collected into villages and utilized fire, has existed as a serious problem under the ever-increasing impacts of exponentially increasing population and of industrializing society. Environmental contamination of air, water, soil, and food has become a threat to the continued existence of many plant and animal communities of the ecosystem and may ultimately threaten the very survival of the human race.

It seems clear that if we are to preserve for future generations some semblance of the biological order of the world of the past and hope to improve on the deteriorating standards of urban public health, environmental science and technology must quickly come to play a dominant role in designing our social and industrial structure for tomorrow. Scientifically rigorous criteria of environmental quality must be developed. Based in part on these criteria, realistic standards must be established and our technological progress must be tailored to meet them. It is obvious that civilization will continue to require increasing amounts of fuel, transportation, industrial chemicals, fertilizers, pesticides, and countless other products; and that it will continue to produce waste products of all descriptions.

What is urgently needed is a total systems approach to modern civilization through which the pooled talents of scientists and engineers, in cooperation with social scientists and the medical profession, can be focused on the development of order and equilibrium in the presently disparate segments of the human environment. Most of the skills and tools that are needed are already in existence. We surely have a right to hope a technology that has created such manifold environmental problems is also capable of solving them. It is our hope that this Series in Environmental Sciences and Technology will not only serve to make this challenge more explicit to the established professionals, but that it also will help to stimulate the student toward the career opportunities in this vital area.

Robert L. Metcalf
James N. Pitts, Jr.
Werner Stumm

PREFACE TO THE
1973 RUSSIAN EDITION

Toxicology as a science is now more than a century old. At first it was of necessity a purely descriptive discipline; but as more and more facts accumulated, there arose an urgent need to make generalizations, and this required an increasing use of various quantitative methods. It is precisely the wide application of these methods, which in recent years have been penetrating into many other biological disciplines, that has imparted to toxicology a truly scientific character by making it possible to derive many important and orderly relationships from an abundance of scattered factual data. It is gratifying to realize that many of these relationships have found practical applicability. Of great importance for the various branches of toxicology, including industrial toxicology, is the growing possibility of predicting the pattern and magnitude of toxic action of chemical agents from the results of simple and rapid tests or even without resorting to experiment at all. Physical and mathematical modeling of the complex interactions between poisons and living organisms is also becoming a reality.

R. P. Feynman, an outstanding physicist and Nobel Laureate, has said, "Science is only useful if it tells you about some experiment that has not been done" (*The Character of Physical Law*, The M.I.T. Press, Cambridge, Mass., 1967, p. 164). It may be stated that quantitative methods are making toxicology such a science to a large extent.

Although the various individual aspects of quantitative toxicology have for a relatively long time been dealt with in journal articles, conference papers and abstracts, contributions to nonperiodical publications, and so on, the relevant information remains widely scattered in the literature. The time seems ripe for an attempt to sum up the results of work accomplished by various authors, to arrange systematically the information amassed, and to demonstrate its possible practical applications. This monograph represents such an attempt.

A book of this size cannot be expected to encompass all the facets of quantitative toxicology that have been worked out in more or less detail. The presentation is therefore confined to selected topics covering what appear to be the more important, though by no means all, developments in quantitative toxicology. Also discussed are some theoretical aspects of toxicology that as yet cannot be dealt with in quantitative terms but are deemed worthy of consideration either because they have served as a basis for revealing sustained quantitative relationships in the action of poisons on the living organism or because they point out some of the paths to be followed by quantitative toxicology.

Chapters 1, 2, and 6 were written by N. A. Tolokontsev; Chapters 3 and 4 by V. A. Filov; Chapter 5 by E. I. Liublina; Chapter 7 by A. A. Golubev, V. A. Filov, and E. I. Liublina; and Chapter 8 by E. I. Liublina and A. A. Golubev.

The authors will welcome any suggestions and criticisms regarding the choice and treatment of the topics included in the book.

PREFACE TO THE
ENGLISH-LANGUAGE EDITION

This book appears to have been the first attempt to present a systematic account of the more important quantitative aspects of toxicology, mainly industrial toxicology. It has been well received in the USSR and some East European countries. We were gratified to be requested to prepare the book for publication in the United States.

The substantial progress made in quantitative toxicology since the book was first published in Russian in 1973 has necessitated its revision and considerable expansion. Since most of the material contained in the original edition has not grown obsolete, the structure of the book has been retained, and the revision has mainly involved corrections, deletions, and short additions, as well as updating of the text where necessary. The bulk of new material is contained in the addenda to the various chapters, where most of the topics discussed in the main text are elaborated on and other aspects not covered there are included. The main text of the book is therefore independent of the addenda and may be read separately.

Addenda have been prepared to all chapters except Chapter 3; the subject discussed therein appears to have been exhausted, and no further developments have occurred. The addendum to Chapter 6 consists of two parts, concerned, respectively, with combined and complex exposures to poisons.

In addition to toxicologists as such, the book is intended for environmental specialists and hygienists and, we hope, may be found useful by pharmacologists, sanitary chemists, biochemists, and indeed by all those interested in the problems of interaction between xenobiotics and the living organism or between pollutants and the biosphere. The latter aspect deserves a few words of special mention.

In the face of the ever-growing pollution of the biosphere with a multitude of chemicals, many of which are detrimental to human health and deteriorate the natural environment, it is inevitable that problems of toxicology draw the attention of many specialists from allied fields of science. A consequence of this "movement into toxicology" has been its mathematization, an increasing reliance on quantitative methods for the tackling of both traditional (dose-time-response relationships, joint action of poisons, etc.) and relatively new problems of toxicology relating to toxicokinetics, cumulation and adaptation, migration of substances in the various components of the environment, evaluation of multiple and complex exposures, determination of permissible burdens on the environment and on man, and many other aspects, including the creation of mathematical models of the environment on which to base scientifically sound strategies of environmental monitoring and quality control. A good illustration of the introduction of quantitative methods into toxicology and of its conversion into a global discipline can be seen in the proceedings of the Soviet-American Symposia on the Comprehensive Analysis of the Environment held in 1974 (Tbilisi, USSR) and 1975 (Honolulu, Hawaii).

One final remark is in order. This book cannot be regarded as an all-embracing account of current theoretic concepts, methods, or results in quantitative toxicology. Also, along with quantitative aspects, it contains some of a qualitative nature, but these have been included solely for the purpose of showing that a given property, mechanism, or condition has to be taken into account in the quantitative study of toxic effect.

Throughout the process of revising the book and preparing the addenda we have constantly missed the logical thinking and expertise of Alexander A. Golubev, one of the authors of the original edition, who died in 1972.

We will consider our objective fulfilled if those wishing to become acquainted with the quantitative aspects of toxicology find the book useful and, perhaps more important, if it provides a stimulus to the advancement of this important and exciting field of study.

The authors wish to express their gratitude to V. E. Tatarchenko for his technical assistance in preparation of the Russian text and for his translation of it into English.

V. A. FILOV
E. I. LIUBLINA
N. A. TOLOKONTSEV

Leningrad, USSR
September 1978

CONTENTS

1. **The Toxic Effect as a Result of Interaction between the Poison and the Living Organism**   1

    1. Species Differences in Sensitivity to Poisons   1
    2. Sex Differences in Sensitivity to Poisons   3
    3. Age and the Toxic Effect   5
    4. Individual Variations in Sensitivity to Poisons   6
    5. Biorhythms and the Toxic Effect   6
    6. Route of Absorption and Exposure Regimen   10
    7. Effect of Some Environmental Factors on the Action of Poisons   13
    Addendum: On Species Differences in Sensitivity to Poisons 15

2. **The Relationship between Amount of Poison and Toxic Effect** 23

    1. Introduction   23
    2. Lethal Doses and Concentrations   26
    3. Threshold Doses and Concentrations   31
    4. The Toxic Action Zone   34
    5. Maximum Permissible Doses and Concentrations   39
    6. Paradoxical Effects   43
    Addendum: Dose-Time Curves   48

3. **The Equilibrium Distribution of Nonelectrolytes between the Environment and the Living Organism**   53

    1. General Considerations   53
    2. Ferguson's Principle; Elements of Thermodynamic Equilibrium   56

3. The Main Corollaries to Ferguson's Principle   60
4. Application of Ferguson's Principle to Studies on Mammals   68
5. The Problem of Real Hazards Presented by Volatile
    Substances Absorbed by Inhalation   76
6. Some Implications of the Thermodynamic Approach to the
    Study of the Absorption and Fate of Substances in the Body
    (Possible Applications of the Activity Concept in
    Biology)   85

**4. Kinetic Aspects of the Absorption and Fate of Poisons in the
    Body   94**

1. General Considerations Relating to the Absorption,
    Transformation, and Elimination of Poisons   94
2. Modeling: Scope and Purpose   104
3. Elements of Mathematical Modeling; Models for
    Absorption   110
4. Elimination   140
5. Some Methods for the Calculation of Rate Constants;
    Factors Influencing the Elimination Kinetics   164

Addendum: Toxicokinetics   170

A1. Methods of Toxicokinetics   171
A2. Nonlinear Effects in Toxicokinetics   172
    A.2.1 Quantitation of Nonlinear Effects   173
    A.2.2 Uptake of Substances by Tissues   173
    A.2.3 The Limit of Nonlinearity and Its Possible Use   181

A3. Factors Modifying Toxicokinetics   182
    A.3.1 Factors That Depend on the Biological Object   183
    A.3.2 Effect of Physiologic Variables   194
    A.3.3 Effect of Disease States   196
    A.3.4 Factors Associated with Dosage Form   201
    A.3.5 Effect of Temperature   202
    A.3.6 Toxicokinetic Aspects of Interaction between
           Xenobiotics   203
    A.3.7 Chemical Structure, Physicochemical Properties,
           and Toxicokinetics   212

A4.   Some More Particular Aspects of Toxicokinetics   218

    A.4.1   Examples of Studies on the Toxicokinetics of
           Heavy Radioactive Elements   218

    A.4.2   The Toxicokinetics of Mercury   220

    A.4.3   Trichloroethylene and Its Metabolites   225

A5.   Environmental Toxicokinetics (Ecological Toxicokinetics)   227

A6.   The Dynamics of Uptake of Xenobiotics into Tissues:
    Elements of a Theory   232

A7.   Tasks and Prospects   243

5.   **Cumulation of Poisons: Quantitative Evaluation**   **252**

  1.   Evaluation at the Lethal Level   252

  2.   Evaluation at the Threshold Level   257

Addendum: Some Further Aspects of Cumulation   266

A1.   Three Types of Cumulative Action   267

A2.   Standardization of Cumulation Coefficients   268

A3.   Quantitative Assessment of Adaptation to Poisons   269

6.   **Quantitative Evaluation of the Toxic Effect from Poisons Acting
Jointly**   **270**

  1.   Introduction (and Some Aspects of Terminology)   270

  2.   Graphic Methods   274

  3.   Analytic Methods   283

  4.   Maximum Permissible Levels of Harmful Substances
      Jointly Present in the Environment   284

Addendum 1: Toxic Effects from Exposure to a Combination
             of Chemicals and from Exposure to Chemical
             and Physical Agents   286

    A.1.1   Single (Acute) Exposure   287

    A.1.2   Chronic Exposure   290

    A.1.3   Effect of Vapor-Gas-Aerosol Mixtures   294

    A.1.4   Exposure to Chemical and Physical Agents   300

Addendum 2: Complex Exposure   305

    A.2.1   Quantitative Evaluation   305

    A.2.2   Examples of Studies on Complex Exposure   307

7. The Relationship between Structure and Toxicity   **312**

1. General Considerations   312
2. The Quantitative Aspects of Structure-Related Changes in
    the Toxicity of Organic Substances   320
3. The Toxicities, Structures, and Physicochemical Properties
    of Inorganic Substances   337
    Addendum: Quantitative Relationships between Structure and
    Biological Activity   345
    A1. Correlations between Toxic Properties and
         Physicochemical Parameters   345
    A2. Further Development of Extrathermodynamic
         Approaches to QSAR Problems   347
         A.2.1 Hammett-Taft's Approach   347
         A.2.2 Free and Wilson's Method   348
         A.2.3 The Extrathermodynamic Approach of Hansch   348
         A.2.4 Comparison of Free and Wilson's and Hansch's
                Methods; New Models   350
         A.2.5 Application of Pattern Recognition Methodology   352
    A3. Structure-Activity Relationships among Inorganic
         Compounds   353

**8. Methods for the Calculation of Toxicity Parameters and
    Maximum Allowable Concentrations, as Well as of Less
    Accessible Constants from Those More Readily Accessible**   **361**

1. Methods Used for the Calculation of Indices of Biological
    Potency in Homologous and Other Series   362
2. Calculation Methods Based on Correlations between
    Physical Properties and Biological Indices of Volatile
    Organic Compounds   367
3. Calculation of Toxicity Indices for Particular Classes of
    Volatile Organic Compounds from Readily Accessible
    Constants   372
4. Calculation of Biological Indices for Nonvolatile Organic
    Compounds   381
5. Calculation of Toxicity Indices and Maximum Allowable
    Concentrations for Gases and Vapors of Inorganic
    Compounds   382

6. Calculation of Approximate Values of Unknown Toxicity
   Indices from Those Which are Known   383
7. Calculation of Less Accessible Physical and
   Physicochemical Constants From Those More Readily
   Accessible   391
Addendum: Recent Progress in Methods for the Calculation of
Toxicity Parameters   397
A1. Nonvolatile Organic Compounds   397
A2. New Methods for Calculating Tentative Safe Exposure
    Levels and Other Toxicity Indices   399
A3. Correlations between Toxicity of Chemicals and Their
    Inhibitory Actions on Isolated Mitochondria   401
A4. Prediction of Skin-Absorptive Properties of Chemicals   404
A5. Transition from LD_{50} Values for One Route of Entry to
    Those for Another Route   405
A6. Calculation of Maximum Allowable Concentrations in
    Ambient Air and in Water   406

Conclusions   **418**

References   **422**

Index   **449**

1

THE TOXIC EFFECT AS A RESULT OF INTERACTION BETWEEN THE POISON AND THE LIVING ORGANISM

The title of this chapter serves to emphasize that any reaction of a living organism in response to any harmful substance results from an interaction of the organism and the substance—a fact which is not always fully appreciated. This means that in any study of the toxicity of particular substances, in designing and conducting any toxicological experiment, and in interpreting its results the fullest possible consideration must be given to the properties and features of both the organism and the chemical agent concerned. Moreover, the toxic effect produced by a poison may be strongly affected by various environmental variables such as temperature, humidity, and pressure. Therefore a toxic effect, strictly speaking, is the result of interaction of three distinct entities, namely, the poison, the organism, and the environment.

It should be stated at the outset that no attempt will be made here to present a review or summary of the literature dealing with each particular aspect of the subject discussed in this introductory chapter. Rather, only a few examples will be given, for the main purpose of illustrating the need to take into proper account the aspect or variable under consideration when studying the toxicity of substances.

1. SPECIES DIFFERENCES IN SENSITIVITY TO POISONS

It has long been known that different species of animals vary in their sensitivity to poisons. A knowledge of the origin, development, and course of intoxications in particular animal species is very important for toxicologists because toxicity data obtained in animal experiments are in most cases to be transferred to man. A reliable extrapolation is not possible unless the qualitative and quantitative characteristics underlying species differences in sensitivity to the poisons concerned are well known. In the USSR the first (and still relevant) summary of the problem of interspecies differences in sensitivity to poisons appears to be the one contained in Lazarev's book, *General Principles of Industrial Toxicology*, published in 1938. Of the more recent works mention may be made, for example, of those by Krasovsky (1967, 1973), Krasovsky et al. (1969, 1970a,b), and Ulanova (1970), wherein a large body of evidence on quantitative interspecific differences is presented.

The mere accumulation of quantitative data, important as they are, is of course insufficient, and attempts have been made to disclose the mechanisms underlying species differences in sensitivity to poisons. Of the studies along this line those of L. A. Tiunov and his associates deserve first mention (e.g., Tiunov, 1967; Tiunov and Keizer; 1966; Tiunov et al., 1969; Liniucheva and Tiunov, 1966; Liniucheva et al., 1969). Among other things these studies have clearly demonstrated that species differences in responses to poisons depend primarily on the way in which the poisons are metabolized. It has been found, for instance, that dogs cannot be used to study poisons capable of acetylation, such as meta- and para-aminobenzoic acids, if the data are to be transferred to man: these substances do not acetylate in dogs, in contrast to man. On the other hand, their fates in man and rabbits are similar. One example illustrating the importance of knowing the qualitative features of the particular biological systems involved in the metabolism of the poison under consideration and responsible for the observed species differences in responsiveness to that poison is provided by a study of liver catalase activities in white mice and rats (Tiunov, 1967). Although the catalase level in mice is normally similar to that in rats, a 2-hr exposure to benzene by inhalation resulted in a noticeable reduction of catalase activity in rats (from 20.0 ± 1.5 to 13.1 ± 1.2 units), whereas in mice the activity remained virtually unchanged (17.6 ± 0.5 before and 17.7 ± 0.5 after exposure).

Among many other important factors contributing to species sensitivity are degree of complexity and differentiation of the central nervous system; level of development of the mechanisms regulating various body functions; characteristics of the skin; body size and weight; and life span. Of these factors let us consider life span, which appears to be of considerable importance in toxicological experiments on animals, especially when the experiment is aimed at arriving at an estimate of the maximum permissible concentration of a poison in the human environment. It is desirable that the duration of such an experiment be determined on the basis of the ratio of the fraction of life span during which man is likely to be exposed to the poison in question, to the whole life span. That life span is indeed an important consideration can be seen from the following.

As shown by Sacher (1960) and other authors, life span correlates well with, and has a significant regression on, a number of important species-related variables. For example, if x is log life span, y is log body weight, z is log brain weight, and w is index of cephalization, then

$$w = z - 0.666y + 0.888 \tag{1}$$

$$x = 0.325z + 0.684 \tag{2}$$

$$x = 0.198y + 0.471 \tag{3}$$

$$x = 0.636z - 0.225y + 1.035 \tag{4}$$

$$x = 0.198y + 0.636w + 0.471 \tag{5}$$

Equations 4 and 5 are very similar, but (5) is more acceptable because w and y are less dependent variables than z. The results will not change if a specified metabolic rate (energy expenditure) is substituted in (5) for body weight because these two variables have a correlation as high as 0.998 (Brody, cited in Sacher, 1960). Denoting the metabolic rate [in cal/(kg day)] by r and substituting Brody's relation $r = -0.266y + 1.050$ in (5) for y, one can obtain a relation of life span to the index of cephalization and metabolic rate:

$$x = 0.636w - 0.744r + 1.252 \tag{6}$$

To conclude this section, it should be noted that in view of the close interrelationship of the various factors underlying species and other differences in sensitivity to poisons, the separation of individual factors is rather artificial and represents only the initial, analytical stage in the study of complex interrelationships between the organism and the poison.

2. SEX DIFFERENCES IN SENSITIVITY TO POISONS

There is still much to be learned about the influence of sex differences on the sensitivity of man and animals to harmful substances. The complexity of this problem was convincingly demonstrated by Lazarev back in 1938. Data from animal experiments are contradictory. Some authors find females to be more sensitive, while others report the reverse to be true. The evidence obtained for human beings in cases of accidental poisoning is also controversial.

In a study on human volunteers (four men and three women) administered Acetophos, it was found (Krasovsky et al., 1969) that women were somewhat more sensitive to the poison (as manifested by both subjective signs and objective findings), but the differences in cholinesterase inhibition (Table 1) were inconclusive and might have been due to individual rather than sex

Table 1. Changes in Blood Levels of Cholinesterase in Men and Women after a Single Administration of Acetophos at a Dose Rate of 2 Mg/Kg (in percent of the baseline level, taken as 100%)

After 30 Min	After 2 Hr	After 5 Hr	After 24 Hr
Males			
84.5	84.5	92.2	103.0
93.3	85.6	79.4	101.3
90.1	92.3	89.7	103.6
94.3	69.2	61.4	85.0
Average: 90.5	83.0	80.7	98.2
Females			
71.2	51.5	52.4	98.9
78.5	75.7	86.5	105.5
91.0	57.6	54.7	91.7
Average: 80.3	61.5	64.5	98.7

Source.   Krasovsky et al. (1969).

differences in sensitivity. (Thus, as can be seen from Table 1, cholinesterase activity after 30 min was 84.5% in one man and 91.0% in one woman; after 2 hr it was 69.2% in one man and 75.7% in one woman; etc.) Similarly inconclusive results were obtained by the above authors for rabbits, mice, and rats.

In a study of the health status and morbidity of male and female workers in synthetic rubber factories (Pokrovsky, 1967) women were found to be more susceptible than men to certain organic poisons. This was true both of the specific actions of the poisons on the reproductive function and of their systemic effects.

Another example is a study on sex differences in the susceptibility to silicosis, where quantitative alterations in the lungs and tracheobronchial lymph nodes were more strongly marked in female than in male rats (Katsnelson and Babushkina, 1969). On the other hand, male mice proved to be less resistant to 30% ethyl alcohol given in daily subcutaneous injections in doses of 0.1 to 0.2 ml: 84% of males but only 30% of females died by the end of the second week; female mice remained more resistant even after castration (cited in Lazarev, 1938).

Although the effects of disease states on the sensitivity to poisons are almost unknown, it is generally recognized that both the risk of poisoning and the severity of intoxication are increased during pregnancy.

3. AGE AND THE TOXIC EFFECT

The effects produced by poisons are age-dependent. Some poisons are more toxic for younger animals, and some for older ones. Generally, young and old animals tend to be more sensitive to harmful substances than are sexually mature adults. There are many deviations, however, from this general trend. Thus young rabbits were found to be much less susceptible to subacute poisoning with benzene given in subcutaneous injections than mature animals, whereas the reverse was true when mice and rats were subjected to acute poisoning with benzene administered by inhalation or by mouth (Savchenkov, 1969). This example shows that the species of animal, route of administration, and exposure conditions are among the factors that need to be considered when studing the effect of age on the sensitivity to a poison.

That the relationship between age and toxic effect is fairly complex is evident, for example, from the results of numerous investigations carried out by Frolkis and summarized in his monograph *Regulation, Adaptation, and Aging* (1970). In studying the age-related sensitivity to and tolerance for various cholinomimetic, cholinolytic, and sympathomimetic agents, he showed among other things that, while in young animals dimethylphenyl-piperazinium causes bradycardia mainly by stimulating the vagus nerve, in old animals it produces bradycardia by acting directly on the parasympathetic ganglia of the heart. This example indicates that different mechanisms may be responsible for functional changes of the same type in animals of different ages.

Considerable age-related differences in sensitivity to poisons are also observable in man. Thus adolescents have been reported in the literature to be two, three, or even ten times as sensitive to industrial poisons as adults (e.g., Doskin, 1969). Most explanations offered to account for such increased sensitivity are of a hypothetical nature. In some cases children are found to be less susceptible to the action of poisons than adults and adolescents; one explanation is that they are much more resistant to hypoxia than are adults or adolescents (Fridliand, 1963).

It seems appropriate to conclude this section by quoting the following passage from Lazarev's book:

A future researcher of the problem of age-related sensitivity to poisons will formulate it in quite specific rather than general, abstract terms, since there can be no single solution to this problem applicable to all poisons: he will have to study the effect of age in relation to particular poisons. This does not mean that there is no hope of arriving at broader generalizations. This only means that any generalizations must be based on facts and will probably require different explanations in different cases (Lazarev, 1938, p. 274).

4. INDIVIDUAL VARIATIONS IN SENSITIVITY TO POISONS

It is common knowledge that different individuals of the same species, sex, and age vary in their responses to the same dose of a given poison. Excellent expositions of this subject can be found in Lazarev's (1938) and Williams' (1956) books. The wide individual variations in sensitivity to substances appear to be based on biochemical individuality:

> ... it will be quite impossible to find a drug that will act with complete uniformity on all human beings. In order for this to be accomplished, variation, the cornerstone of evolution, and biochemical individuality would have to be abolished (Williams, 1956, p. 117).

This fully applies to poisons as well.

In toxicology, as in a number of other biomedical disciplines, biological variability is often looked upon as an inevitable evil, and, to reduce it, a variety of methods for statistical treatment of empirical data have been developed. In the quest for common principles underlying the processes being investigated, information about the individual features of each member of the population under study is sometimes completely ignored. At the same time, as justly pointed out by Gorn (1966), individual variations in sensitivity to toxic agents, the limits of these variations, and the selection of criteria to assess these limits, as well as the underlying causes and mechanisms of individual variability—all these questions still remain among those that have been explored least. The reason for this is the great complexity of the problem. It is hardly an exaggeration to say that many of the qualitative and quantitative characteristics of toxic effect cannot be understood unless the factors determining biochemical individuality are taken into consideration.

5. BIORHYTHMS AND THE TOXIC EFFECT

Although the importance of differences in sensitivity to poisons related to species, sex, age, and individual variability, as well as to some other factors such as nutrition, has been recognized for a long time, it was only recently that the attention of toxicologists was drawn to yet another cause of variation—the one associated with the internal biological clocks responsible for various rhythmic responses of the living organism. Oscillations in the internal environment known as biorhythms differ in frequency, amplitude, and phase. The most clearly marked are seasonal and diurnal, or circadian, rhythms.

Table 2.   Effect of Medinal (Sodium Barbital) and of Caffeine in the Presence of Medinal on the Sleep of Intact Mice in Different Seasons

Season	Drug	Number of Mice	Time Taken to Induce Sleep (min)	Sleep Duration (min)
Winter	Medinal	10	66.5 ± 8.2	360 ± 33.0
	Medinal + caffeine	10	104.0 ± 2.3	317 ± 20.0
Spring	Medinal	10	56.1 ± 11.0	470 ± 34.0
	Medinal + caffeine	10	79.1 ± 3.2	470 ± 17.0
Summer	Medinal	10	93.5 ± 11.3	242 ± 14.3
	Medinal + caffeine	10	86.7 ± 3.7	384 ± 12.0
Fall	Medinal	10	120.0 ± 19.0	190 ± 18.7
	Medinal + caffeine	10	156.0 ± 1.4	177 ± 15.0

Source.   Golikov (1968).

5.1.   Seasonal Rhythms

In the USSR the first major review of the literature concerned with the influence of seasonal biorhythms on pharmacological action was the monograph by Golikov (1968). Although the data collected by the author concern mainly drugs, they fully apply to various toxic agents as well. An example of seasonal differences is given in Table 2.

It can be seen from this table that the hypnotic effect of Medinal (0.175 g/kg) and the antihypnotic effect of caffeine (4 mg/kg) varied with the seasons. The time taken to induce sleep in mice was shortest in the spring and much longer in the summer and fall. The duration of sleep changed in the opposite direction, being longest in the spring and shortest in the fall.

Seasonal differences in sensitivity to poisons may have serious practical implications in toxicology. Indeed, a toxicological experiment on animals aimed, for example, at establishing the maximum allowable concentration of a harmful substance in the human environment (in the air of cities or of workplaces, in bodies of water, etc.) usually lasts 3 to 4 months during a year, and it may well happen that the minimal effective (threshold) concentration has not been established in the course of one such experiment, so that a second experiment is called for. Clearly, this repeat experiment is likely to be carried out in a different season and to give inconclusive or unexpected results unless seasonal variations are taken into proper consideration.

5.2. Circadian Rhythms

No less important in the problem of interaction between the organism and poisons appear to be the circadian rhythms, that is, biorhythms with a period of approximately 24 hr. Although no publications dealing specifically with the effect of circadian rhythms on the sensitivity of man or experimental animals to poisons could be found in the available literature, some studies having relevance to this subject have been published. As an example, Table 3 shows results from a study by Sarkisov et al. (1969a) on the relationship between the cellular and extracellular forms of regeneration in the liver of white mice with liver dystrophy caused by carbon tetrachloride given in subcutaneous injections. The highest absolute rise in mitotic activity occurred at 6.00 hr in both the control and the test mice, while at 4.00 hr the mitotic activity in the test group was five times that in the control. Liozner et al. (1959) found the mitotic activity of hepatocytes to be highest between 3.00 and 9.00 hr. It may be presumed that various liver function tests used in toxicological experiments (see, e.g., Elizarova, 1971) will give different results in morning than in evening hours.

According to Agadzhanian (1967), circadian variations are known for at least 40 physiological functions. A comprehensive treatment of the subject of circadian rhythms can be found, for example, in *Biological Clocks* (1961), *Rhythmic Functions in the Living System* (1961), Emme (1962), Sollberger (1963), Komarov et al. (1966), Bünning (1964), Agadzhanian (1967), and *Biological Rhythms in Psychiatry and Medicine* (1970). It has been found, for instance, that glycogen tends to accumulate in the liver between 15.00 and 3.00 hr and to be expended in the remaining 12 hr. Blood sugar is at the highest level at 9.00 hr and at the lowest at 18.00 hr. The internal environment of the body is predominantly acid in the first half of the day (between 3.00 and 15.00 hr) and is mainly basic in the second half (15.00 to 3.00 hr). Blood pressure is lowest at 9.00 and highest at 18.00 hr. Hemoglobin level is highest from 11.00 to 13.00 and lowest from 16.00 to 18.00 hr.

Many more examples can be cited. New evidence continues to accumulate rapidly, calling for most serious attention by toxicologists. Regrettably, the the problems of toxicology that may be linked to biorhythms appear not to have been even formulated, let alone studied, although they may be of not only academic but also practical interest. Take night or shift work in certain industries, for example. If, in a toxicological-hygienic survey, the working conditions in an industry are evaluated in terms of physiological parameters or working efficiency, wrong conclusions may well be reached if circadian rhythms are not taken into consideration.

The question of the role of biorhythms in toxicology bears a direct relationship to Wilder's law of initial value, formulated around 1930. This law,

Table 3. Diurnal Variations in the Mitotic Index (Number of Mitoses per 1000 Hepatocytes) of Hepatocytes of Mice between 0.00 and 10.00 Hr after 10 Injections of 40 % Carbon Tetrachloride Solution in Doses of 0.2 Ml on Alternate Days

Group	Time of Day (hr)							
	0	2	4	6	7	8	9	10
Test								
$M \pm m$	2.4 ± 1.2	2.6 ± 1.2	1.02 ± 0.17	4.11 ± 0.27	0.26 ± 0.06	1.36 ± 0.25	0.66 ± 0.25	0.57 ± 0.08
n	9	6	9	9	6	6	3	9
Control								
$M \pm m$	2.8 ± 1.86	2.6 ± 0.16	0.2 ± 0	6.3 ± 1.48	0.46 ± 0.07	0.26 ± 0.07	0.97 ± 0.05	0.06 ± 0.04
n	3	3	8	3	3	3	4	3
P (%)	84	68	0.8	20	2	0.3	28	0.1

Source. Sarkisov et al. (1969a).

which in some cases may help not only to explain the observed differences in magnitudes of toxic effect but also to predict these differences, is an empirical-statistical rule for the quantitative relation between stimulus and response. According to this rule, the extent and direction of response of a physiological function depend to a large measure on its initial level: the higher the initial level (value) of the function, the smaller the response to function-raising stimuli and the larger the response to function-depressing stimuli (Wilder, 1967). The author validates this rule, in particular, by citing data on the effects of atropine, pilocarpine, adrenaline, and nicotine on blood pressure and pulse rate in man. Basimetry (the study and application of the law of initial value) and rhythmometry (the quantitative study of rhythms) are closely related in that both are concerned with changes in physiological performances as a function of time (Wilder, 1967). Wilder's plea to study body activity as a function of time applies to toxicology as well.

In conclusion it should be noted that, although the results obtained so far with toxic chemicals in relation to biorhythms are uncertain, divergent, and not well understood, research into biorhythms may eventually lead to the development of methods for the detection and, especially, the evaluation of various toxic effects, both in experiment and in real industrial environments. Thus disturbance of circadian rhythms, which reflect variations in the otherwise relatively constant internal environment of the organism, may well prove to be one of the most reliable criteria of the unfavorable influence exercised by the chemical agent under investigation.

6.   ROUTE OF ABSORPTION AND EXPOSURE REGIMEN

6.1.   Route of Absorption

It is well known that one and the same poison may produce quite dissimilar effects, depending on the route by which it enters the body. This question is the first to be discussed in nearly all textbooks and manuals of toxicology. The mechanism underlying the specific effect produced when the poison is absorbed by a particular route is also known in many cases. Thus a person loses consciousness within 1 to 3 min of inhaling vapors of hexane or of the nonene-nonane fraction of petroleum but can drink as much as several dozens of milliliters of either of these poisons without any noticeable effect. The reason for this difference is that both these chemicals are very sparingly soluble in the blood and have a low blood/air partition coefficient (see Chapter 4, and also Lazarev, 1964; Filov, 1967). Having entered the stomach, they are absorbed into the bloodstream, pass through the liver and the right heart, and enter the pulmonary circulation; once in the lungs, they come in contact with alveolar air and, because of their very low blood/air partition coefficient, leave the blood to be expelled in the expired air.

Attempts have been made to establish quantitative correlations between the toxicity parameters of poisons absorbed by different routes. One example is the study by Pozzani et al. (1959), in which the relationship between inhalation and oral dose data was considered for a large number of poisons.

6.2. Exposure Time

A given quantity of a harmful substance may enter the body rapidly or slowly, at one time or on several separate occasions. The toxic effect may be different in each of these cases.

The first quantitative generalization relating the toxic effect of a respirable substance to its concentration and the time of exposure appears to be Haber's formula: $W = c \cdot t$ or $c \cdot t = $ constant, where W (for $Wirkung$) is the magnitude of the toxic effect, c is the concentration, and t is the exposure time. It has long been known that this formula is valid only for a limited number of substances and for certain medium ranges of their concentrations and of exposure times.

An example of a poison for which Haber's relation holds more or less satisfactorily is phosgene (Flury and Zernic, 1931). A poison for which it is inapplicable is hydrogen cyanide; when its highly lethal concentration (killing animals within a matter of minutes) is reduced two- or threefold, hydrogen cyanide fails to produce any lethal effect even on many hours' exposure (Lazarev, 1938).

Heubner (cited in Lazarev, 1938) divided all harmful substances into two different groups, depending on whether their toxic action are time-dependent or time-independent (*zeitgebundene Giftwirkungen* and *zeitlose Giftwirkungen*). A typical poison whose toxic effect is time-dependent is phosgene; this group includes many poisons causing metabolic disturbances, for example, those which block enzyme systems. Among the poisons whose toxic action are almost independent of time are hydrogen cyanide and many volatile narcotics and local anesthetics (e.g., curare and cocaine). This distinction holds only when the absorption occurs very rapidly and at a constant rate. Actually, as shown in Chapter 4, the process of absorption may be fairly complex. In fact Haber's formula given above appears in most cases to define merely the amount of the substance that has entered the body rather than to describe the relation between effect, concentration, and exposure time. Nevertheless, it may be added, it is valid not only for poisons whose effects are time-dependent, such as irritant gases, but also for some of those whose effects are almost independent of time, namely, those for which the "capacity" of the body is very large in relation to their concentrations in air and whose rates of change in the body are comparatively slow (e.g., ethanol). Moreover, as pointed out by Lazarev (1938), this formula is even applicable to some poisons for which the body capacity is not very large. Thus it was found to be valid, within limits, in animal experiments with exposure to some aromatic hydrocarbons for which the approach to saturation occurs at a constant rate and very slowly, since much of the poison entering the body is destroyed there.

6.3. Intermittent Exposure and Exposure to Variable Concentrations

The evaluation of health hazards associated with intermittent exposure and, especially, exposure to fluctuating concentrations of airbone toxic agents is a very important, but as yet relatively little studied, problem from the viewpoint of both practical toxicology (e.g., for deciding whether the maximum permissible concentration of a toxic substance in the work environment should be the maximum concentration never to be exceeded or the average concentration per hour, during the shift, etc.) and general, including quantitative, toxicology (Lazarev, 1940b; Volkova, 1965; Samedov, 1967; Sidorenko and Pinigin, 1969; Liublina et al., 1971).

The first experimental study to compare toxic effects from exposure to constant and to variable concentrations was carried out by Klenova (1949). In this study, where the duration of exposure to and the dose of acetone or ethanol vapors tolerated by white mice before the onset of narcosis were used as criteria of toxic effect, continuous exposure to acetone vapors at a constant concentration was found to be more effective than discontinuous (intermittent) exposure to the same concentration but less effective than exposure to variable concentrations of the same average size. The toxic effect from ethanol was virtually the same whether the concentration was held constant or was varied.

Similar results were obtained by Tolokontsev (1960a, b) for chloroform and ethanol in inhalation experiments on rabbits. With exposure to variable concentrations, the blood level of chloroform followed closely the fluctuations in inspired concentration, and the toxic effect was more strongly marked than with exposure to a constant concentration even when the peak concentrations in the blood were not higher. The picture was different with ethanol: its blood levels showed no fluctuations during exposure to variable concentrations, and its toxic effect was virtually the same in both exposure regimens. It was shown that the difference between the speeds of passage of chloroform and ethanol through the rabbit body and, consequently, between their toxic effects is due to their different solubilities in the blood (high for ethanol and low for chloroform). The greater toxic effect from chloroform in the case of exposure to variable concentrations was presumed to have been due to disruption of the process of habituation (a phenomenon well known in toxicology and pharmacology; see Chapter 5) as a result of fluctuations in chloroform concentration in the arterial blood. The question of habituation to poisons with intermittent exposure is discussed by Liublina et al. (1971) and Liublina (1973a).

In experiments on rats the toxic effect (as judged by the rate of methemoglobin accumulation and the degree of pulmonary edema) was stronger from intermittent than from continuous exposure to oxides of nitrogen (Paribok and Ivanova, 1965a). Intermittent exposure to carbon monoxide likewise produced a greater toxic effect than did continuous exposure in a chronic experiment with rats (Gadaskina et al., 1961). Similar results were obtained by Burkatskaya and Matiushina (1968) for pesticides and by Samedov (1967) for hydrocarbons from petroleum oil.

7. EFFECT OF SOME ENVIRONMENTAL FACTORS ON THE ACTION OF POISONS

It should be noted first of all that, in practice, only on relatively rare occasions does a change in environmental conditions strongly affect the toxic effect directly, that is, by altering the physicochemical properties of the poison (although temperature, humidity, and other environmental variables sometimes have a substantial impact on these properties). Much more frequently, environmental changes modify the toxic effect by altering the body responsiveness to the poison. After this preliminary remark, let us discuss briefly two environmental variables: ambient temperature and barometric pressure.

7.1. Ambient Temperature

As with most other environmental factors, changes in the toxic actions of poisons seen to occur under altered temperature conditions are nearly always secondary to changes produced by the temperature factor in the functional state of the organism, such as impairment of heat regulation, water loss, respiratory or circulatory disturbances, acceleration or retardation of biochemical processes, and alteration of metabolic level.

The toxic actions of most poisons increase or decrease with environmental temperature, depending on the poison and a number of other factors. For each poison there is a temperature range within which its toxic action is smallest.

Of the studies that have appeared in the USSR since 1938 (i.e., after the publication of Lazarev's book, where effects of the temperature factor are discussed in a comprehensive way), mention may be made of the following: combined effect of high temperatures and various poisons (Pokrovsky, 1946; Pakhomychev et al., 1959); impact of temperature on the toxic actions of narcotics in low concentrations (Liublina, 1955); effect of temperature on the toxic actions of oxides of nitrogen (Paribok and Ivanova, 1965b); influence of temperature variation on the toxicity of mercury (Trakhtenberg et al., 1965); combined exposure to high temperature and thiolic poisons (Savitsky, 1967); toxicity of gasolines prepared from Baku oil in relation to temperature (Abasov, 1967); effects of elevated temperatures on the toxicities of trichlorfon (Denisenko et al., 1968), α-methylstyrene (Kapkayev and Sukhanova, 1968), and carbon monoxide (Tiunov and Kustov, 1969).

As an example, here are the main results of the above-mentioned studies by Denisenko et al. (1968), where rats received trichlorfon in a subcutaneous injection just before, in the course of (1 or 3 hr after the beginning of heating), or immediately after exposure to heat for a total of 4 hr. While exposure to heat was found to increase the toxicity of trichlorfon in all four treatments, the toxic effect (1) was greater when trichlorfon was administered before than after heating; (2) was particularly marked when it was given in the course of heating; and (3) was approximately the same whether the insecticide was given 1 or 3 hr after the beginning of the 4-hr heating period. These results well illustrate the point that the toxic effect is the result of interaction between three main factors: the organism, the poison, and the environment.

7.2. Barometric Pressure

In 1938 Lazarev noted that studies on the toxic action of poisons under altered barometric pressure "are still at the incipient stage." The situation has changed little since then, although this question is no longer one of merely academic interest. In particular, the extensive programs of oceanographic research and continental shelf exploration, as well as the rapid development of aviation and outer space exploration, have created the need for practical recommendations in this area.

The impact of reduced atmospheric pressure on toxicity was discussed, for instance, by Tiunov and Kustov (1969) with reference to carbon monoxide. Among other things they indicated that a reduction of pressure down to 600 and 500 mm Hg enhances the toxic effect of this poison. No examples of the influence of elevated barometric pressure could be found in the available literature, except those given by Lazarev in his monograph *The Biological Action of Gases under Pressure* (1941). One thing is perfectly clear, however; increased barometric pressure (hyperbarism), which causes abrupt changes in many physiological functions, is bound to modify the toxic effect as well.

This chapter has dealt, in a fairly fragmentary way, with some of the more important factors and has given some examples purporting to show that any toxic effect is always the result of a very complex interplay in time of the triad of organism, poison, and environment. Each of these "components" is highly complex and variable in itself, in terms of both quality and quantity. Clearly the result of their interaction—the toxic effect—is also subject to variation.

That is the reason why Starkenstein wrote that "no substance, whatever its quality or quantity, can be called a total poison, for its toxic action will always depend on the conditions under which it acts on the organism" (quoted in Lazarev, 1938).

That is the reason why the data on any toxic effect must always be treated not in absolute terms but rather in terms of probability, that is, in the sense that, when an exposure or experiment is repeated under identical conditions, the effect from the poison will be "probably the same," that is will be the same only "on the average."

That is the reason why the mathematical-statistical methods, which originated in biology and then developed to a high degree in the fields of mathematics, physics, and technology, have now made a comeback to biology and, in particular, are employed on an ever greater scale in toxicology.

In conclusion, it should be reiterated that the foregoing discussion has been superficial and incomplete. Thus no mention has been made of the roles of diet or of fatigue and other body states, or of the significance of different states of aggregation of the poison, or, for that matter, of many important environmental variables such as humidity, noise, vibration, and various kinds of radiation. Even a very cursory consideration of each of these factors would have greatly increased the size of this introductory chapter without, however, adding anything new in the way of substantiating the main thesis propounded here, namely, the need to study with care and take into account all relevant factors in evaluating the toxicity of a substance.

ADDENDUM: ON SPECIES DIFFERENCES IN SENSITIVITY TO POISONS

Among the many problems dealt with by quantitative toxicology, one of the most important and difficult is that of extrapolating from animals to man the various kinds of data on body-poison interactions (passage of poison through

Table A1.   Summary of Benzidine Biotransformation in Various Species

Species	Metabolites
Mouse	Monoacetylated 3-OH-ethereal sulfate Monoacetylated 3-OH-glucuronide N-Hydrogen sulfate and/or glucuronide 3-OH-Benzidine glucuronide
Rat	3,3′-Dihydroxybenzidine (?) 4′-Acetamido-4-amino-3-diphenylyl hydrogen sulfate 4′-Amino-4-diphenylylsulfamic acid 4′-Acetamido-4-diphenylylsulfamic acid
Guinea pig	4′-Acetamido-4-aminodiphenyl-N-glucuronide 4′-Acetamido-4-amino-3-diphenylyl hydrogen sulfate
Rabbit	3′-OH-Benzidine sulfate and glucuronide 4′-Acetamido-4-amino-3-diphenylsulfonic acid 4′-Amino-4-diphenylyl hydrogen sulfate N-Glucuronides 4′-Acetamido-4-aminodiphenyl 3-OH-Benzidine
Dog	3-OH-Benzidine 3-OH-Benzidine hydrogen sulfate 4-Amino-4-hydroxybiphenyl Mono- and diacetylbenzidine 4,4′-Diamino-3-diphenyl sulfate and glucuronide
Monkey	Monoacetylbenzidine
Man	3,3′-Dihydroxybenzidine (?) Mono- and diacetylbenzidine 3-OH-Benzidine N-Hydroxyacetylaminobenzidine

Source.   Haley (1976).

the body, modes and sites of action, toxicity parameters, etc.). It is natural therefore that this matter was discussed at the recent Soviet-American Symposia on the Comprehensive Analysis of the Environment held in Tbilisi (Bochkov, 1975; Newill, 1975) and Honolulu (Haley, 1976; Hoel, 1976). It is with such extrapolation in mind that the question of species differences in sensitivity to poisons was touched upon in Chapter 1, where some examples were given to illustrate the dependence of toxic effects on species-specific metabolic features. Of interest in this respect are the data of

Table A1 showing differences in the biotransformation of benzidine among several species.

Clearly, the mechanism of substance action and the clinical features of ensuing intoxication may vary greatly from one species to another, depending on the way in which a given poison is metabolized. It is highly desirable, therefore, that the metabolic profiles of the species concerned be known when selecting animals for a toxicological experiment if its results are to be extrapolated to man.

Experimental evidence on species differences is accumulating fast, and a number of generalizations have already been made. One example is the work of Krasovsky and his associates (Krasovsky, 1973), devoted to the modeling of intoxications and providing rationales for animal data extrapolation to man when establishing hygienic standards for toxic substances. Krasovsky has collected and scrutinized a very large body of data on inter-species variations in sensitivity to poisons and has established a number of consistent relationships. Some of these are illustrated below.

Table A2 needs no comment except that cholinesterase activity in the blood was used as criterion in the comparisons. The data of Table A3 on chronic toxicities of six inorganic substances were selected by Krasovsky from 40 publications of various authors (all substances were ingested in drinking water). It can be seen that the differences in sensitivity between man, dog, and rat are within one order of magnitude.

Krasovsky has concluded that these and other, similar results do not support the hypothesis that, with repeated exposure to poisons, the toxicodynamic process tends to be more intensive in man, or that the functional

Table A2. **Equally Effective Doses of Acetophos** ($ED_{50} \pm S_{ED_{50}}$ in mg/kg) for Man and Animals

Test Object	Observation Time	
	1 Hr	5 Hr
Man	5.0 ± 2.5	3.5 ± 1.4
Rabbit	2.7 ± 2.6	4.4 ± 4.2
Guinea pig	6.4 ± 4.2	6.0 ± 3.4
Rat	10.0 ± 4.8	12.5 ± 8.2
Mouse	24.0 ± 13.7	28.5 ± 18.0

Source. Krasovsky (1973).

Table A3.   Differences in the Sensitivity of Man and Animals to Toxic Substances (sensitivity of man is taken as unity)

	Difference as Measured		
Substance	From LD_{50} Ratio	From Ratio of Threshold Concentrations in Water	Species
Fluorine	2.5	1–3	Rat
Calcium	—	1	Rat
Nitrites	1.7–3.0	2.5	Rat, dog
Arsenic	3.5	1–10	Rat
Lead	1.5	1	Rat
Mercury	4.0	3–50	Rat

systems are more rapidly overstrained and exhaused in man than in animals; therefore there are no grounds for postulating any "special" susceptibility of man to the chronic action of poisons. This conclusion has obvious implications for both the theory and the practice of quantitative toxicology.

In Chapter 1 attention was called to the high degree of correlation between life span and such important variables as body weight, brain weight, and index of cephalization. This should make it possible to use life span as one of the main criteria in experiments on animal models designed to supply data for extrapolation to man. Of course other criteria can also be employed for this purpose. (Primarily, it seems, those that show high correlation with life span.) A valuable criterion is body weight, as has been clearly demonstrated by Krasovsky (1973). In providing a theoretical basis for his method of animal data extrapolation to man, Krasovsky formulated what he calls the "determining principle of body weight." He calculated, with the aid of a computer, about 700 regression equations relating toxicity parameters to body weight for several species. Interspecies differences in sensitivity were studied using acute toxicity data for more than 400 substances and data on magnitudes of pharmacologic doses for another 250 substances. The results showed a linear correlation between the toxicity parameters and body weight for 80 to 85% of the substances. The magnitude of the change in the species differences to poisons was, however, expressed in each case by an individual value of the regression coefficient b. The results are presented in Figure A1.

This figure shows virtually all possible variants of change in toxicity parameters of the different substances as a function of body weight in

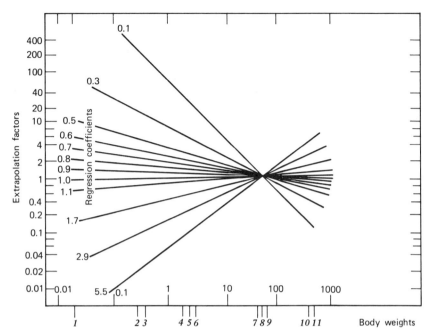

Figure A1.   Fan of species differences in sensitivity of mammals to toxic substances. *Abscissa*, body weights (kg) of various animals and man: *1*, mouse; *2*, rat; *3*, guinea pig; *4*, cat; *5*, rabbit; *6*, monkey; *7*, small cattle; *8*, pig; *9*, man; *10*, large cattle; *11*, horse. (From Krasovsky, 1973.)

mammals. The family of lines depicted in the figure is believed by Krasovsky to reflect the distribution pattern of the obtained values of the regression coefficient b (from 0.1 to 5.5), with the greatest density of variates in the range from 0.5 to 1.0. The 700 substances analyzed included some whose toxicity indices fell sharply ($b = 0.1$) or rose sharply ($b = 5.5$) in a series of mammals. For the large majority of substances, however, the values of the coefficient b lay between 0.9 and 0.5, that is, the sensitivity of the animals to these poisons increased as a linear function of body weight. Almost 20% of the substances had regression coefficients close to 1, that is, the toxicities of these substances were practically identical for all the animal species studied. For about 10% of the compounds, the toxicity indices did not increase but, on the contrary, decreased linearly in going from small to large animals ($b > 1.0$). The results of these investigations thus show that the toxicity parameters of individual substances obey the "determining principle of body weight," and that the species differences among animals can be described by first-order equations in most cases (for 80 to 85% of the substances). On this basis, a method for extrapolating toxicological data from animals to man was developed and tested. The agreement between calculated and empirically established values was quite satisfactory.

Toxicologists cannot fail to appreciate the importance of this "body weight rule." One should not, however, forget about the 15 or 20 % of substances that do not obey it. Generally, the problem of interspecies scaling needs to be given closer study. In this context an example given by Schmidt-Nielsen (1972, pp. 86–87) is so very instructive and eloquent as to be worth quoting *in toto*:

> Among mammals in general, perhaps, the most conspicuous difference is their size. A 4 ton elephant is a million times as large as a 4 gram shrew, and the largest living animal, the blue whale, can be another 25-fold larger. Twenty-five million shrews put together are very difficult to imagine, and since they eat about half their body weight of food per day, they would be very hard to feed. We can conceive of twenty-five elephants put together, although it is a formidable mass of elephants.

> If we just consider size of an elephant, we can easily make some serious mistakes. A few years ago the journal *Science* published a note which described the reaction of a male elephant to LSD. The investigators wanted to study the peculiar condition of the male elephant known as "musth." A male elephant in "musth" is violent and uncontrollable, but he is not in rut (and, although some people think so, "musth" doesn't mean that he "must" have a mate). Shortly after the publication of this note a letter to the editor of *Science* described the calculation of this dose of LSD as "an elephantine fallacy" (Harwood, 1963*). The authors had calculated the dose, based on the amount that puts a cat into a rage, and had multiplied it up by weight until they arrived at 297 mg of LSD to be given to the elephant. The long description of what happened can be shortened by saying that after the injection of 297 mg (enough for 1500 "trips," for a single human dose is about 0.2 mg), the elephant immediately started trumpeting and running around, then he stopped and swayed; five minutes after the injection he collapsed, went into convulsions, defecated, and died. The authors concluded that elphants are peculiarly sensitive to LSD.

> I am using this example to illustrate the tragic event that may result from a lack of appreciation of the problem of scaling. How should we calculate the drug dosage? Of course, if we want to achieve equal con-

---

* P. D. Harwood, Therapeutic dosage in small and large mammals (Letter to the Editor), *Science*, **139**, 684–685 (1963).

centrations in the body fluids of a small and a large animal, we should calculate in simple proportion to their weights. If this calculation is done from a 2.6 kg cat and its dose of 0.1 mg LSD per kg, we arrive at the now obviously lethal dose of 297 mg LSD for the elephant. If instead, as the letter-writer in *Science* said, we calculate on the basis of metabolic rate, we find that a much smaller dose of 80 mg is needed. This makes some sense, for we can expect that detoxication of a drug or its excretion may be related to metabolic rate. But there could be other considerations or special circumstances. For example, LSD could be concentrated in the brain, and in that event we would have a much more complex situation and might want to consider brain weight.

We could also use as a basis for the calculation an animal which is not so notoriously tolerant to LSD as cats; for example, we could use man. The weight of a man is 70 kg, and a dose of only 0.2 mg LSD gives him severe psychotic symptoms. On a weight basis this suggests that the elephant should receive 8 instead of nearly 300 mg LSD. Based on metabolic rate, which in man is $131 \, l \, O_2 \, h^{-1}$ and in the elephant, 210, we get a 3 mg dose for the elephant. If we consider the brain size, which in man is 1400 g and in the elephant about 3000 g, we arrive at only 0.4 mg ....

For comparison, LSD doses for the elephant calculated on different bases are shown in the following table:

Possible Calculations of a "Suitable" Dose of LSD to Give to an Elephant

(a)	Based on body weight of elephant and dose effective in cats	297 mg
(b)	Based on metabolic rates of elephant and cat	80 mg
(c)	Based on body weight of elephant and dose effective in man	8 mg
(d)	Based on metabolic rates of elephant and man	3 mg
(e)	Based on brain sizes of elephant and man	0.4 mg

I don't intend to say how much LSD should have been injected, if any; I only wish to point out that scaling obviously is not a simple problem. There are, however, many situations in which deviations from strict similarity are more obvious and easier to analyze.

In conclusion, it should be remembered that, in the last analysis, the reliability of extrapolations will always depend on the selection of appropriate test objects. It is well known from the field of experimental pathology how careful and cautious one must be in simulating any pathologic process occurring in man.

ADDENDUM REFERENCES

Bochkov, N. P., Data extrapolation in the evaluation of mutagenic actions of environmental factors on man, in *Vsestoronniy Analiz Okruzhaiushchei Prirodnoi Sredy. Trudy Sovetsko-Amerikanskogo Simpoziuma, Tbilisi, 25–29 Marta 1974 g.* [*Comprehensive Analysis of the Environment. Proceedings, Soviet-American Symposium, Tbilisi, March 25–29, 1974*], pp. 152–157, Gidrometeoizdat, Leningrad, 1975.

Haley, T. J., Extrapolation of animal data to human response. An assessment of the factors involved, in *Vsestoronniy Analiz Okruzhaiushchei Prirodnoi Sredy. Trudy II Sovetsko-Amerikanskogo Simpoziuma, Gonolulu, Gavayi, 20–26 Oktiabria 1975 g.* [*Comprehensive Analysis of the Environment. Proceedings, Second Soviet-American Symposium, Honolulu, Hawaii, October 20–26, 1975*], pp. 92–104, Gidrometeoizdat, Leningrad, 1976.

Hoel, D. G., Human risk assessment based on laboratory animal studies, in *Vsestoronniy Analiz Okruzhaiushchei Prirodnoi Sredy. Trudy II Sovietsko-Amerikanskogo Simpoziuma, Honolulu, Gavayi, 20–26 Oktiabria 1975 g.* [*Comprehensive Analysis of the Environment. Proceedings, Second Soviet-American Symposium, Honololu, Hawaii, October 20–26, 1975*], pp. 57–63, Gidrometeoizdat, Leningrad, 1976.

Krasovsky, G. N., "Modelirovaniye Intoksikatsiy i Obosnovaniye Usloviy Ekstrapoliatsii Eksperimentalnykh Dannykh s Zhivotnykh na Cheloveka pri Reshenii Zadach Gigiyenicheskogo Normirovaniya" ["Simulation of Intoxications and Extrapolation of Animal Data to Man in Solving Problems Involved in the Establishment of Hygienic Standards"], unpublished doctoral dissertation, Moscow, 1973.

Newill, V. A., Maximum permissible human stress, in *Vsestoronniy Analiz Okruzhaiushchei Prirodnoi Sredy. Trudy Sovetsko-Amerikanskogo Simpoziuma, Tbilisi, 25–29 Marta 1974 g.* [*Comprehensive Analisis of the Environment. Proceedings, Soviet-American Symposium, Tbilisi, March 25–29, 1974*], pp. 121–137, Gidrometeoizdat, Leningrad, 1975.

Schmidt-Nielsen, Knut, *How Animals Work*, Cambridge University Press, London, 1972.

2

THE RELATIONSHIP
BETWEEN AMOUNT OF
POISON AND TOXIC EFFECT

1. INTRODUCTION

The first question facing the toxicologist—whatever the purpose of the study he is undertaking—is that of the indices (parameters, criteria) of toxicity of the poison or poisons under study. In other words, he is seeking to know what concentrations of the poison in the environment (or what doses if the poison can enter the body, e.g., by the oral route) may cause poisoning. The information that he gains about the toxic properties of the poison is of interest not only per se; more often than not, the toxicologist wants to know the relative toxicity of the substance with a view to determining its position among other toxic substances whose toxicities are already known. Clearly, a reliable conclusion on this point can be reached only if the criteria of toxicity used are quantitatively precise and certain.

It should be emphasized that the quantitative certainty of toxicity parameters is important not only from a purely toxicological point of view (e.g., for the establishment of maximum allowable concentrations of chemicals in the environment), but also from a more general biological standpoint. Reliable quantitative data on toxicity may be very useful for the clarification of relationships between the structures of substances and their biological actions—a problem of great interest also to members of many other professions, including biochemists, biphysicists, and synthetic chemists. Since, as already mentioned in Chapter 1, the toxic effects of poisons always result from their interaction with living systems, establishment of the quantitative relationships governing this interaction, along with clarification of the underlying mechanisms, may be of great importance for elucidating the structures and functions of the biological systems themselves.

In revealing differences or similarities in the biological actions of poisons having different or similar physiocochemical properties, one must be certain that these differences or similarities can be established with sufficient reliability. This is possible only if the indices of toxicity, which are expressions of relationships between the amount of poison and its effect, are stated in precise and unequivocal quantitative terms.

Although, as its title implies, this chapter is concerned with amount-effect relationships, any toxic effect, generally speaking, also depends on the time of exposure to the poison. Therefore, environmental conditions being held constant, the toxic effect is the result of interaction between three factors: the organism, amount of poison, and time.

The relationship between dose, time, and effect (response) may be represented by a surface in three-dimensional space. When this surface is cut by planes parallel to the coordinate planes, three families of curves, relating in pairs the dose, time, and effect, are obtained. Accordingly, three types of toxicological experiment are possible in principle with each poison:

1. Experiments to establish the relationship between dose or concentration and toxic effect. These experiments are the most common. They include, for example. tests aimed at determining median lethal doses or concentrations.
2. Experiments to establish the relationship between time of exposure and toxic effect. These are of course meaningful only in the case of poisons whose action is time-dependent (see Chapter 1). Although such experiments are rarely conducted in toxicology, a knowledge of time-response relationships may be of great importance in certain cases, for instance, in establishing maximum allowable concentrations for different durations of exposure (this is discussed in Section 5).
3. Experiments to establish the relationship between dose or concentration and time of appearance of some selected toxic effect. As an example, experimental studies of cumulative properties of poisons may be cited, though with reservations. The reservations are, first, that exposure in this case is not continuous and, second, that the effect selected (e.g., death of 50% of test animals) may not be attained at all if the daily dose used constitutes only a small fraction (e.g., 0.01) of the total dose producing this effect.

The amount of poison is expressed in various suitable units. Thus concentrations may be stated in terms of weight per unit volume (mg/m^3, mg/liter), in percent, or in parts per million. Doses may be stated in terms of units of weight or volume of the poison per unit of (usually) body weight (mg/kg, ml/kg). Concentration or dose may be also expressed as a fraction of the concentration or dose causing some selected response, such as death of 50% of the test animals ($0.5\ LD_{50}$, $0.1\ LC_{50}$, etc.). Furthermore, concentration is sometimes stated as a fraction of the saturation concentration value (a thermodynamic expression; see Chapters 3 and 8).

The amount of effect (response) can be estimated in two ways: (1) by measuring the proportion of test animals which show some selected response to the poison (e.g., a given percent mortality within the first 24 hr after administration of the poison); and (2) by measuring the amount of change in some index (e.g., decrease in weight, or time to achieve a specified response). These two kinds of response are known as all-or-none (quantal) and graded, respectively. In a quantal response assay the response of each test animal is recorded as positive or negative (yes, no; $+$, $-$; 1, 0). In a graded response test the response is measured not in terms of incidence but in some unit of response elicited in each individual animal (in milliliters, minutes, grams, degrees, etc.). In this case the result of each individual measurement may be expressed in integers or fractions and may be positive or negative. The effect is thus measured on a continuous scale in contrast to quantal response assays, where it is measured on a discontinuous scale.

Whereas in a quantal response assay it is sufficient merely to determine, for every animal, whether or not the selected response (effect) has occurred, a graded assay requires measuring the extent of the response shown by each animal. Clearly, more refined experimental procedures and individual approaches to the test animals have to be used in graded response assays.

It is common practice in toxicology to study dose-effect relationships in acute, subacute, and chronic tests. The main criteria of toxicity are death of animals, changes in indices of particular bodily functions, threshold effects, and absence of any alterations in the state of test animals. In accordance with this set of biological indicators, the parameters of toxicity most frequently used include lethal, effective, threshold, and maximum permissible doses or concentrations, as well as toxicity zones. In addition, cumulative and other more specific (e.g., carcinogenic, teratogenic) properties of poisons are evaluated.

This chapter is concerned chiefly with some quantitative aspects relating to the establishment of criteria for toxic effects. The quantitative evaluation of cumulative properties of poisons is the subject of Chapter 5.

To conclude this introduction, the following point needs to be emphasized. It is believed by some toxicologists that quantitative assessment of toxicity may at times be of less importance than its qualitative evaluation. Such a view is hardly justifiable. For one thing, it does not make much sense to *oppose* qualitative and quantitative aspects in the action of toxic substances. The magnitude of an effect (the quantitative characteristic) and its specificity (the qualitative characteristic) are the two aspects of the same result of interaction between the organism, the poison, and the factors of the environment in which the interaction takes place. For another thing, the qualitative features of toxic effect invariably have quantitative parameters and must therefore be expressed in a quantitatively unambiguous form. If, for instance, one substance impairs tissue respiration while another blocks the transmission of nerve impulses, both of these actions must be expressed in quantitatively definite terms.

2. LETHAL DOSES AND CONCENTRATIONS

The whole range of doses and concentrations of any poison that elicit some response on the part of biological test objects may be conditionally divided into two zones: the zone of lethal values (LD, LC) and the zone of nonlethal (effective) values (ED, EC),

The quantitative expression of dose (concentration)—response relationships has long been the subject of intensive researches that have led to considerable theoretical developments. These, however, are not always applied in the practice of toxicology. Thus, for example, such criteria as the LD_0 and LD_{100} are still employed by some authors to characterize the toxicity of chemicals in the zone of lethal doses and concentrations,* even though these criteria are known to be neither conclusive nor sufficient.

It was convincingly shown long ago (e.g., Moshkovsky, 1941) that the LD_0 and LD_{100}, that is, the dose that causes no fatalities in a population of test animals and the dose that kills all the test animals, respectively, do not convey satisfactory information about the toxic properties of the substance and are too uncertain quantitatively. This may be illustrated by considering the LD_{100}, the minimal lethal dose that is fatal to all test animals. It is sometimes called the absolute lethal dose (Pravdin, 1947). However, in view of the biochemical individuality and biological variability mentioned in Chapter 1, it should be considered not as an absolute dose but at best as the one most likely to be fatal for a given number of test animals. In another sample of animals or in an experiment staged in a different season one or more animals may (and often do) survive. This explains the possibility of considerable differences between the values of a given toxicity parameter as determined for the same poison in different laboratories.

The point involved here can be readily seen from a theoretical consideration. If p is the probability (however close to unity) that each animal (or any other biological test object) will die upon exposure to the LD_{100}, then the probability that this dose will kill all test animals (n) will be p^n. The probability of occurrence of an opposite event, namely, that not all animals will die (e.g., that one animal will survive), will be $(1 - p^n)$. The value of $(1 - p^n)$ will increase with increasing n and will tend to unity:

$$(1 - p^n) \to 1, \qquad n \to \infty$$

---

* Hereafter, only the word "dose" will be used in most instances for the sake of brevity.

It follows, then, that the larger the test group the greater the probability that at least one animal will survive and therefore the smaller the probability that all will die. This means that the value of the LD_{100} will invariably increase as the number of test animals is increased. The same reasoning applies to the LD_0, but its value will decrease with increasing sample size. The reason for these variations are individual differences in the sensitivity to poisons. It is thus clear that the parameters LD_{100} and LD_0 are inadequate, for they fail to take account of the variation in tolerance within a population of test subjects.

A much more satisfactorily defined characteristic of toxicity in the zone of lethal doses is given by the LD_{50}, that is, the dose that is fatal to 50% of the test animals. This parameter is used by the majority of researchers to characterize the toxicity of substances, and there are a number of detailed procedures for its calculation (Bliss, 1935; Van der Waerden, 1957; Kulikov and Malashenko, 1966; Belenky, 1963; Livshits, 1966; Rybak et al., 1966; Prozorovsky, 1967; Weber, 1972). However, the LD_{50} alone does not fully and reliably describes the toxicity of the substance. Let us take one example (Moshkovsky, 1936).

Suppose that there are three substances: a, b, and c. Their toxicities are represented by the respective curves in Figure 1. These are typical S-shaped dose-response curves.

In the LD_{50} zone (III) the substances are arranged in the order of toxicity as follows: $b > c > a$. In each of the other zones, however, their order will be different:

$$a > b > c \quad \text{in zone I}$$

$$b > a > c \quad \text{in zone II}$$

$$c > b > a \quad \text{in zone IV}$$

Thus, if the toxicity is judged from the magnitude of effect (percent mortality) produced by a given dose, the order in which the substances are arranged in terms of their toxicities may be quite different when some other dose level is used. On the other hand, if the toxicity is judged from the size of the dose required to produce a selected percentage mortality, then, again, the substances may be arranged in a still different order when some other response level (effect) is selected.

The quantity LD_{50} in fact expresses the probability that 50% of the test animals will die. Some methods for its estimation are based on the assumption of normality of the dose-response curve; this assumption proves valid in most cases encountered in practice. It follows from this that in addition to the parameter of position (LD_{50}) the statistical population of data used to determine lethal doses must be also characterized by a parameter of scatter.

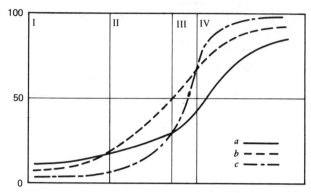

Figure 1. Dose-response curves for substances *a*, *b*, and *c*. *Abscissa*, doses; *ordinate*, percent mortality. I, II, III, and IV denote different toxicity zones for *a*, *b*, and *c*. (After Moshkovsky, 1936.)

Such a parameter is the mean square error, $S_{LD_{50}}$. Therefore the most certain and, perhaps, also the best quantitative characteristic of toxicity in the lethal dose zone is the LD_{50} stated together with its mean square (standard) error. Nevertheless, while the LD_{50} is determined in most cases, only on rare occasions is its standard error stated, with the result that many of the toxicity data reported for a given poison are not used by the authors themselves nor can they be used by others.

As shown in Chapter 8, the LD_{50} and LC_{50} correlate well with many physicochemical properties of substances. Further studies of the relationship between the structures and the biological activities of substances may be expected to yield more reliable correlations of physicochemical parameters with toxicity indices if the latter are certified by stating their standard errors.

The parameter LD_{50} is of course not the only one that may be used to characterize lethal doses. Thus, as pointed out by Horsfall (1945), practical experimenters working with fungicides wonder why the LD_{50} is often used rather than some higher and more practical value like the LD_{95} or LD_{100}. The advantages of the LD_{50} over the LD_{95} are well known. It can be estimated with greater precision and on a smaller number of animals; also, it can be determined by interpolation, and this is more reliable than extrapolation, which sometimes has to be resorted to in estimating the LD_{95}. Nevertheless, the parameter LD_{95} is often more useful for practical workers than the LD_{50}, even though it may not be determined with quite as much precision. In cases where dose-response lines have different slopes, the LD_{95} is a much more significant level of response than the LD_{50}. For this reason, notes Horsfall, "the trend is toward LD_{95} and away from LD_{50} despite the groans of some of our statistically minded brethren" (Horsfall, 1945, p. 31).

That the quantities LD_0 and LD_{100} are too uncertain has already been mentioned. However, if they are considered for the 0.95 or 0.99 level of significance (by determining them on a probit-log-dose line for the probits 6.64 and 3.36 or 7.33 and 2.67, respectively), they will become quite certain from a quantitative point of view. The LD_{100} will then become the LD_{95} or LD_{99}, and the LD_0 will become the LD_{05} or LD_{01}. Thus, although there exist well-developed methods for determining the LD_{50} along with its standard error, and most toxicologists use it to evaluate lethal doses, other indices such as the LD_{01}, LD_{05}, LD_{95}, and LD_{99} may also be considered with a view to their application for practical purposes. In some cases (e.g., in evaluating the toxicities of insecticides), they may serve as quite unequivocal quantitative criteria and thus can assure the comparability of experimental data obtained for particular substances in different laboratories using different-sized groups of animals.

The sigmoid shape of dose-response curves is in most cases accounted for by biological variation. Such interpretation is validated by the satisfactory approximation of these curves by a normal curve. Clark (1933) and some other authors suggested, however, that the S-shaped form of dose-response curves not only reflects individual differences in sensitivity to drugs and poisons but also depends on the relationship between the concentrations of the chemical agent at the point of application and the point of attack and on specific features of its binding by the biological substrate. Beginning with Ehrlich, researchers have accumulated a large body of evidence agreeing well with this hypothesis (Druckrey, 1957; Saunders, 1957; Barlow, 1964; Albert, 1973).

A knowledge of dose-response relationships may help in elucidating the mechanism of action of the substance (e.g., may explain why a given curve has a particular shape). This, however, is a complicated problem since many a dose-response relationship can be well approximated not only by a normal distribution but also, as Clark (1937) has shown, by the following:

the hyperbola (Langmuir's adsorption isotherm):

$$kx = \frac{y}{100 - y} \qquad (k = 1)$$

the exponential curve (empirical Weber–Fechner law):

$$ky = \log(ax + 1) \qquad (k = 0.0166, a = 5.3)$$

the parabola (Freundlich's adsorption isotherm):

$$kx^n = y \qquad (k = 49, n = 0.5)$$

The numerical solution of these expressions with their coefficients given in parentheses shows that the differences between them are much smaller than the errors in even the most accurate biological experiments. This of course complicates the use of dose-response curves for elucidating the mechanisms of toxic action. And yet, although an analysis of the dose-response relationship for some one poison does not yield reliable information about the mechanism of toxic action, an analysis of such relationships for several substances (e.g., in a comparative toxicity assay) may provide some useful insights into this mechanism. A study of dose-response curves obtained in experiments using the method of the limiting factor can bring to light even the most subtle mechanisms of toxic effect (Barlow, 1964; Albert, 1968).

In toxicology dose-response relationships are studied more commonly than any others. Somewhat less frequently studied are time-response relationships, which show how much of an effect is produced by a given dose in a population of test subjects at different times after administration of the toxic agent. The resulting time-response curves are also S-shaped and resemble a truncated normal distribution (Bliss, 1937). This was interpreted by Bliss as being due to individual variations in susceptibility to the poison. However, no less important here may be the kinetic features of the absorption and distribution of the substance, as well as the specifics of its binding by the biological substrate.

As regards dose-time curves (i.e., those relating dose to time of appearance of a selected response), they are somewhat different from dose-response curves and in some cases resemble Hoorweg–Weiss's strength-duration curves. Sometimes they can be fairly well approximated by a Poisson distribution. This suggests the possibility of using for their analysis the concepts of the target and hit theories developed in quantitative radiobiology (Zimmer, 1961; Timofeev–Resovsky et al., 1968). Attempts to apply these concepts to the analysis of dose-time-response relationships seem to be justified, in particular, by the following consideration. Comparison of the sizes of the molecule of a common chemical agent, the molecule of muscle protein, and the muscle cell gives the following ratio:

$$1 : \frac{1.8 \times 10^2}{1.1 \times 10^4 \times 3.6 \times 10^3}$$

This size relationship indicates that the probability of the chemical agent hitting a desired receptor is extremely small. However, as Albert (1968) has shown, even under such circumstances the receptor may be reached and combined with at a dilution as high as 10^{-9} mole/liter. Perhaps the concepts of the hit theory will prove workable when used for a quantitative interpretation of dose-time-effect relationships in the case of specifically acting poisons (Tolokontsev, 1963).

Everything that has been stated above about the quantitative uncertainty of toxicity criteria and about the dose-time-response relationships in the range of lethal values applies to the zone of nonlethal doses and concentrations as well. It should be noted that, irrespective of whether the effect is recorded in terms of quantal or of graded actions, toxicity parameters are usually given in the literature as mean effective values (ED_{50}), and only on very rare occasions are their standard errors ($S_{ED_{50}}$) stated.

3. THRESHOLD DOSES AND CONCENTRATIONS

Doses and concentrations that are not lethal are usually called toxic or effective. In the USSR the minimal values of doses and concentrations at the lower limit of the toxicity zone are referred to as threshold. Outside the USSR the term "threshold" is sometimes used with reference, not to minimal effective values, but to those at the lower limit of the lethal action range (Gaddum, 1933; Horsfall, 1945).

The establishment of threshold values is a very important task of practical toxicology. Pravdin (1947, p. 135) pointed out that "the toxicological significance of threshold concentrations is determined by the fact that they provide a starting point for establishing permissible concentrations of toxic gases, vapors, and dusts in the air of workplaces."

This view is shared by other Soviet toxicologists and hygienists concerned with the establishment of maximum permissible values for harmful substances not only in the air of the work environment but also in the atmosphere of populated areas, in bodies of water, and in foods.

The concept of "threshold dose," however, is still more tentative and indefinite than that of "lethal dose." The threshold dose depends not only on species and individual differences in sensitivity, properties of the poison, and various other factors mentioned in Chapter 1, but also, and perhaps first and foremost, on the method used to establish it. The sensitivity of methods (physiological, biochemical, morphological, etc.) employed in toxicity studies is virtually unlimited, and it is even more difficult to fix the boundary between doses causing and not causing particular changes in a given system or organ than between doses that kill the animal or other biological test object and those that fail to do so. The difficulty is compounded by the lack of agreement about what is to be considered a threshold effect. Indeed, what is a threshold dose? Is it a dose that brings about any change in a particular reaction, or a dose that elicits a response which goes beyond the limits of what is normal (physiologically, biochemically, etc.)? But then one is faced with the highly complex problem of the limits of normality. These limits are very difficult to establish for many body responses (see, e.g., Williams, 1956).

The above-mentioned difficulties in giving an unequivocal definition of the concept of threshold dose, as well as the difficulties involved in the interpretation of experimental results at the threshold level, appear to explain why methods for the quantitative estimation of threshold effects have been developed to a much lesser degree than those for the evaluation of effects in the zone of lethal doses. Gaddum, who worked very fruitfully in the field of quantitative evaluation of biological actions of drugs and poisons, considered that the concept of "threshold dose of toxicity" has no value (cited in Horsfall, 1945). Horsfall, who shared this view, remarked wittily that "the fallacy of the threshold dose of toxicity has the resilience of a tree made of rubber. It cannot be pushed over" (Horsfall, 1945, p. 36).

Such an attitude on the part of prominent researchers could not of course be conducive to the development of quantitative methods for assessing the effects of poisons in the vicinity of the lower boundary of the toxic action zone. Clearly, this situation stands in striking contrast to the importance of threshold doses and concentrations for practical toxicology. Nevertheless, it seems that, however complicated the problems involved may be, they should not be considered unsolvable.

Whereas in the zone of lethal doses the effect of a poison on each test animal is necessarily recorded in the quantal form (i.e., "dead" or "alive"), in the zone of threshold doses the toxic effect can be recorded either quantally or as graded actions (i.e., not only as "occurring" or "not occurring" but also by measuring the amount of change in some response). This may complicate the quantitative treatment and subsequent assessment of experimental data. Although almost any graded response can be measured as an all-or-none effect, one cannot agree with those (Belenky, 1963) who propose to record responses quantally whenever possible, for the measurement of graded responses may yield more useful information about the poison than do quantal records, and special methods for the measurement of graded responses have been developed (one such method is described by Belenky himself, 1963; see also, e.g., Khadzhai, 1965).

Depending on the nature of the experimental material and the purpose of the study, different methods can be used for the quantitative evaluation of threshold doses and concentrations. Two main cases are possible.

Case 1.   The toxic effect produced by the poison may be expressed in terms of changes in some reaction or activity as compared to the baseline level, that is, the level before exposure to the poison. Typical examples are alterations in the flexor reflex, blood pressure, oxygen consumption, and similar indices measured on the same animals before, during and after the experiment. In such experiments the threshold dose of the poison causing a change in the index being measured is determined for each test animal, and the mean dose is then computed from the individual doses thus obtained.

This mean value is taken as the threshold dose for the index in question. This procedure, however, cannot be regarded as satisfactory. For one thing, threshold doses are usually determined on a small number of animals (much smaller than for lethal doses); for another, the desire or even requirement that an effect be obtained in all test animals may strongly affect the magnitude of the established threshold dose, for the reasons stated above in discussing such criteria as the LD_0 and LD_{100}.

It is preferable to establish threshold doses using the same procedure as for the estimation of the LD_{50} and its standard error. The dose producing the desired effect in 50% of the test animals (ED_{50}), as well as the ED_{99}, ED_{95}, or ED_{01}, can then serve as unequivocal quantitative criteria. The parameter $ED_{50} \pm S_{ED_{50}}$ is to be preferred whether the response is to be recorded quantally or as graded actions. This, however, is not the only possible quantitatively definite criterion of toxicity in the zone of threshold doses and concentrations. In some cases other methods of data treatment may be employed, in particular, certain nonparametric techniques.

Thus some paired tests such as the sign test may be used to considerable advantage to characterize the threshold effect under study. The use of rank-order tests allows one to assess the probability of occurrence or nonoccurrence of an effect in response to a given dose of a poison. In this case the size of the threshold dose will not depend much on the number of test animals, and (what is more important) it will be expressed not in absolute but in probabilistic and quantitatively definite terms. The question of the level of probability to be used can be settled in different ways. Evidently the minimal dose producing an effect with a probability of .95 will be smaller than, say, such a dose for the .99 level of significance. It is, however, very difficult to establish a dose that will produce an effect with a specified probability. It is much simpler to determine the dose that will produce an effect with a probability lying within a certain range, for example, between .99 and .95. In practice, when the sign test is used (for bilateral boundaries), this will mean that a positive effect should occur 8 to 9 times for 10 animals ($n = 10$), 10 to 16 times for $n = 20$, 20 to 22 times for $n = 30$, and so on. Alternatively, it is of course possible to consider an effect as positive only if the probability of its occurrence will be no less than .99; that is, when the sign test is used, the effect should occur in 9 cases out of 10 no less frequently than in 16 cases out of 20, and so on. An even more rigid level (e.g., .997) may be set. All these are particular cases, however. What is important is that rank tests make it possible to state the magnitude of the threshold dose of the poison in terms of probability, in a quantitatively unequivocal way.

Case 2. There are situations in which the baseline level of the index (or indices) under study and changes in that index brought about by the poison cannot be measured on the same biological test objects, either because of the nature of the index itself (some biochemical, cytochemical, and morphological indices are examples) or because of the possibility that the bodily functions under study may strongly change with time (e.g., seasonal variations) even without exposure to the poison, as is often the case in long-term (chronic) experiments. In such situations a control group is introduced, and the occurrence or otherwise of a threshold effect is judged by comparing the test and control groups. The results may be expressed in quantal or graded form. By properly designing the experiment and by selecting a suitable method of measuring the threshold effect, the $ED_{50} \pm S_{ED_{50}}$ may be calculated in this case also. No less effective may be the use of Wilcoxon's test, the X test, and some other rank tests. Because of the nature of experimental data, paired nonparameteric tests (e.g., the sign test) cannot be applied in this case. The most effective appears to be the X test, particularly since it can be used to estimate the degree of the threshold effect and not merely to record its occurrence or nonoccurrence. The possibility of establishing a quantitatively much less uncertain threshold value is thereby greatly increased. The question of the level of probability at which the effect should be considered as having taken place can in principle be settled in the same way as in Case 1.

4. THE TOXIC ACTION ZONE

As far as the improvement of working conditions and, in particular, the establishment of maximum allowable concentrations of chemicals in the air of workplaces are concerned, the toxic action zone is a more meaningful index than any other single index of toxicity such as, for example, the lethal concentration (Pravdin, 1947, p. 135).

One cannot but agree with this statement. The toxic action zone (or toxicity zone) is an important characteristic of the potential hazard presented by the poison, and it is extensively used in the USSR in evaluating the relative toxicities of various substances, in developing methods for the calculation of maximum allowable concentrations of poisons in the environment, and for some other purposes. Liublina and Golubev (1967) have shown, for example, that the permissible concentrations calculated from a formula that takes account of the toxicity zone are particularly close to the experimentally established values.

The concept of "toxicity zone" appears to have been borrowed by toxicologists from pharmacology. It is related to the concept of "therapeutic range," which has been variously defined as the distance between the initially effective dose and the one that is unequivocally toxic (Gramenitsky, 1931); as the range between the minimal effective and minimal toxic doses (Anichkov and Belenky, 1954); and as the ratio of the toxic to the therapeutic dose (Shadursky, 1961). Since the authors just cited did not define the doses themselves and did not specify the methods by which they are to be determined, the term "therapeutic range" as defined above remains vague and quantitatively uncertain. The proposal by Moshkovsky (1936) to make this concept clear-cut and quantitatively unambiguous by expressing the effective and tolerable doses in terms of the ED_{50} and the TD_{50}, respectively, was not generally accepted in toxicological practice. It was only comparatively recently that Belenky (1959, 1963) and his associates (Belenky et al., 1960) began to use the quantities LD_{50} and ED_{50} for the calculation of the therapeutic range. For example, they introduced an index of the narcotic action range, defined as the ratio of LD_{50} to ED_{50} narcotic, and an index of the anticonvulsive action range, defined as the ratio of LD_{50} to ED_{50} anticonvulsive. Belenky (1963) has devised special procedures for the graphic analysis and quantitative evaluation of the thereaputic action range.

From the quantitative point of view, the concept of "toxicity zone" is as uncertain as that of "therapeutic range." Thus the "toxicity zone" was defined by Pravdin (1947) as the range of doses and concentrations from threshold to lethal (LD_{100} or LC_{100}); Liublina and Golubev (1967) used this term to mean the ratio of the LC_{50} to the threshold value; Sanotsky (1962) and Ulanova (1970) introduced the concepts of an "acute action zone" (Z_{ac}), given by the ratio LC_{50}/Lim_{ac}, and of a "chronic action zone" (Z_{chr}), given by the ratio Lim_{ac}/Lim_{chr}. Thus the indices used to define the toxicity zone are threshold doses (concentrations) and the quantities LD_{50} and LD_{100} (or LC_{50} and LC_{100}). Since different indices are used in different laboratories for the determination of the toxicity zone, since these indices themselves lack definitiveness and certainty, and since, in general, there are no universally recognized methods for the quantitative estimation of threshold doses and concentrations, it is not of course possible to give an unequivocal definition of the toxicity zone either. This situation cannot be considered as satisfactory. But it can be remedied only by discarding the existing concepts of the toxicity zone and the methods used for its estimation.

The toxicity zone as an index of the potential hazard presented by a given poison is substantially different from other indices such as the LD_{95}, LD_{50}, and LD_{05}. Whereas the latter indices may be referred to as absolute (in the sense that they are objective and can be established only directly in experiment), the toxicity zone may be called a relative indicator. Its magnitude is established to a large extent arbitrarily, that is, depending on the doses or concentrations used to calculate it (LD_{95}, LD_{50}, LD_{05}, ED_{50}, ED_{05}, etc.). Obviously, the toxicity zone defined, say, by the LD_{50}/ED_{50} ratio will be smaller than that given by the LD_{50}/ED_{05} ratio. The criteria LD_{95}, LD_{50}, LD_{05}, ED_{50}, and other, similar indices may be called quantitative. In a relative toxicity assay, for example, these indices make it possible to evaluate the substances in terms of their toxic potencies (by comparing the doses that produce a given effect). Differences between their toxicity zones calculated by the same method and using the same criterion may be indicative of the mechanisms of action of the substances compared (Horsfall, 1945; Cornfield, 1964). It appears therefore that the toxicity zone may be tentatively called a qualitative index—but only tentatively, of course, for it is clear that the indices that have been called quantitative above are also dependent on the mechanism and kinetics of interaction between the organism and the poison. Without discussing this question at any length (it requires a special study), it should be noted here that, unfortunately, the information about the magnitudes of toxicity zones obtained in comparative toxicological studies is still rarely used in analyses of the mechanism of action of harmful substances.

If the collection of data used to calculate the LD_{50}, ED_{50}, or some other index of toxicity is treated as a statistical distribution (as is done by many investigators when establishing the toxicities and pharmacological activities of poisons and drugs), the toxicity zone will be a parameter of the distribution, namely, a measure of scatter. As stated above in discussing the quantitative aspects of toxicity indices in the zone of lethal doses and concentrations, the best characteristic of position is the arithmetic mean (LD_{50}), while the best characteristic of scatter, that is, of the slope of the dose-response curve, is the standard error ($S_{LD_{50}}$). Therefore the parameters LD_{50} and $S_{LD_{50}}$ appear not only to characterize adequately the toxic properties of chemicals for lethal doses and concentrations but also to provide a quantitatively unequivocal estimate of the toxicity zone in general. For a further discussion of the magnitude of the toxicity zone let us consider Figure 2 and Table 4.

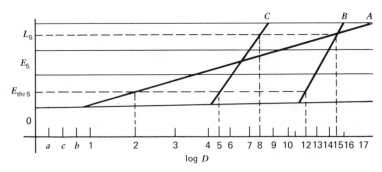

Figure 2. Dose-response lines for substances A, B, and C on a logarithmic-probit grid. *Abscissa,* log doses in arbitrary units; *ordinate,* the intervals L, E, and E_{thr} denote the zones of lethal, effective, and threshold doses; respectively, 0 designates the no-effect zone; a, c, and b are maximum permissible values.

Table 4.   Arbitrary Values of the Log Doses for
Substances *A*, *B*, and *C* in Figure 2

Doses[a]	Substance		
	A	*B*	*C*
Lethal			
LD_{100}	17	16	9
LD_{50}	15	15	8
LD_0	10	14	7
Threshold			
$ED_{thr\ 100}$	3	13	6
$ED_{thr\ 50}$	2	12	5
$ED_{thr\ 0}$	1	11	4
Maximum permissible value	*a*	*b*	*c*

[a] LD_{100} and $ED_{thr\ 100}$ are probable at the .99
level of significance (probit = 7.33), and LD_0
and $ED_{thr\ 0}$ at the .01 level (probit = 2.67).

Figure 2 shows three dose-response lines for the hypothetical substances
A, *B*, and *C*. Consider the toxicity line for *A*. Obviously the magnitude of the
toxic action zone will depend on the ratio of the doses used to calculate it.
Thus the ratio of the LD_{100} (its value is equal to 17 in the figure; see Table 4)
to the $ED_{thr\ 50}$ (it is equal to 2) will be greater than, say, the ratio $LD_{50}/ED_{thr\ 50}$
(17/2 > 17/3). Thus, although the position of the dose-response line remains
constant, the magnitude of the toxicity zone depends on the method used to
calculate it. Clearly, the usefulness of such a toxicity index is highly limited.
    The dose-response lines of Figure 2 are straight because they are shown
in log-probit coordinates. The probit method of analysis developed by
Gaddum (1933) and expounded in final form by Bliss (1935) has been widely
applied because it makes possible the description of dose-response relationships by straight lines. The possibility of describing the process under study
by an equation of a straight line offers important advantages by simplifying
the analysis of data and making it more effective. There exist a number of
methods for rectifying curves (see, e.g., Worthing and Geffner, 1946; Yakovlev,
1953). One such method is the probit analysis, whose underlying concept
is that a logarithmic dose-response curve is a graph of a function of the normal
distribution. Although, in some cases, the dose-response relationship in
probit-log coordinates is not linear either, the experimental points can still
be smoothed out by properly transforming the variables, as demonstrated,

for example, by Bliss in 1962 in a paper he read before the Leningrad Society of Naturalists (the paper discussed general biological models from the standpoint of statistics).

Expressing the dose-response relationship by a straight line offers an objective and unequivocal criterion for estimation of the toxicity zone. Thus this zone may be characterized in terms of the tangent of the angle made by the straight line with the abscissa in the zone of lethal doses or concentrations, that is, in terms of the slope of that line. Then the magnitude of the toxicity zone will not depend on the will of the investigator but will be constant for a given substance. In the first quadrant the slope will vary from 0 to ∞. The boundary values may obviously be excluded from consideration, and the slope in most instances will be somewhere between 0.18 and 5.67 (i.e., the angle will be not less than 10° and not more than 80°). In addition, this will afford a simple and reliable means of estimating the significance of differences between the toxicity zones of several substances and thus yield useful insights into their mechanisms of action.

From the viewpoint of mathematical statistics, the dose-response curve is a regression line and its slope is a regression coefficient. By comparing the regression coefficients (e.g., Fisher, 1954; Ezekiel and Fox, 1959; Aivazian, 1968) of several substances in a comparative toxicity assay, it is therefore possible to determine the significance of differences between the slopes of their regression lines. A qualitative description of the differences between the toxicity zones of the substances ("greater," "smaller," "greater by so much," etc.) can then be replaced by a quantitative estimate, that is, by a statement of the probability of the differences.

Since the toxicity zone is related to the therapeutic range, it may be thought that everything said above about the toxicity zone applies to the therapeutic range as well. This is not so. Being an indicator of the potential hazard from a particular poison, the toxicity zone shows how the effect produced by that poison varies with its dose within the range of lethal values. In this sense the toxicity zone may be considered as an indicator of the potential danger of the poison in general. The therapeutic range has a somewhat different essence. Practically, there are no "general" drugs, but only those for the treatment and prevention of particular diseases or pathologic processes. The therapeutic range may likewise be expressed by the slope of the dose-response line. This, however, raises the question as to the zone within which the slope is to be calculated. If, for instance, one is concerned with a group of anticonvulsive agents, the slope can be calculated either for the zone of lethal doses or for that of anticonvulsive doses. In Figure 2 the slope of each dose-response line for the substances A, B, and C remains constant in all zones. In reality the lines may have different slopes in different zones. Thus it may be presumed that the distribution of sensitivities of animals or other biological test objects in respect to lethal doses will differ from that of their sensitivities in respect to nonlethal doses (in a quantal response test) by the parameter of position and will not differ by the parameter of scatter. Whether or not this presumption will prove valid and, if so, how often, is not clear. This question, which is of interest not only for pharmacology and toxicology, but also from a general biological point of view, can be answered only by conducting specially designed experimental studies.

The concept of "toxicity zone" has been discussed here in terms of the statistical parameters of toxicity, in an abstract quantitative aspect. In the next chapter it is considered from a different angle—in terms of the thermodynamic approach to the fate of poisons in the organism, using the concept of thermodynamic activities of substances.

5. MAXIMUM PERMISSIBLE DOSES AND CONCENTRATIONS

In many cases the ultimate goal of estimating toxicity indices such as the LD_{50}, ED_{50}, threshold values, and toxic action zones is the establishment of maximum permissible doses and concentrations of harmful substances in the human environment. The permissible concentration as a criterion of toxicity (or, rather, as a criterion of nonaction, of zero toxicity) is an index which differs from those discussed above by being particularly dependent on the will and attitude of the investigator. "Sober scientific analysis . . . shows how little justified is the hope of obtaining a precise value of the permissible concentration directly from experiment, without inevitable calculations and comparisons" (Lazarev, 1940b). These calculations and comparisons are aimed at finding the transition (or correction, or safety) factor that would make it possible to reduce the threshold value to the maximum permissible level. In searching for such a factor, the physicochemical properties of the substance, the mechanism of its action, its fate in the body, its lethal and threshold doses and concentrations, its cumulative properties, and other factors are usually taken into consideration. Great importance is attached to the magnitude of the toxic action zone. In the USSR the following recommendation has been generally accepted:

> When the toxic action zone is narrow, the permissible concentration should be as much as possible below the toxic action threshold, that is, as far as possible from the threshold concentration. Conversely, the broader the toxic action zone of the substance, the smaller is the hazard of acute poisoning and therefore the closer the permissible concentration may approach to the threshold concentration (Pravdin, 1947, p. 136).

The question of the satefy factors to be used in passing from effective (threshold) down to permissible doses and concentrations is a very important one, and it has been given close attention by a number of investigators (e.g., Sanotsky, 1962, 1964; Kagan, 1970; Ulanova, 1970). However, it is very difficult to establish sufficiently objective and unequivocal safety factors because of the lack of agreement in regard to the concepts and definition of toxicity parameters and the absence of generally used standard procedures for the estimation of these parameters (and for the treatment of experimental data in general). This particularly concerns the identification of threshold effects and the calculation of toxicity zones. As a result, the safety factors and, consequently, the maximum allowable doses or concentrations established for similar substances and identical conditions of exposure, or even for one and the same substance by different authors, may be very different.

Let us consider a hypothetical situation by turning again to Figure 2 and Table 4. Suppose that it is necessary to establish the maximum permissible doses for substances A, B, and C. Let us compare first B and C. All the doses of C (9, 8, 7, 6, 5, and 4) are lower than the corresponding doses of B (16, 15, 14, 13, 12, and 11). It follows from this that the maximum permissible dose for C (c) should be smaller than that for B (b), as is shown in the figure.

Consider now the data for A and B. The positions of the values a and b on the abscissa is this case are not so obvious as in the case of B and C. Indeed, the LC_{100} of A is greater than that of B, and their LC_{50} values are equal, while all threshold doses of A (3, 2, and 1) are smaller than those of B (13, 12, and 11). The toxic action zone of A is much larger than that of B. What, then, should be the maximum permissible values for A and B? Should the permissible value of A (a) be smaller (as is shown in Figure 2) than that of B (b)? No conclusive arguments can be advanced to answer this question in the affirmative. Even more difficult to resolve appears to be a situation similar to that shown in Figure 2 for substances A and C. All lethal doses of C are smaller than those of A. Yet all threshold doses of C are larger than those of A. The toxic action zone of A is greater than that of C. The maximum permissible value for A (a) is smaller than that for C (c). If Pravdin's recommendation is to be followed, the permissible value (a) should be much closer to the threshold value (1) for A than the permissible value (c) to the threshold value (4) for C. Would this be a correct solution for this situation? It appears that no general considerations or recommendations can be stated. In practice, the solution of such problems often depends on the previous experience of the investigator, his intuition, and other, similar factors.

The existing methods of planning experimental studies aimed at establishing permissible values for poisons in the environment and the commonly used methods of quantitative analysis of their results do not enable one to establish in a definite and definitive manner the permissible doses or concentrations of harmful substances in the environment. This can be done, however, by applying certain quantitative methods for the treatment and analysis of experimental data. Some of these methods have been discussed above.

The progress made in the development of highly sensitive physiological and biochemical tests that can detect very early and slight alterations in the human and animal organism, as well as the experience gained in establishing standards for atmospheric pollutants, suggests that the permissible level of a toxic substance in the environment can be arrived at not only by reducing the threshold value by a given number of times but also by establishing the maximum no-effect dose or concentration of the substance with respect to some limiting index (Cherkinsky, 1964). The value of the maximum no-effect dose or concentration (ED_0 or EC_0) should be stated not in absolute terms but in terms of probability. If methods of nonparametric statistics are to be used to estimate threshold effects, then the probability of no effect apparently should not be less than .99. Such a threshold value can well be accepted as the maximum permissible one for many toxic nonelectrolytes that do not produce marked specific actions.

When the threshold dose (concentration) is expressed as $ED_{50} \pm S_{ED_{50}}$, the difference $ED_{50} - 2S$ (where S is the standard deviation for the population of values used to establish the ED_{50}) may be taken as the maximum permissible value. In this case the probability of occurrence of a threshold effect will be about .05. Even more rigid limits may be set, for example, by taking $ED_{50} - 3S$ as the maximum permissible value, in which case the probability of a threshold effect will be only .003. This is of course quite an acceptable level. This principle of calculating the safe dose from LD_{50} data was proposed by Gaddum (1956), who considered as safe a dose equal to $LD_{50} - 6S_{LD_{50}}$, which gives as the probability of a fatal outcome a value as small as 10^{-9}. An example illustrating the relationship between lethal and safe doses calculated from this difference is shown in Figure 3, where the safe doses of the hypothetical substances A and C are a and c.

This method compares favorably with other methods used to establish safe (permissible) doses and concentrations, since the calculated safe values are quantitatively unequivocal. If this principle is to be used in practice for the establishment of maximum permissible doses and concentrations of toxic substances in the environment, however, it would be better to rely not on lethal but rather on effective doses and concentrations, for example, narcotic or those producing a twofold decrease in cholinesterase activity. Then the maximum permissible value might be, for example, $ED_{50} - 3S$. Such an index of the potential hazard from the poison would appear to be quite unambiguous from a quantitative point of view.

This section has dealt briefly with some theoretical aspects of estimating unequivocal maximum permissible values for harmful substances in the environment. Whether the methods mentioned here and other methods may

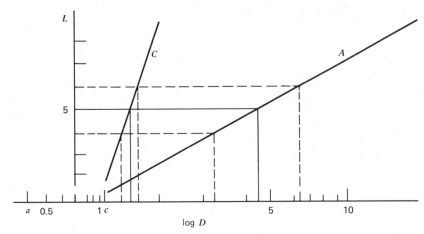

Figure 3.   Dose-response lines for substances A and C on a logarithmic-probit grid. The $LD_{50} \pm S_{LD_{50}}$ is 4.6 ± 0.70 for A and 1.4 ± 0.05 for C, the safe doses are 0.4 (a) for A and 1.1 (c) for C. The dose ratios for A and C are the same as in Figure 2.

be valuable and suitable for practical purposes cannot be judged until they have been thoroughly tested. It would be desirable, for example, to determine the maximum allowable concentrations by several different methods and then to compare them. In this way it may be possible to find a principle for establishing maximum permissible values that would be less subjective than those presently used. Unfortunately, the toxicity data reported by different authors for the same substances are rarely equivalent and unambiguous; such quantities as $ED_{50} \pm S_{ED_{50}}$ are encountered only as exceptions.

In conclusion mention should be made of another promising line of research, namely, the study of dose-time relationships. An interesting example is the equation relating the maximum allowable concentrations (MACs) of carbon monoxide to the times of exposure for which they were set up (Tolokontsev, 1967). In the USSR, Sanitary Standard CN–245–71 lays down five different permissible levels of carbon monoxide—for 15-min, 30-min, 60-min, and 7-hr exposures and for the atmosphere of populated areas (long-term exposure). Initially it was thought that the MAC-time curves for these exposure times might be fitted by Hoorweg–Weiss' equation, widely used in physiology for relating time and effect. Yet an attempt to find suitable coefficients met with failure (probably because this equation is applied only to short time intervals). Later a simple polynomial equation was computed:

$$\log C = 1.8 - 0.7 \log t + 0.068 \log t^2$$

where C is the MAC (in mg/m^3), and t is the time (in hr).

This formula in fact makes it possible to estimate the value of the MAC for any duration of exposure. Because of improvements in chemical technology and working conditions, in many cases it is no longer necessary for workers in the chemical industry to stay continuously at their workplaces during the shift so that the time of their contact with harmful substances is reduced. Accordingly, the MAC can be set at a somewhat higher level under such conditions. For this reason it would seem useful or, in some cases, even necessary to have similar equations for other toxic substances. The number of MACs or corresponding threshold values required for a given substance may be different depending on its properties, but experience has shown that it should not be less than three and is unlikely to be more than five. The data required for drawing up such an equation may be obtained in a single properly designed experiment.

6. PARADOXICAL EFFECTS

As already mentioned in Section 2, most dose-response curves are S-shaped when plotted on an ordinary arithmetic grid. They usually turn into straight lines on a logarithmic or logarithmic-probit grid. For most substances the sigmoid shape of the curves is accounted for by individual variations in sensitivity to the poison under study and, in the final analysis, biochemical individuality. Clark (1933, 1937), Lazarev (1938), Karasik (1944), and a number of other authors (see, e.g., the "Discussion" published in *Proc. R. Soc.*, Ser *B*, **121**, pp. 580–609, 1937) examined in detail the various curves describing the relationship between dose and biochemical effect and discussed the possible underlying mechanisms.

Other kinds of dose-response relationships are also known. Thus some heavy metals have stimulatory actions in low concentrations but produce inhibitory effects when present in higher concentrations. A concentration-action curve for such substances, known as oligodynamic, is shown in Figure 4.

The other curve of Figure 4 exemplifies a paradoxical effect—a phenomenon commonly defined as a reversal of the usual direction of change, a turn in the opposite direction, of some response. As far as toxicology is concerned, the unique aspect of paradoxical effects is that toxicity actually increases as the dose or concentration decreases. Most of the examples of paradoxical effects given below were taken from an interesting review by Schatz et al. (1964), where this subject is treated in a comprehensive manner.

There are substances which may be more toxic at lower than at higher concentrations over a given concentration range. Two examples are adenine and thymine (Schatz et al., 1964). In some cases there is a bimodal or even multimodal dose-effect relationship wherein toxicity first increases, then

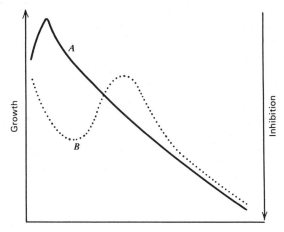

Figure 4. Curves in arithmetic coordinates showing oligodynamic (*A*) and paradoxical (*B*) effects. (From Schatz et al., 1964.)

decreases, and increases again as the dose of the substance increases. In the above authors' view such effects are much more frequent than one would ordinarily assume and are of widespread importance in the biochemistry and physiology of many living systems under many different conditions. Their theoretical and practical importance has not yet been fully appreciated.

Paradoxical effects sometimes remain unnoticed simply because they occur above or below the concentration range tested, or at intermediate concentrations which are not considered (Buffel and Vendrig, 1963; Reiner, 1955; cited in Schatz et al., 1964). In other cases, where paradoxical effects were clearly evident, they are not mentioned when the experimental results are discussed. According to Schatz et al., dips in dose-response curves are often disregarded. They write:

Statistical methods can most effectively prevent recognition of paradoxical effects because the mathematics employed in statistical analyses do not consider these phenomena. With scattered points, statistical methods are used to determine where the straight line or smooth line should be drawn. The whole statistical approach assumes that these would be the ideal curves. Deviations or irregularities caused by paradoxical effects are treated as experimental errors or experimental variation. It is therefore paradoxical that statistics, employed to minimize or avoid mistakes, can be responsible for concealing paradoxical effects.

This passage has been specially quoted as an antithesis of what has been repeatedly emphasized in the preceding pages of this chapter—the need for establishing unequivocal indices of toxicity. The rather antimathematical and antistatistical statement of Schatz et al. has, however, some justification. As known, statistics is a double-edged tool, for it can both promote and hinder the establishment of truth. And yet, if properly applied, present-day statistics may uncover paradoxical effects (e.g., by demonstrating the quantitative heterogeneity of the test material) and evaluate them in quantitative terms. The advances made in quantitative systematics and taxonomy and in the field of pattern recognition provide striking demonstrations of the potentialities of statistics for dealing with qualitative problems by quantitative methods.

Schatz et al. adduce many examples of paradoxical responses by microorganisms, plants, and animals to a large number of substances. In most of these examples each dose-response curve has two optima. One example is the growth curve for *Amoeba proteus*, which shows two distinct peaks in the numbers of amoeba as the concentration of $MgCl_2$ is increased (Pace, 1933; cited in Schatz et al., 1964). This example is mentioned here with the sole purpose of suggesting that statistics and mathematics, if used to analyze such a curve, might have helped in unraveling the mechanism of the paradoxical effect involved by accounting for the bimodal character of the curve and determining its parameters.

In this connection it seems fitting to cite an example which, though unrelated to toxicology, demonstrates well the possibilities of mathematics in solving biological problems. In studying data on observed variations in brightness discrimination as a function of the brightness itself, many investigators failed to detect any indication of a kink or break in the corresponding curve, but an attempt to describe this relationship by a single equation was unsuccessful. However, Hecht (cited in Worthing and Geffner, 1946), having shown mathematically the presence of significant breaks in the data for each observer, succeeded in describing this curve by two equations on the assumption that the curve was the result of interaction of two types of visual processes corresponding, respectively, to the cone and rod receptors of the retina. Subsequently the validity of this assumption was fully confirmed.

A detailed discussion of the mechanisms underlying dose-effect relationships is beyond the scope of a book devoted to quantitative toxicology. There is probably no need to dwell on mechanisms of paradoxical effects either. Nevertheless it seems appropriate to give a few examples of mechanisms where these have been elucidated. Thus some enzymes may vary in their sensitivity to a poison or to intermediate products which accumulate as a result of interaction with the poison, so that the activity of the biochemical system involved may vary paradoxically as the dose of the poison increases

(Slater and Hulsmann, 1959; cited in Schatz et al., 1964). In some cases a purely quantitative increase of the toxic substance may lead to the formation of qualitatively new molecular species which may have completely different properties resulting from the substance that is added. Thus the paradoxical effects of fluorine were attributed to the formation of toxic polymers (Tsubol and Reiner, 1954; Reiner, 1955; London, 1955; all cited in Schatz et al., 1964). Another example concerns the paradoxical effect of dithiocarbamate on the growth and respiration of various fungi. It was found that, as the concentration of dithiocarbamate increases, the toxic 1:1 copper complex is formed first; the addition of more inhibitor results in a smaller inhibitory effect because the 1:1 complex is converted to the insoluble 1:2 copper:dithiocarbamate chelate; further addition again produces inhibition because of the formation of zinc, manganese, iron, and other heavy metal complexes which are less stable than those of copper (Goksyor; cited in Schatz et al., 1964).

Although, as already mentioned, most of the examples of paradoxical effects discussed in this section were taken from the review by Schatz et al. (1964), it should be noted that this subject has been given considerable attention by a number of authors, both inside and outside the USSR. Thus a highly interesting discussion of paradoxical reactions is contained in Wilder's (1967) book. In the USSR several original studies shedding important light on the mechanisms of various paradoxical effects have been published. Here are some examples.

Golubev (1956) has shown that the pulmonary edema brought about in mice by exposure to vinyl esters (vinyl propionate and vinyl butyrate) has a clear-cut paradoxical nature. The threshold concentration of vinyl propionate was found to be 2 mg/liter. At concentrations above 4.6 mg/liter, the edema progressively increased with increasing concentrations to attain a maximum level at 8 mg/liter, a concentration that produced particularly marked convulsions and led to rapid death. The mice given the poison at a concentration of 10 mg/liter (the minimal concentration causing narcosis) had, however, a much less marked edema than those given 8 mg/liter. All higher concentrations (16, 32, and 48 mg/liter) increased the depth of narcosis with a proportionate decrease in the degree of edema, so that the least marked edema was seen in mice given the highest narcotic concentration (48 mg/liter). Similar results were obtained for vinyl butyrate. Golubev has explained this phenomenon and has shown that the degree of pulmonary edema strongly depends on the state of the nervous system. Preliminary narcotization with sodium amytal diminished or abolished the paradoxical effect.

Sarkisov et al. (1969b, c) encountered a paradoxical effect in their studies of liver regeneration in mice following the damage caused by carbon tetrachloride. The poison was much less toxic and killed fewer mice when injected on alternate days than when given in the same dose (0.2 ml of 40% CCl_4) once in a fortnight in a total dose equaling only about one sixth of that administered in the first case. The authors attributed this paradoxical effect to different intensities of regeneration with different dosing intervals. When CCl_4 was administered fortnightly, the intensity of regeneration was much lower than with more frequent injections. The mechanism and the general medical significance of this phenomenon are specifically discussed in a monograph by Sarkisov and Vtiurin (1969) and in a review by Sarkisov (1970).

Generally similar results were reported by Tiunov et al. (1970) for furfural, which caused lower mortality among mice and rats when given on successive days than on alternate days in the same dose, even though the total dose in the former case was twice that in the latter. Biochemical studies of enzyme systems revealed the activity of xanthine oxidase to be increased when the poison was given daily and greatly reduced when it was given on alternate days.

A rather curious effect that may also be regarded as paradoxical was obtained by Kagan (1968, 1970) in studying the cumulative effects of harmful substances in relation to the sizes of their daily doses. The cumulative effects of some substances (e.g., DDT) was found to increase as the daily dose was lowered. The specific mechanisms underlying this phenomenon appear to be very complex. The cumulative action of a substance is the result of many processes, including among others the absorption, distribution, chemical transformations, accumulation in the more vulnerable systems, organs, and tissues, and elimination of the substance; important factors are degree of reversibility of the toxic process and habituation—a phenomenon not yet fully understood.

In conclusion, let us turn again to Schatz et al. (1964), who note that it is paradoxical that paradoxical effects are not always reproducible. One cannot but agree with them. This is paradoxical indeed—but only in respect of effects whose mechanisms have not been explored. Some of the "paradoxical" effects described in the above review, as well as those revealed by Golubev, Sarkisov et al., and Tiunov et al., are not in fact paradoxical, for they are reproducible and (more important still) their mechanisms are understood. In reality a paradox indicates that there is a problem—and nothing more.

Finally, it should be pointed out that paradoxical reactions are of general biological interest. They may occur not only in response to chemical agents, but also under the action of various nutrients, physical factors, and, indeed, any other component of what is known as the external environment. The most important factor responsible for paradoxical effects is of course the living organism itself, its internal environment.

ADDENDUM: DOSE-TIME CURVES

On p. 42 an empirical concentration-time relationship was presented for maximum allowable concentrations of carbon monoxide, and the desirability of establishing similar relationships for other toxic substances was indicated. In the past few years research into dose (concentration)-time relationships for purposes of environmental hygiene has been pursued on a wide scale in the A. N. Sysin Institute of General and Community Hygiene under the USSR Academy of Medical Sciences (Chernukha and Yakushevich, 1974; Pinigin, 1970, 1974, 1976; Pinigin et al., 1974; Sidorenko and Pinigin, 1976a, 1976b). The relationships found have proved to be very useful for solving many problems in quantitative toxicology. They are used in predicting threshold toxicities with continuous and discontinuous exposure to harmful substances; evaluating cumulative effects; forecasting long-term toxic effects from the data of short-term tests (an application of particular relevance to the development of rapid methods of establishing MACs); quantifying and predicting the results of combined and complex exposures to harmful substances; determining maximally permissible total body burdens of toxic substances on man; and classifying toxic substances by degree of hazard.

By determining the times of onset of toxic effects under various conditions of exposure to toxic substances (ethanol, methanol, acetone, benzene, acrolein, butyl acetate, chloroform, sulfur dioxide, carbon monoxide), the authors cited above have demonstrated that concentration-time relationships can be quite satisfactorily described by equations of hyperbolas. On a logarithmic grid they are well approximated by straight lines of the type

$$\log T = \log T_0 - \tan \alpha \cdot \log C \qquad (A1)$$

where T is the time of onset of a given toxic effect on inhaling the substance in concentration C, T_0 is the time of appearance of the same effect with concentration C_0 and is taken as the unit of time measurement, and α is the angle of inclination of the straight line to the abscissa (concentration). Examples of such relationships, taken from Sidorenko and Pinigin's paper (1976b), are given in Figures A1 and A2.

With respect to the concentration, (A1) can be written as

$$\log C = \log C_0 - \tan \alpha \cdot \log T \qquad (A2)$$

Taking the antilogarithm of (A2), we have

$$C = \frac{C_0}{T^k} = C_0 T^{-k} \qquad (A3)$$

where $k = \tan \alpha$. This equation expresses an empirical relationship between the concentration of a substance in air eliciting a given effect and the time of

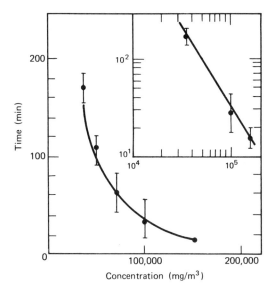

Figure A1. Dependence of the time of death of mice on benzene concentration in the air with continuous inhalation on a normal scale and (inset) logarithmic scale. (From Sidorenko and Pinigin, 1976b.)

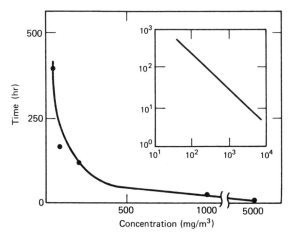

Figure A2. Dependence of the time of onset of inverse antagonist muscle-chronaxie relationship in white rats on benzene concentration in the air with continuous inhalation on a normal scale and (inset) logarithmic scale. (From Sidorenko and Pinigin, 1976b.)

continuous inhalation. Comparison of concentration-time relationships for various substances has shown the slopes to be different for different substances. According to Pinigin (1970), this is due to differences in physico-chemical and toxic properties and in toxicodynamic characteristics among the substances compared, as well as to differences in the processes of their cumulation and of compensation for the toxic effects they produce. The greater the angle of inclination or the smaller its tangent, the more dangerous is the substance, because the toxic effect will occur sooner on reducing the concentration (Sidorenko and Pinigin, 1976a). Furthermore it has been shown that, other factors being equal, the angle of inclination for one and the same substance will be smaller the closer its effect is to the threshold level. For lethal concentrations, for example, this angle will be greater than for those causing only slight alterations in some biochemical or physiological indices.

This feature appears to be a very important one, and it has enabled Sidorenko and Pinigin (1976a) to classify toxic substances according to hazards (Table A1).

The hazard rating of substances on the basis of concentration-time curves for prolonged continuous exposure (in conditions simulating atmospheric pollution) has been shown to agree satisfactorily with the hazard rating of the same substances for intermittent exposure (i.e., in conditions of 4- to 6-hr exposure daily, simulating industrial settings).

Expressing the concentration-time relationship in the form of an equation or on a logarithmic grid has enabled Pinigin (1976) to propose a method for predicting the threshold of chronic action from data of a short-term (up to 1 month) test, using four or five different concentrations and then transferring the results into a prediction for a period of up to 5 months. He writes, "There

Table A1.   Rating of Hazards from Toxic Substances Based on Parameters of the Concentration-Time Curve

Class of Hazard	Parameters of Curve		Increase in Time of Onset of Effect with Tenfold Reduction of Substance Concentration in Air
	Slope	Tangent of Slope	
1 (Extremely high)	>155	<0.466	3-fold
2 (High)	155–137	0.466–0.932	9-fold
3 (Moderate)	137–125	0.932–1.428	27-fold
4 (Slight)	<125	>1.428	>27-fold

Source.   Sidorenko and Pinigin (1976a).

are grounds for stating that predictions of chronic action thresholds based on the concentration-time relationship are more reliable from a quantitative point of view than arriving at these thresholds in a modern experiment involving the establishment of no-effect concentrations" (Pinigin, 1976). This statement, based as it is on experimental evidence, carries important implications, primarily for the quantitative validation of the safety factors used in arriving at daily average MACs for atmospheric pollutants and for the extrapolation of animal data to man.

Since the concentration-time relationship can be described by straight lines, it may be used to estimate equally effective concentrations of different substances in air or of one and the same substance entering the body by different routes from different media. The criterion of equal effectiveness will then be equal times of onset of the selected effect. It has been proposed to use this principle in assessing combined and complex exposures to harmful substances, as well as in hygienic evaluations of the actual burden of chemical pollution (Pinigin, 1976; Sidorenko and Pinigin, 1976a). The papers referred to in this addendum also give other examples of possible applications of the dose (concentration)-relationship.

In conclusion it seems appropriate to quote a passage from the preface to the book *The Natural Philosophy of Time* by the British cosmologist G. J. Whitrow:

> In a recent article (*The New Scientist*, 19th February, 1959, p. 410) Professor J. I. Synge, F.R.S., wrote that, in his view, of all measurements made in physics the measurement of time is the most fundamental and "the theory underlying these measurements is the most basic theory of all." He argued that Euclid put us on the wrong track by taking space as the primary concept of science and relegating time to a poor second (Whitrow, 1961, p. vii).

It is to be hoped that Euclid meant no harm. Returning to our subject, it seems that Synge's and Whitrow's view regarding the importance of time is also relevant to toxicology, primarily quantitative toxicology, and that toxicological studies taking the time factor into full consideration hold much promise.

ADDENDUM REFERENCES

Chernukha, T. M., and Yu. E. Yakushevich, On the biological equivalence of doses and concentrations of benzene administered *per os* and by inhalation, in E. I. Korenevskaya, Ed., *Gigiyenicheviskiye Aspekty Okhrany Vneshnei Sredy. Sbornik*

Nauchnykh Trudov, pp. 52–58, Institut Obshchei i Kommunalnoi Gigiyeny im. A. N. Sysina, Moscow, 1974.

Pinigin, M. A., Quantitative expression of the dose-time relationship for exposure of animals to chemical agents, in G. I. Sidorenko, Ed., *Materialy Konferentsii po Itogam Nauchnykh Issledovaniy za 1969 god (8–9 Iyunia) AMN SSSR*, pp. 26–28, Institut Obshchei i Kommunalnoi Gigiyeny im. A. N. Sysina, Moscow, 1970.

Pinigin, M. A., Pressing problems in communal toxicology due to air pollution by chemicals, in *Farmakologiya. Khimioterapevticheskiye Sredstva. Toksikologiya. Problemy Toksikologii*, Vol. 6, pp. 83–132, VINITI: *Itogi Nauki i Tekhniki* Series, Moscow, 1974.

Pinigin, M. A., Forecasting in the field of air pollution control: scope and methods, in G. I. Sidorenko and M. A. Pinigin, Eds., *Metodicheskiye i Teoreticheskiye Voprosy Gigiyeny Atmosfernogo Vosdukha (Sbornik Nauchnykh Trudov)*, pp. 3–10, Institut Obshchei i Kommunalnoi Gigiyeny im. A. N. Sysina, Moscow, 1976.

Pinigin, M. A., Yu. E. Yakushevich, and Kh. S. Markarian, Evaluation of intermittent action of volatile nonelectrolytes, in E. I. Korenevskaya, Ed., *Gigiyenicheskiye Aspekty Okhrany Vneshnei Sredy. Sbornik Nauchnykh Rabot*, pp. 45–52, Institut Obshchei i Kommunalnoi Gigiyeny im. A. N. Sysina, Moscow, 1974.

Sidorenko, G. I., and M. A. Pinigin, Hygienic criteria of the maximum permissible stress, in *Vsestoronniy Analiz Okruzhaiushchei Prirodnoi Sredy. Trudy II Sovetsko-Amerikanskogo Simpoziuma, Gonolulu, Gavayi, 20–26 Oktiabria 1975 g. [Comprehensive Analysis of the Environment. Proceedings, Second Soviet-American Symposium, Honolulu, Hawaii, October 20–26, 1975]*, pp. 119–128, Gidrometeoizdat, Leningrad, 1976a.

Sidorenko, G. I., and M. A. Pinigin, Concentration-time relationship for various regimes of inhalation of organic compounds, *Environ. Health Perspect.*, **13**, 17–21 (1976b).

Whitrow, G. J., *The Natural Philosophy of Time*, Thomas Nelson, London and Edinburgh, 1961.

3

THE EQUILIBRIUM DISTRIBUTION OF NONELECTROLYTES BETWEEN THE ENVIRONMENT AND THE LIVING ORGANISM

1. GENERAL CONSIDERATIONS

The basic principles governing the entry of foreign substances into the body from the environment may be conveniently considered on a mental model where the living organism is reduced to the level of a multiphase biological system. Such simplification is justified for reasons which will not be stated here, in the belief that they have been sufficiently well demonstrated elsewhere (e.g., Rashevsky, 1964; Filov, 1967). In our model the multiphase biological system (a living organism) resides in an environment (medium) which may be treated as a single multicomponent phase.

This model is the most general one and corresponds to the situation, most pertinent to occupational toxicology, where a living organism is in a medium containing a toxic compound. The most simple and (in a majority of cases) valid assumption will be that the concentration of the compound remains roughly constant. This is often the case, for example, when a person stays in a room containing vapors of harmful substances or when one is concerned with the action of solutes on fishes or aquatic animals.

A different situation, more pertinent to forensic and food toxicology, prevails when a known amount (dose) of a foreign substance has been introduced into the body. The model will also be different: a definite quantity of a new component has been applied directly to one or more phases of the biological system. Other, less general situations may also be encountered.

Here attention will be focused on the first-mentioned model. When the principles underlying the distribution of substances in this case are understood, it should not be difficult to visualize models for other situations. We will not do this here, and the discussion that follows solely concerns a biological system placed in a medium containing a toxic substance whose concentration varies only slightly with time.

Given this situation, the absorption of the substance into the biological system from the external medium can be described by the laws of diffusion. The substance is accumulating in all phases of the organism (biophases), and its fate there will depend on its chemical structure and on the characteristics of the phases. Two main alternatives are conceivable here: (1) either the substance accumulates in organs and tissues which behave as inert biophases, or (2) it reacts chemically with components of the biophases so that its molecules undergo changes, that is, the substance is metabolized. Metabolism occurs in most cases, but its rate may vary widely. When the metabolic rate is sufficiently slow, the first alternative is mainly realized, and vice versa. The kinetic aspects of these processes are dealt with in Chapter 4. Here it should be noted that stable compounds continue to be absorbed until a thermodynamic equilibrium is reached, after which the parameters of the system no longer change with time (this is discussed in greater detail below).

Once a state of equilibrium is attained, the concentrations of the substance remain constant in all phases of the biological system provided that the external concentration remains constant also. If such an equilibrium system is placed in a medium free of the substance concerned, the substance will be lost from the system through a process which obeys the same laws of diffusion as the process of absorption.

A foreign compound that has penetrated into the biological system produces some effect which, if marked, can be usually described as toxic. Toxic actions are fairly diverse, each group of compounds or even each individual compound having a distinctive pattern of action. Nevertheless all extraneous compounds can be divided into two broad categories according to the nature of their biological action. These categories are closely related to the behavior of substances in the biophases. The inert substances that are eliminated unchanged or are transformed slowly tend to act nonspecifically. The principal feature of nonspecific action is general inhibition of functions peculiar to the living organism. This type of action is variously known as narcotic, physical, structurally nonspecific, and so on. Here, however, the term "nonelectrolytic," proposed and validated by Lazarev (1944), will be adhered to.

On the other hand, there are many compounds capable of specific actions resulting from particular (but different for different compounds) chemical reactions with biophase components. The specifically acting substances are therefore those which invariably undergo transformation in the body. Sometimes much of a specifically acting substance is eliminated unchanged. The specific effect is then apparently determined by the part of the substance which has reacted with biological components. Understandably, a combination of nonelectrolytic (i.e., nonspecific) and specific actions is encountered more commonly.

Nonelectrolytic action is shown by an enormous number of substances in respect to most diverse biological objects of animal and plant origin, being, in fact, one of the most general phenomena in nature. Specifically acting substances often produce some nonelectrolytic effects along with specific ones. In such cases the nonelectrolytic effect is manifested first and is most conspicuous, being later attended or followed by specific effects. The nonelectrolytic effects of potent poisons are often indetectable, but this does not mean that they are nonexistent. It is logical to suppose that they do occur but are too weak, or do not have enough time, to become evident because of the rapid onset of characteristic poisoning. One example is the narcotic action of vinyl propionate, which is demonstrable only with massive doses and is masked by the specific action, to remain unnoticed, with smaller doses (Golubev, 1957).

Such a pattern of effects appears to be related to the initial penetration into the organism of unchanged molecules of the substance, which exhibit nonelectrolytic action at this stage. However, the presence in the organism of a certain substrate with which the substance interacts chemically leads to specific biological effects.* A good example is the action of ethyl alcohol. The relatively slow rate of its breakdown conditions a strongly marked narcotic effect, followed by the well-known specific signs of poisoning associated with the oxidation of ethanol to acetic aldehyde.

The universality of nonelectrolytic action, which is manifested in similar physiological responses to substances having quite dissimilar molecular structures, appears to be associated with some common mechanism of action. This mechanism is still unknown, but substances with nonelectrolytic action are thought to produce biological effects by accumulating in some vitally important parts of a cell and thus disorganizing a chain of normal metabolic processes (Albert, 1973). In other words, they are acting simply as foreign bodies. Hence one can conclude that the principal property of such substances responsible for their biological action is their capacity to be accumulated by cells. It will be recalled here that this capacity depends on the balance of the molecular structural features that determine the hydrophobic and hydrophilic properties of the atoms of the substance.

The accumulation of substances in biophases unaccompanied by chemical transformations is associated with weak interactions between the substance and the biological substrate involving van der Waals forces or hydrogen

---

* This is of course a fairly simplistic view of the process under consideration. Much more complicated relationships obtain when, for example, the main effect is caused by a metabolite.

bonds. These and other forces of interaction and their biological roles are discussed in detail by Mullins (1954) and Albert (1973).

A certain degree of specificity in action seen with various nonelectrolytes may be related not only to the superimposition of specific effects but also to the capacity of particular nonelectrolytes to be predominantly absorbed into particular biophases of the organism where they disrupt a chain of metabolic processes. This question will not be discussed here.

Other things being equal, the degree of nonelectrolytic action depends entirely on the concentration of the nonelectrolyte in the biophase or biophases responsible for this action. The assertion, which is occasionally encountered in the literature, that narcosis (i.e., nonelectrolytic action) is a function of equilibrium (implying an equilibrium distribution of the substance between the circumambient medium and the organism) is misleading and appears to be due to terminological confusion. Actually, an effective concentration of the nonelectrolyte may be attained in the sensitive biophases considerably before an equilibrium is set up. When the effective concentration and equilibrium are reached simultaneously, this is an extreme case: a given nonelectrolytic effect cannot then occur before an equilibrium is attained simply because not enough of the substance will have been accumulated for the effect to take place. This explains why the concentration of a nonelectrolyte which corresponds to the establishment of equilibrium and brings about a particular toxic effect can be conveniently used as a criterion of the potency of that nonelectrolyte.

2.   FERGUSON'S PRINCIPLE; ELEMENTS OF THERMODYNAMIC EQUILIBRIUM

In toxicology it is common practice to compare the toxic potencies of volatile nonelectrolytes by measuring the external concentrations of these substances that produce equal biological effects. The conditions of exposure are so selected as to ensure the maximum possible equilibrium between the concentration in the external medium and that in the test organism. The equitoxic equilibrium concentrations then characterize the toxicities of the compounds and so can serve for comparative purposes.

This approach long remained the only one used, despite its obvious shortcomings. The main shortcoming is that the toxic action produced by the molecules of a compound inside the organism is judged from its concentration outside the organism. It became possible to remedy the situation because of Ferguson's idea (1939) of characterizing the toxicities of substances by their chemical potentials rather than their external concentrations.

The chemical potential (μ) is a thermodynamic function very convenient for describing the equilibrium states of multiphase systems. The physical meaning of this function is as follows: the chemical potential of a substance in a given phase shows how much the energy of that phase will change when the number of molecules of the substance reversibly changes by 1. A strict description of the chemical potential need not be given here, for it can be found in any textbook on thermodynamics (e.g., in the excellently and popularly written book by Ter Haar and Wergeland, 1966). Here the discussion will be confined to the thermodynamic consideration of equilibrium as applied by Ferguson to toxicology.

From the viewpoint of thermodynamics, the condition for the equilibrium distribution of a substance among any number of phases of a given system is that its chemical potential is the same in all phases:

$$\mu_1 = \mu_2 = \cdots = \mu_n$$

where the subscripts refer to the different phases.

In the case of a substance acting on a biological object, the system comprises the medium in which the object has been placed, and the object itself. Clearly, this is a multiphase system, for an indeffinitely large number of phases can be singled out in any organism. At equilibrium the substance is so distributed in the system that the ratio of its concentrations in any two phases is equal to its partition coefficient between these phases. A knowledge of the concentration of the substance in the external medium gives no indication of its concentration in a given phase of the organism so long as the partition coefficient for that phase remains unknown. This coefficient can be determined by experiment if the phase is known. Since the phase (or phases) responsible for the toxic action is in most cases not known, the partition coefficient is also unknown, so that knowledge of the external concentration does not yet furnish any direct information about the substance at the point of attack.

The problem presents itself in a different light when one considers the chemical potential of the substance rather than its concentration. By determining the chemical potential in the external medium in equilibrium with the organism, one thereby determines this potential in any phase of the organism where equilibrium actually exists, including the site of action. Knowledge of the chemical potentials of substances in equilibrium between the medium and the organism thus makes it possible to evaluate the relative potencies of the substances on the basis of a quantity which characterizes them directly in the site of attack, and not only in the circumambient external medium.

The difficulty stemming from the fact that the chemical potential, like energy, is not susceptible to direct numerical determination can be obviated by using the thermodynamic expression

$$\mu = \mu_0 + RT \ln A$$

where R is the gas constant; T is the absolute temperature; μ_0 is the chemical potential in the standard reference state, from which increments in chemical potential are reckoned just as electrical potentials are always measured with respect to earth, whose potential is arbitrarily taken as zero; and A is the thermodynamic activity, or just the activity, of the substance.

As pointed out by Ferguson, in determining the chemical potential for biological purposes, it is convenient to take the state of the pure substance as the standard reference state. Then the μ_0 becomes standard, and μ values will be defined by the expression $RT \ln A$ or, since R and T remain constant, by the activity only.

Activity is a function of the concentration so chosen that the ideal-gas laws remain valid for real systems when the activity has been substituted for the concentration. (This activity is sometimes termed the "effective concentration"; outside the USSR it is called the "thermodynamic concentration" by a number of biologists.)

In the case of gaseous substances that do not deviate strongly from ideal-gas behavior, as is true for most situations within the province of toxicology and pharmacology, activity is given by the equation

$$A = \frac{P}{P_0}$$

where P_0 is the saturated vapor pressure at 20°C, and P is the partial vapor pressure corresponding to the selected effect.

When this relationship holds, the physical meaning of activity is that it is the relative saturation of the medium expressed as a fraction of unity. This simple expression immediately transfers the thermodynamic consideration from the realm of theory to the field of readily accessible practice.

Activity can be determined from the above relationship in a vast majority of situations involving the action of gaseous substances on living organisms. In some cases, however, for example when narcosis is effected by inert gases at high pressures, the formula is inapplicable (Lazarev, 1941; Lazarev et al., 1948; Lawrence et al., 1946; Cullen and Gross, 1951) because the deviations from ideality are too large. To make it usable the pressures must be replaced by fugacities so that

$$A = \frac{f}{f_0}$$

Fugacities are corrected pressures so defined as to maintain the ideal-gas laws when substituted in them (fugacity is introduced with the same conditions as activity). Fugacity values for gases at different pressures are given in the thermodynamic literature; they are amenable to calculation and experimental determination (e.g., Mullins, 1954; Shakhparonov, 1956). The first to use the fugacity concept for the calculation of activities corresponding to the production of narcosis by gases strongly deviating from ideality were Ferguson and Hawkins (1949).

A more complex situation is encountered when substances are applied to biological objects in solution, for instance, in toxicity studies on aquatic animals. Activity can then be calculated only if the solution obeys Henry's law (at least approximately) over the entire range of possible concentrations, that is, if $C = kP$, where C is the concentration of the substance and P is its pressure over the solution. Then $P = C/k$ and $P_0 = C_0/k$, where C_0 is the solubility, so that

$$A = \frac{P}{P_0} = \frac{C}{C_0}$$

This relationship is valid only for substances with limited solubility.

To determine the activity of a substance in solution, it seems convenient to introduce a gaseous phase in equilibrium with the liquid phase and to find the value of activity from the vapor pressure in the gaseous phase. The same activity will then also characterize the substance in the liquid phase as well as in any biophase in equilibrium.

It is important that at equilibrium the activity will be the same in all phases if the same standard reference state is selected for the different phases. Indeed, since

$$\mu_1 = \mu_i$$

(where the subscript i refers to any phase in equilibrium), $\mu_0 + RT \ln A_1 = \mu_0 + RT \ln A_i$, which is possible only if $A_1 = A_i$.

Thus nonelectrolytic action can be characterized by activity instead of chemical potential. The principle here is the same, and the only difference is a numerical one, since $(\mu - \mu_0)$ differs from A only in that, to obtain the chemical potential, it is necessary to take the logarithm of A and to multiply it by RT. This will apply to all cases because the taking of logarithms and the values of T (room temperature) and R are standard.

As already indicated, a stricter and much more extensive treatment of thermodynamic equilibrium can be found in textbooks on thermodynamics and physical chemistry. For a detailed acquaintance with the relationships given above, the book by Shakhparonov (1956) and a special biological paper by Mullins (1954) are recommended.

Ferguson, who proposed making use of thermodynamics for toxicological purposes and who discussed the implications of such thermodynamic consideration, did not formulate any principle. The term "Ferguson's principle" appears to have established itself in the literature after the publication of Albert's book (1968). Although various authors attach different meanings to it, this concept is usually taken to mean the use of activity as an index of toxic action. In our view a formulation of Ferguson's principle should embody its essence, namely, that it is expedient to compare the potencies of nonelectrolytes on the basis of their activities corresponding to a selected effect, since the activity characterizes the substance not only in the external or any internal medium but also in the site of its action.

3. THE MAIN COROLLARIES TO FERGUSON'S PRINCIPLE

In 1921, in treating experimental data on the narcotic effects of 29 substances on the isolated frog heart, Fühner compared their potencies by using the ratio

$$\frac{\text{Concentration in the solution}}{\text{Solubility in the solution}}$$

that is, he made an empiric use of activity without being aware of the concept of activity, which appeared later. This ratio proved to lie within the narrow range of 0.30 to 0.35. Later he characterized the hemolytic concentrations of a number of substances by the reciprocal of their activities (Fühner, 1923), whose values lay, as a rule, between 2 and 3; urethane and chloral hydrate were exceptions to the rule, having much higher values. Fühner's results remained ignored for a long time.

After the publication of Ferguson's paper (1939) which demonstrated the advantages of using activities as indices of toxicity over any other method of expressing the toxicities of nonelectrolytes, there appeared studies which compared effective concentrations with effective activities of toxic substances in various homologous series (Gavaudan et al., 1944a, b; Badger, 1946; Gavaudan, 1947; Ferguson and Pirie, 1948; Johnson et al., 1951; Ferguson, 1951; Ivens, 1952; Ross and Ludwig, 1957; Byrde et al., 1958).

These studies, which used mainly insects, unicellular organisms, and plants as the biological material, led to some general conclusions. By way of example, typical results from Ferguson's studies are reproduced in Tables 5 and 6. These tables indicate that, while the biologically effective concentrations of substances in homologous series exhibit a wide range of variations (ten-, hundred-, and thousandfold), the corresponding activities differ only severalfold in most cases.

In a homologous series the activities required to produce equal effects increase with increasing molecular size, attaining unity where traceable. The member with an activity equal to or approaching unity is the last member

Table 5. Equitoxic Concentrations and Activities of Various Substances for the Grain Weevil

Substance	Minimal Lethal Concentration (mg/liter)	(moles/liter $\times$ 10^{-6})	Minimal Lethal Activity
Pentane	897	12,500	0.45
Hexane	353	4,100	0.50
Heptane	137	1,370	0.56
Decane	12	85	1
Benzene	210	2,690	0.53
Toluene	96	1,040	0.68
Ethylbenzene	50	470	0.90
Propylbenzene	30	250	1
Methyl chloride	166	3,280	0.014
Ethyl chloride	1124	17,400	0.28
Propyl chloride	428	5,460	0.30
Butyl chloride	200	2,160	0.38
Amyl chloride	73	690	0.40
Methyl bromide	3.3	35	0.0004
Methylene bromide	90	520	0.20
Bromoform	16	64	0.22
Methanol	100	3,130	0.47
Ethanol	85	1,850	0.59
Propanol	50	830	0.77
Butanol	30	360	1
Methyl formate	15	250	0.0007
Ethyl formate	35	480	0.035
Propyl formate	28	320	0.072
Fluorobenzene	180	1,880	0.46
Chlorobenzene	45	400	0.63
Bromobenzene	20	125	0.56
Methyl iodide	2	14	0.0007
Ethyl iodide	11	71	0.01
Propyl iodide	5.9	34	0.014
Butyl iodide	5	27	0.036
Amyl iodide	4.6	23	0.1
Isopropyl iodide	65	380	0.11

Source. Ferguson and Pirie (1948).

Table 6.   Bactericidal Concentrations and
Activities of Alcohols for *B. typhosus*

Alcohol	Concentration (moles/liter)	Activity
Methanol	10.8	0.33
Ethanol	4.86	0.32
Propanol	1.50	0.34
Butanol	0.45	0.37
Pentanol	0.13	0.52
Hexanol	0.039	0.63
Heptanol	0.012	0.74
Octanol	0.0034	0.88

Source.   Ferguson (1939).

of the series which is effective on the selected criterion of toxicity. Such behavior of activity in homologous series fits into the well-known Richardson rule relating the decrease in effective concentrations of homologues (i.e., the increase in their toxicities) to the increase in their molecular weights (see Lazarev, 1938, or Ferguson, 1939, for details). The increase in toxicity does not, however, continue indefinitely: there invariably occurs a cutoff of toxicity as the series is ascended so that the higher homologues are ineffective when judged by the selected toxicity criterion. Richardson's rule receives a clear interpretation in thermodynamic terms: a cutoff occurs wherever the activity approaches unity since, by definition, it cannot exceed unity.*

* The position of this cutoff depends on the toxic effect selected. The more severe the selected effect, the sooner the last effective member whose activity approaches unity is reached in a homologous series. Conversely, the less severe the effect, the higher up the series the cutoff will occur. The phenomenon of cutoff is of general biological importance; in fact it is one of the prerequisites for the existence of life itself (Lazarev, 1944). Cutoff is accounted for by the fact that the physicochemical properties directly involved in the toxic actions of substances (e.g., vapor pressure) vary in a homologous series at rates different from the rates of change in the corresponding constant properties (e.g., saturated vapor pressure).

The different rates of change in such physicochemical properties inevitably lead to their intersection in a homologous series. Since one óf these properties (saturated vapor pressure in our example) is maximal, changes in the other are limited. The limit for the vapor pressure of vapors of a substance is the saturated vapor pressure. A cutoff signifies that such a limit has been reached.

Generally speaking, the "cutoff rule" is valid not only for homologous series, but also for many other series of substances arranged on the basis of uniformly varying physicochemical characteristics. This rule sets a limit to the increase in toxicity whatever the type of toxic action —nonelectrolytic or any specific.

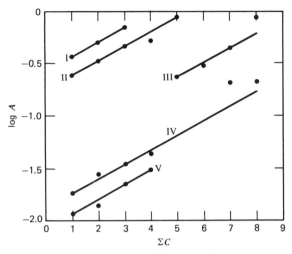

Figure 5. Relationship between the logarithm of the thermodynamic activity required for equieffective biological action and the length of carbon chain in homologous series. I, alkyl acetates: hemolysis of ox blood; II, alcohols: bactericidal action; III, aliphatic hydrocarbons: narcosis of mice; IV, alcohols: inhibition of development of sea-urchin eggs; V, alcohols: tadpole narcosis. (From Badger, 1946.)

Badger (1946), using his own data and those of Ferguson, plotted the logarithms of activities required for equal effects as a function of the number of carbon atoms [log $A = f(\sum C)$] for several homologous series; the plots proved to be straight lines with equal slopes (Figure 5). This means that the last effective member of a series is defined by the point of intersection of the corresponding plot with the line log $A = 0$. (Indeed, since when log $A = 0$, $A = 1$ and $P = P_0$, and P cannot be greater than P_0.)

Table 5 lists various substances whose toxic effects were assessed by one and the same criterion. It can be seen from this table that, with two exceptions, the activities in different series vary within a similar range—from 0.2 to unity. The exceptions are, first, the series of formates and alkyl iodides, where activities are very small and vary widely, and, second, methyl chloride and methyl bromide, which deviate from their respective series in having activities much lower than one would expect.

Ferguson (1939) suggested that thermodynamic activity be used as a criterion of the type of action of substances producing a particular biological effect. When the activity values required for the same effect in a homologous series are high and show little variation, the homologues have the non-electrolytic type of action (referred to as physical toxicity by Ferguson). On the other hand, when such equieffective activities do not lie within a narrow range, or the activity value of some one member is much lower than the compactly grouped activity values of other members, the action is specific (chemical, according to Ferguson). An ill-defined behavior of activities required for equal effects points to a combination of these two types of action. Thus, in the series of alkyl iodides, a typically specific action of lower members is succeeded by a combined one as the series is ascended to amyl iodide and isopropyl iodide.

Ferguson and Pirie (1948) concluded from their experiments with the grain weevil that the mode of toxic action is predominantly nonelectrolytic at an activity of 0.1 and higher and is mainly specific at lower activity values. Gavaudan et al. (1944a), in their studies on the inhibition of mitoses, reported activities ranging from 0.08 to unity for the nonelectrolytic type of action. From a theoretical consideration based on the lipoid theory of narcosis they concluded that the lowest activity compatible with this type of action is of the order of 0.05. Albert (1973) has given an even broader range, from 0.001 to 1.0. These estimates of the activity range do not agree with data of the present authors obtained on mammals (see the next section).

Ferguson's results (1939) have an additional aspect. It can be seen from Table 7, where substances from various homologous series are listed in an arbitrary order, that the activities have a ninefold range of variation, giving an average figure of approximately 0.5. If one agrees with such averaging, one can say that a toxic compound produces a lethal effect when the ambient air is about half saturated with its vapors (in the case of substances with the nonelectrolytic type of action). It is this kind of averaging which underlies occasionally encountered statements that nonelectrolytes have equal activities for equal toxic effects.

It should be noted here that equilibrium distribution between the external medium and the living organism is attainable only in the case of substances with the nonelectrolytic type of action. A given biological effect can then be characterized by the activity of the substance responsible for that effect, implying that all the relationships involving the activity function are valid, that is, that the activity has a thermodynamic meaning. In the case of substances having the specific type of action, such equilibrium is possible, if at all, only at a level corresponding to a situation where some of the substance disappears in the organism as the result of specific reactions and where more of the substance enters the organism by a process of compensatory absorption. For such situations the activity has not been determined, and the figures which are given for the activity (from vapor pressure determinations) do not represent activity as such, for they are devoid of thermodynamic meaning. From a biological viewpoint, however, such figures are meaningful in that they are indicative of the type of action of the substances concerned. This question is dealt with at greater length in Section 5 of this chapter.

Table 7. Values of Activities Corresponding to Lethal Effects of Vapors on the Wireworm (exposure time = 1000 min at 15°C)

Substance	Activity
Monomethylaniline	0.3
Dimethylaniline	0.4
Pyridine	0.1
Bromoform	0.5
Tetrachloroethane	0.6
Chlorobenzene	0.5
Toluene	0.4
Nitromethane	0.6
Benzene	0.2
Heptane	0.5
Chloroform	0.2
Trichloroethylene	0.4
Carbon tetrachloride	0.4
Hexane	0.6
Dichloroethylene	0.2
Pentane	0.9

Ferguson's principle was employed in a number of studies where substances were described as acting specifically or nonelectrolytically (nonspecifically) according to their thermodynamic activities at the time of action (Gavaudan et al., 1944b; Gavaudan and Poussel, 1947; Ferguson et al., 1950; Shirk et al., 1951; Richardson, 1952; Paribok, 1957; Lindenberg et al., 1957; Ross and Ludwig, 1957; Byrde et al., 1958). This principle was also referred to by Horsfall (1956), and its use has been advocated by Barlow (1964) and Albert (1968) for purely practical purposes in the initial evaluation of the toxicity and mechanism of action of a substance.

Indeed, if the substance tested for a particular biological effect is found to produce that effect at an external concentration corresponding to a thermodynamic activity commensurable with unity, the likelihood of its having a nonspecific (nonelectrolytic) mode of action is high. Hence one would not expect it to show particularly novel biological properties and would not initiate a program in which the molecule was to be altered only slightly, for example, by inserting a methyl group in various positions (Albert, 1968).

It is worth noting that Hassal (1953, 1955) questioned the validity of dividing substances into nonelectrolytically and specifically acting depending on the magnitude of their activity values at the time of action. He pointed out that a specific effect was possible even at relatively high activity values. He suggested that the type of action in a homologous series could be judged from the slope of a plot of a logarithmic function of the equieffective concentration against the number of carbon atoms.

On the basis of the thermodynamic hypothesis of Ferguson and of the modern physicochemical theories of solubility, McGowan concluded that the biophases responsible for nonelectrolytic actions appear to be identical or very similar in all organisms. This conclusion was first derived from his work with nonelectrolytes in the gaseous state (McGowan, 1951a) and then also with nonelectrolytes in aqueous solutions (McGowan, 1951b, 1952a). Subsequently, having assumed that the biophases responsible for nonelectrolytic actions of different compounds on various organisms were identical, McGowan (1952b, 1954, 1955) proposed formulas for calculating the toxicities of nonelectrolytes. This line of studies has been reviewed in detail by Liublina et al. (1967).

Ferguson's view that the thermodynamic activities required to produce equal effects increase progressively in a homologous series—a generalization which has been validated by a number of the authors cited above, as well as by our studies—was challenged by Brink and Posternak (1948), who concluded from their own and some other studies that a far more general rule is that of constant activity for equal effect. They supported this contention by data from many experiments with different biological objects exposed to the action of aqueous solutions of alcohols. They believed this rule to be valid not only inside but also outside of homologous series.* They also pointed out deviations from the rule, for example, in the case of acetic esters. They classed Ferguson's data among such deviations.

According to Brink and Posternak (1948) and Posternak and Larrabee (1951), both the rule and the deviations from it could be accounted for by the differential suppression of nerve impulse transmission by toxic substances. These authors worked with the isolated stellate ganglion of the cat, in which part of the preganglionic nerve fibers make synaptic connection on post-ganglionic nerve cells, while others pass through the ganglion without synapses intervening. They recorded electric impulse conduction via synaptic and nonsynaptic pathways in ganglia perfused with fluids containing various alcohols. The rule of equal activity for equal effect was found to be valid for synaptic but not for nonsynaptic pathways of nerve impulse conduction, as shown schematically in Figure 6.

---

* In their experiments with larvae of aquatic animals Crisp and Marr (1957) likewise failed to notice any well-defined, increasing trend in activity in homologous series. However, since they used different exposure times for different substances, it is probable either that equilibria had not been attained or that the figures they obtained were incomparable for some other reason.

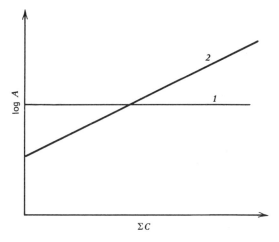

Figure 6. Schematic representation of the relationship between the log A and the number of carbon atoms (ΣC) of alcohols for two different pathways of nerve conduction. *1*, synaptic conduction; *2*, nonsynaptic conduction. (After Posternak and Larrabee, 1951.)

Somewhat later, the view that the above rule was valid for effects involving synaptic conduction was supported by several authors (e.g., Larrabee and Holaday, 1952; Larrabee and Posternak, 1952). However, as early as 1953, Posternak admitted that the "rule" had too many exceptions to be called a rule.

A more detailed discussion of this subject would involve us in a consideration of the physiological mechanisms of narcosis, which is far from our purpose here. We will merely note one criticism of Brink and Posternak's hypothesis of equal activity for equal effect, made by Ferguson (1951). The latter author pointed out that, for one thing, Brink and Posternak substantiated their hypothesis by data drawn almost entirely from work on narcosis produced by alcohols and, for another, that they did not discriminate between the normal and branch-chained alcohols, an omission which might give a false impression of the constancy of activity value.

Indeed, alcohols do often produce equal effects at equal activities. Most of the examples (some of which are given by Brink and Posternak) concern narcosis in tadpoles and isolated frog heart. From their detailed analyses of the activities of various isomers of different alcohols equally effective for the *Gobio* fish, Lindenberg and Gary–Bobo (1951, 1952) and Gary–Bobo and Lindenberg (1952) concluded that the activity varied slightly, but without any regular trend. Subsequently Lindenberg (1956) found Brink and Posternak's hypothesis to be valid for aqueous solutions of alcohols in *Gobio* fish.

The data of Ferguson (1939, 1951) and of Bradbury and Armstrong (1955), as well as our results presented in the next section of this chapter, indicate that the activities required for equal effects increase in the series of normal alcohols both for insects and for mammals.

In comparing these two contradictory sets of data, it may be noted that the former come from experiments on narcosis in water, whereas the latter are from those on narcosis in air. This distinction is immaterial from the physical point of view, for the overall result will be the same, whatever the medium from which the nonelectrolyte enters the organism (the medium can affect only the rate of entry). It is possible that different types of narcotic action are involved, as was suggested by Posternak and Larrabee (1951).

Ferguson's principle has been employed to evaluate the mechanism of action of substances. Examples are the studies of Lindenberg (1955, 1956), which led to the suggestion that phenol, cresols, and benzene and its homologues act by the same mechanism; the study of Molinengo (1963), whose results make it possible to judge the permeability of biomembranes for compounds with different chemical structures; and the work of Laffort (1966), who studied the mechanism of action of odorous substances at the olfactory threshold level.

4. APPLICATION OF FERGUSON'S PRINCIPLE TO STUDIES ON MAMMALS

As stated in Section 3, the bulk of available data on the comparative toxicities of substances in relation to their thermodynamic activities comes from studies on insects, bacteria, and plants. Much more pertinent to the purposes of industrial toxicology, of course, would be the results of investigations on animal models close to man. Of the studies mentioned above, mammals were used in only two or three. The material was very limited in these studies, and their results were similar to those obtained for lower animals. More recently, mammals were employed in more extensive studies (Filov, 1962, 1963a) which led to further conclusions. Before proceeding to discuss these results, it is appropriate to consider in more detail the equilibrium distribution of nonelectrolytes between the external medium and the organism and the time taken to attain this distribution.

When vapors of a nonelectrolyte are inhaled, the establishment of equilibrium can be ascertained, for example, from their concentrations in the inspired and expired air, provided that the transformations undergone by the nonelectrolyte are not too rapid and that the expired concentration progressively increases, eventually to become equal to the inspired concentration. This indicates that an equilibrium has been reached, that is, that the organism has been completely saturated. The time taken to attain this saturation will of course vary from one substance to another, depending on the capacity of the body in respect to the substance concerned. The greater the capacity, the longer is the time required to reach the equilibrium.

The exposure periods considered suitable for the equilibration of threshold concentrations are usually rather long and variable. Thus in the USSR 2-hr exposures are used by most investigators; Bradbury and Armstrong (1954, 1955), in their work with weevils, used exposures of 2 and 4 hr; Ferguson (1951), working with the same test object, evaluated the narcotic potencies of substances after a 3-hr exposure; Hassal (1953, 1955) considered 5 hr to be the optimal time; and so on. Such a standard empirical approach may lead to divergent results not suitable for comparison.

It must be remembered that any living organism is a multiphase system and, as such, shows highly complex equilibrium relationships. The different phases (tissues) vary widely in their capacity to be saturated with particular substances and have different blood supplies. Nonelectrolytic action is believed to depend on the accumulation of a substance in some one phase or in a limited number of phases. It would therefore be interesting to know the time required for an equilibrium to be reached in the phases which are responsible for nonelectrolytic action. Strictly speaking, an equilibrium can only occur in all phases of the organism simultaneously. But this may be ignored because it is difficult for the nonelectrolyte to gain entry into some of the phases. The transport-distribution relationships may, however, be a source of error if the phase or phases responsible for nonelectrolytic action are not definitely known.

With these reservations in mind, let us consider the thermodynamic activities of a broad range of nonelectrolytes corresponding to different kinds of nonelectrolytic action.

Table 8 contains data from a single laboratory (Laboratory of Industrial Toxicology of the Leningrad Institute of Industrial Hygiene and Occupational

Table 8.   Isonarcotic Concentrations, Pressures, and Activities (A) of Vapors Causing 50% of White Mice to Fall on One Side with 2-Hr Exposure

Number	Substance	C (mg/liter)	P (mm Hg)	P_0	A	Type of Action[a]
1	Pentane	250	63.4	420	0.15	N
2	Hexane	100	21.2	122	0.17	N
3	Heptane	40	7.3	35.5	0.21	N
4	Octane	25	4	10.7	0.37	N

(Continued)

Table 8. (*Continued*)

Number	Substance	C (mg/liter)	P (mm Hg)	P_0	A	Type of Action[a]
5	Nonane	15	2	3.4	0.6	N
6	Nitromethane	26	7.8	27.8	0.28	N
7	Nitroethane	20	4.9	15.6	0.31	N
8	1-Nitropropane	24	4.9	7.5	0.66	N
9	2-Nitropropane	26.5	5.4	12.9	0.42	N
10	Methanol	120	68.5	89	0.77	N
11	Ethanol	50	20	44	0.52	N
12	Propanol	30	9	14.5	0.63	N
13	Isopropanol	40	12	35	0.35	N
14	Butanol	17	4.3	5	0.86	N
15	Isobutanol	12.5	3	8.8	0.35	N
16	Amylene (mixture)	110	29	500	0.058	NS
17	Hexylene	100	22	139	0.156	N
18	Heptylene	60	11	38	0.3	N
19	Dimethyl ketone	50	15.7	178	0.088	NS
20	Methyl ethyl ketone	25	6.3	77	0.082	NS
21	Methyl propyl ketone	15	3.2	30	0.106	NS
22	Acetaldehyde	14.6	6.1	760	0.008	NS
23	Propionaldehyde	9.8	3.1	300	0.01	S
24	Butyraldehyde	11.8	3	250	0.012	S
25	Methyl acetate	45	11	166	0.07	S
26	Ethyl acetate	40	8.4	65	0.13	N
27	Propyl acetate	45	8	25	0.32	N
28	Butyl acetate	30	4.7	14	0.34	N
29	Isoamyl acetate	30	4.2	5.5	0.76	N
30	Dimethyl ether	226	90	6300	0.014	NS
31	Diethyl ether	92	23	440	0.052	NS
32	Dibutyl ether	10	1.4	6.4	0.22	N
33	Cyclopentane	110	29	262	0.11	N
34	Methylcyclopentane	107	23.4	109	0.21	N
35	Ethylcyclopentane	42.5	8	32	0.25	N
36	Cyclohexane	50	11	77	0.14	N
37	Methylcyclohexane	35	6.5	35	0.19	N
38	Dimethylcyclohexane	22.5	3.7	15	0.24	N
39	Ethylcyclohexane	30	4.5	10.3	0.44	N
40	Benzene	15	3.5	75	0.043	NS
41	Toluene	11	2.2	22.5	0.097	N
42	Ethylbenzene	15	2.6	7	0.37	N
43	Propylbenzene	15	2.3	2.5	0.9	N
44	Methyl bromide	115	22	1250	0.018	NS
45	Ethyl bromide	90	15	388	0.04	NS
46	Propyl bromide	50	7.4	118	0.063	NS

Table 8. (*Continued*)

Number	Substance	C (mg/liter)	P (mm Hg)	P_0	A	Type of Action[a]
47	Methyl iodide	10	1.3	331	0.004	S
48	Ethyl chloride	140	39.6	996	0.04	NS
49	Propyl chloride	81	19	282	0.067	NS
50	Ethylene bromide	7	0.7	10.3	0.066	NS
51	1,1-Dichloroethane	32.5	6	180	0.033	NS
52	1,2-Dichloroethane	17.5	3.3	70	0.046	NS
53	1,2-Dichloropropane	10.5	1.7	42	0.04	NS
54	1,1,1-Trichloroethane	45	6.15	100	0.06	NS
55	1,1,2-Trichloroethane	10	1.4	19	0.07	NS
56	1,1,2,2-Tetrachloroethane	8.5	0.9	4.9	0.19	NS
57	Pentachloroethane	7.5	0.7	2.5	0.27	N
58	Methylene chloride	32.5	7	349	0.02	NS
59	Chloroform	20	3	160	0.02	NS
60	Carbon tetrachloride	50	6	91	0.065	NS
61	Vinyl chloride	64	19	3620	0.0052	S
62	Vinyl 1,1-dichloride	40	7.5	500	0.015	NS
63	Vinyl 1,2-dichloride	40	7.5	167.5	0.045	NS
64	Vinyl trichloride	25	3.5	60	0.058	NS
65	Vinyl tetrachloride	20	2.2	15	0.15	NS
66	Chlorobutadiene	5	1	176	0.006	S
67	Vinyl acetate	21	4.5	82	0.055	NS
68	Vinyl propionate	16	3	40	0.073	NS
69	Vinyl butyrate	48	7.7	15	0.2	N
70	1,3-Butadiene	200–300	67–70	2300	0.03–0.04	NS
71	Monovinylacetylene	60	21	1420	0.015	NS
72	Divinylacetylene	15	3.5	70	0.05	NS
73	Methyl acrylate	18	3.8	65	0.06	NS
74	Methyl methacrylate	17.5	3.2	3.5	0.09	NS
75	Acrylonitrile	0.35	0.12	90	0.0013	S
76	Methacrylonitrile	0.85	0.23	55	0.0042	S
77	Furfural	5	0.93	5	0.19	N
78	Thiofuran	10	2.2	60	0.036	NS
79	Pyridine	10	2.3	15	0.155	N
80	Dioxane	40	8.3	29.5	0.28	N
81	Styrene	12.5	2.2	5.5	0.4	N
82	Mesityl oxide	15	2.8	6.9	0.4	N
83	Formalglycol	75	18.6	80	0.23	N
84	α-Pinene	15	2	4.6	0.44	N

[a] N = predominantly nonelectrolytic action, S = predominantly specific action, NS = intermediate action.

Diseases) on the concentrations of vapors in the air causing 50 % of noninbred white mice to fall on one side as the result of 2-hr exposure (narcotic concentrations). Table 9 lists similar data for the concentrations having threshold action on the unconditioned reflex activity of rabbits with 40-min exposure.

Activity was calculated as the ratio of the vapor pressure (P) required for equal effects to the saturated vapor pressure (P_0):

$$A = \frac{P}{P_0}$$

Table 9. Equieffective Concentrations and Activities of Substances for Threshold Action on Unconditioned Reflex Activity in Rabbits with 40-Min Exposure

Number	Substance	C (mg/liter)	Activity
1	Methanol	4.5	0.029
2	Ethanol	5.0	0.052
3	Propanol	2.25	0.047
4	Butanol	4.0	0.198
5	Nitromethane	1.0	0.011
6	Nitroethane	0.5	0.008
7	1-Nitropropane	0.5	0.014
8	2-Nitropropane	0.5	0.008
9	Dimethyl ketone	1.6	0.0028
10	Methyl ethyl ketone	1.9	0.0062
11	Methyl propyl ketone	1.9	0.0134
12	Formaldehyde	0.015	0.000002
13	Butyraldehyde	0.1	0.0001
14	Chloroform	1.0	0.001
15	Carbon tetrachloride	1.5	0.002
16	Benzene	0.76	0.0024
17	Toluene	0.62	0.0055
18	Xylene	0.23	0.0067
19	Chlorobenzene	0.66	0.00124
20	Vinyl acetate	0.25	0.0006
21	Vinyl propionate	1.0	0.005
22	Vinyl butyrate	2.0	0.02
23	Methylamine	0.3	0.00007
24	Dimethylamine	0.425	0.00013
25	Butylamine	1.0	0.0024
26	Aniline	0.025	0.0136
27	Methylaniline	0.03	0.013

Table 9.   (*Continued*)

Number	Substance	C (mg/liter)	Activity
28	Toluidine (ortho)	0.05	0.0305
29	Xylidine (meta)	0.06	0.0364
30	Pyridine	0.4	0.062
31	Methylpyridine	0.3	0.086
32	Octane	0.9	0.0135
33	Ethyl acetate	2.1	0.0067
34	Diethyl ether	10.0	0.0056
35	1,2-Dichloroethane	0.65	0.0013
36	Trichloroethylene	0.7	0.0016
37	Styrene	0.9	0.029
38	Cyclohexanone	8.0	0.455
39	Furfural	0.25	0.0096
40	Monochlorotrifluoroethylene	0.17	0.000004
41	1,1-Dichloroethylene	1.0	0.000376

The P_0 values were taken mostly from *Tables of Physical and Chemical Constants* (Kaye and Laby, 1957). The equieffective pressures were calculated from the concentrations in accordance with the ideal-gas laws. With rare exceptions the use of these laws was justified because the pressures corresponding to experimental concentrations were less than 1 atm and the deviations from ideality for gases are of consequence only at pressures of several atmospheres. The pressure at a given effect was therefore calculated from the formula

$$P = \frac{760 \cdot C \cdot R \cdot T}{1000 \cdot M}$$

where C is the concentration (mg/liter) of the substance in the air required to produce a given effect, M is the molecular weight of the substance, T is the absolute temperature, R is the gas constant [liter-atm/(deg mole)], and P is the pressure (mm Hg). Since the only variables are the effective concentration and the molecular weight, the formula can be simplified to

$$P = 18.28 \frac{C}{M} \text{ mm Hg}$$

It should be noted that 2 hr is quite sufficient for an equilibrium to be established for most of the substances listed in Table 8; therefore, when narcosis is caused by a nonelectrolytically acting substance, the calculated activity also characterizes the substance at the site of action.

The data presented in Table 8 are generally in line with the results of Ferguson and other authors. Thus the activities required for equal effects tend to increase in homologous series; there are grounds for classifying substances into two main categories: nonelectrolytic and specific, and the range of activity variation in series of substances with the nonelectrolytic type of action is much narrower than the range of corresponding concentrations.

The data of Table 8 are of special interest because they characterize the toxicities of many substances and series of substances for mammals (mice). These data enable the substances studied to be classified according to type of action, as shown in the last column of the table, where N denotes predominantly nonelectrolytic, S mainly specific, and NS intermediate action.

The predominantly nonelectrolytic type of action is displayed by aliphatic hydrocarbons (1–5) and their nitro derivatives (6–9); aliphatic alcohols (10–15); acetic esters (25–29), with the possible exception of methyl acetate; cyclopeptane and cyclohexane and their derivatives (33–39); and some members of other series. The mainly specific type of action is shown by aldehydes (22–24), methyl iodide (47), vinyl chloride (61), chlorobutadiene (66), and acrylonitrile and its methyl derivative (75 and 76, respectively). The substances with the intermediate type of action include the diene hydrocarbons (16–18), ketones (19–21), ethers (30–32), bromide and chloride derivatives of hydrocarbons (44–46, 48–55, 58–60, 62–65), vinyl esters (67, 68) and other vinyl derivatives (70–72), and acrylates (73 and 74).

In our view such a "Fergusonian" classification is highly tentative and can serve only as a rough guide. Ferguson derived his inferences from work with insects, where the cessation of movements was a sole and unequivocal criterion of effect. In the case of mice and, especially, other, more highly organized mammals, any effect caused by a substance, including narcosis (falling on one side), is accompanied or succeeded by other readily detectable effects which may often be critical for judging the type of action shown by the substance. The following two examples should suffice to illustrate this point.

Methanol had to be assigned to substances with the nonelectrolytic type of action as far as its activity required to produce narcosis in mice was concerned. However, it is also known to produce a characteristic specific effect manifested some time after its narcotic action. Vinyl acetate and vinyl propionate were classed among substances with intermediate action; vinyl butyrate, among those with nonelectrolytic action. On the other hand, acetaldehyde was assigned to the specifically acting substances. But it has been proved (Filov, 1959b) that vinyl esters are instantaneously saponified in the body with the formation of acetaldehyde. The latter is the substance mainly responsible for the toxic properties of vinyl esters. For this reason the vinyl esters and acetaldehyde should be rated as substances having the same type of action.

As can be seen from Table 9, not all of Ferguson's inferences are valid in the case of threshold action in mammals. Thus, while the equieffective activities in homologous series increase, their range is often wider than that of the corresponding concentrations expressed in milligrams per liter. An attempt to group the substances according to type of action would describe most of them as having the specific type of action, and this is certainly not true to fact.

One possible explanation for this discrepancy may be the failure of many substances to reach saturation concentrations in the course of 40-min exposure, but the main reason appears to be a decrease in effective activities on passing from more severe to less severe and more delicate effects. It follows, then, that one should not relate definite values of thermodynamic activity to the type of action while ignoring the biological effect.

An important consideration appears to be the course of activity changes in homologous series. Figure 7 shows plots of log activities corresponding to narcosis in mice as a function of molecular size in various homologous series. In constructing these plots we excluded the values of obviously non-equilibrium activities characterizing substances (e.g., methanol and dimethyl ketone) which failed to saturate the mice within the space of 2 hr.

Figure 7 indicates that the log activities generally tend to change uniformly in a homologous series (exceptions are possible because of inaccurate determinations of the quantities used to calculate the activity). Similar plots of log activities were obtained by Badger (1946) (see Figure 5). Badger's plots, however, differ from ours in having identical slopes for different series.*

The data of Figure 7 can be used to estimate, by linear inter- or extrapolation, the unknown effective activity of a member of a homologous series from the known activities of other members. It is also possible to predict the last member of a series that is effective on a given criterion (the cutoff) by continuing the corresponding straight line until it intersects the line $\log A = 0$ (cf. p. 63).

The question dealt with in this section will be further discussed below in the light of the broader aspects to which Sections 5 and 6 are devoted.

---

* It seems that Badger was too casual in plotting his straight lines, for many of the points lay outside them. With a stricter approach some of the lines could have different angles or would not have been straight lines at all.

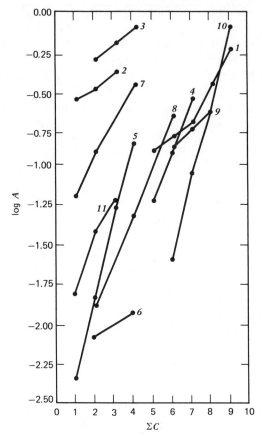

Figure 7. Logarithms of activities corresponding to narcotic concentrations for mice plotted against the length of carbon chain (ΣC) in various homologous series. Figures given below in parentheses refer to the numbers of substances in Table 8 for which the plots are shown here. *1*, paraffins (1–5); *2*, nitro derivatives of paraffins (6, 7, 9); *3*, alcohols (11, 12, 14); *4*, olefins (16–18); *5*, chloro-substituted vinyls (61, 62, 64, 65), the series having been constructed for chlorine; *6*, aldehydes (22–24), *7*, acetic esters (25, 26, 28); *8*, ethers (30–32); *9*, cyclohexane and its homologues (36–38); *10*, benzene and its homologues (40–43); *11*, bromo-substituted paraffins (44–46).

5. THE PROBLEM OF REAL HAZARDS PRESENTED BY VOLATILE SUBSTANCES ABSORBED BY INHALATION

This problem exists primarily in various industrial settings, notably in the chemical industry. Let us consider first one of the main aspects of the problem—the criteria of true hazard. After that we will try to relate these criteria to the thermodynamic activity and will then proceed to discuss the feasibility of constructing a scale of substances arranged according to the hazards presented by the inhalation of their vapors. We are not aware of any previous attempts to develop such a scale, although its desirability has been indicated on several occasions. We will be concerned mainly with acute toxic action, without considering the possible consequences of poisoning.

To be able to judge whether or not acute poisoning can result from inhaling vapors of a toxic substance, it is necessary first of all to have a concept of its toxic concentrations. In industry, however, where large numbers of more or less toxic substances are used, knowledge of their toxic concentrations often proves insufficient; it is also necessary to know the factors that promote or prevent the development of such concentrations in the industrial atmosphere. If the ambient air is polluted by a gaseous substance, the factors to be considered are the leak tightness of the process or equipment concerned, the volume of the workroom, the extent and design of ventilation, and so on. In the case of a liquid (solid) substance, an important additional consideration is the evaporating capacity of the substance, that is, its volatility, as well as the evaporating surface and temperature.

The effective toxicity of a substance, as determined from the toxic concentrations of its vapors in the respiration zone, is thus a function of many and highly variable factors. For this reason the problem of determining the effective toxicity under industrial conditions cannot be solved in general terms, on theoretical grounds alone. It is amenable to solution only for a particular industrial situation where the conditions remain constant or vary in a regular manner. In practice, the problem is solved by studying the ambient air in the respiration zone and comparing the results with data from animal experiments on the determination of toxic concentrations or with data, if available, on the effects of various concentrations on man.

The latter method is clearly insufficient for practical purposes because it cannot yield information of predictive value. To remedy the situation, at least partly, Lehmann (1919) introduced into toxicology the concept of "two-phase toxicity." He believed that in addition to "theoretical toxicity," expressed in milligrams per liter, an important factor to be considered in judging the actual toxicities of vapors of liquids is the volatility, that is, the relative magnitude of evaporation. The product of theoretical toxicity and volatility would represent the two-phase toxicity. Lehmann justified the use of this term by pointing out that both phases—gaseous and liquid—are of significance in cases of poisoning.

In the strict language of mathematics the concept of two-phase toxicity may be formulated as follows (Filov, 1957b; Lazarev, 1958): the theoretical toxicity, as Lehmann called it, or the absolute toxicity, is inversely proportional to the inspired concentration of the substance responsible for the toxic effect, while the concentration is proportional to the vapor pressure of the substance. Therefore the first cofactor of two-phase toxicity (let us denote it by F) is a function of the type $f_1(1/C)$ or $f'_1(1/P)$. Volatility, or evaporativity, is directly proportional to the saturated vapor pressure or to the maximum possible concentration in air corresponding to that pressure, that is, $\sim f_2(P_0)$ or $f'_2(C_0)$. In general,

$$F = f_1\left(\frac{1}{C}\right) \cdot f'_2(C_0) = f\left(\frac{C_0}{C}\right) = f'\left(\frac{P_0}{P}\right)$$

If the concentrations or pressures are expressed in the same units, we can write

$$F = \frac{C_0}{C} = \frac{P_0}{P}$$

The concept of two-phase toxicity makes it possible to assess, though within limits, the true occupational hazard presented by liquids (solids) and, more important, their relative hazards. The limiting factor here is the requirement that the conditions of action of the gaseous substance be standard. The substance must be allowed to evaporate freely from a constant or regularly varying surface in a room of constant volume, other factors also being constant.

In some industrial situations, where the possibility of free evaporation is ruled out and the toxic substance can enter the respiration zone by some other route, for example, by way of faulty gas pipes, the concept of two-phase toxicity becomes meaningless. The actual hazard from a substance will be then determined by factors other than volatility. In view of all this it is not possible to agree with those who identify effective toxicity with two-phase toxicity. Two-phase toxicity can be a measure of effective toxicity only under the conditions specified above in cases where this toxicity is judged from the concentration causing acute poisoning. Under such conditions, when the principal factor is free evaporation, the numerical value of two-phase toxicity may form a good basis for constructing a scale of the real risk of poisoning by volatile substances. It is this possibility which determines the vitality and importance of the two-phase toxicity concept (Lazarév and Filov, 1964).

It is known that two-phase toxicity tends to decrease slowly in a homologous series of organic compounds with the increasing size of the hydrocarbon radical; in contrast, absolute toxicity increases at a comparatively rapid rate (Lazarev, 1938). The limit for the decrease in two-phase toxicity is set by the completely nontoxic member of the series (with all the subsequent members), whose ineffectiveness is due to its low volatility and the associated inability to develop in the air the concentration necessary to produce a toxic effect.

The physical meaning of two-phase toxicity is fairly simple and is immediately apparent from its mathematical expression. Numerically, two-phase toxicity is equal to the quantity which shows how many times the saturation concentration of a substance is greater than the inspired concentration of it that will cause poisoning.

Two-phase toxicity has another sense: its numerical value is the reciprocal of the thermodynamic activity. Indeed,

$$A = \frac{P}{P_0} = \frac{C}{C_0}$$

Hence

$$F = \frac{1}{A} \quad \text{and} \quad A = \frac{1}{F}$$

It is important to bear in mind, however, that the numerical equality of activity and reciprocal two-phase toxicity does not mean that the two are equivalent. The concept of activity is thermodynamically meaningful only when an equilibrium exists between the external medium and the biophase responsible for the nonelectrolytic effect under consideration. As already stated, no true equilibrium is possible in the case of specifically acting substances. For such substances activities have not been determined, and the values obtained as ratios of the respective vapor pressures do not represent activities, for they are devoid of thermodynamic meaning. But these values are meaningful from a biological viewpoint in that they characterize two-phase toxicity and are indicators of the potencies of specifically acting substances (and also, of course, of nonspecifically acting substances).

Since the activity or, to be more precise, its reciprocal characterizes the real hazard presented by a freely evaporating substance, an attempt was made to construct activity-based scales of industrially used poisons that would provide an indication of their relative toxicities (Filov, 1959a). In each scale the substances were arranged in the decreasing order of their equally effective activities, regardless of the type of action. A scale like this is of fundamental importance for the effect selected and the animal species used, for it gives a precise idea of how readily and rapidly the effect will be attained in the case of a freely evaporating substance. Table 10 presents one such scale, based on the narcosis data for mice contained in Table 8.

Along with activities (true or fictitious), Table 10 gives values characterizing the real hazard from substances $(1/A)$, as well as the logarithms of these

Table 10. A Scale of the Real Hazards Presented by Freely Evaporating Substances
(*Criterion:* falling of white mice on one side)

Number	Substance	A	$1/A$	$Log(1/A)$
1	Propylbenzene	0.9	1.11	0.045
2	Butanol	0.86	1.16	0.064
3	Methanol	0.77	1.30	0.114
4	Isoamyl acetate	0.76	1.32	0.120
5	1-Nitropropane	0.66	1.52	0.182
6	Propanol	0.63	1.59	0.202
7	Ethanol	0.52	1.92	0.284
8	Nonane	0.5	2.00	0.300
9	α-Pinene	0.44	2.27	0.356
10	Ethylcyclohexane	0.44	2.27	0.356
11	2-Nitropropane	0.42	2.38	0.376
12	Styrene	0.4	2.50	0.398
13	Mesityl oxide	0.4	2.50	0.398
14	Octane	0.38	2.63	0.420
15	Ethylbenzene	0.37	2.70	0.432
16	Isobutanol	0.35	2.86	0.456
17	Isopropanol	0.35	2.86	0.456
18	Butyl acetate	0.34	2.94	0.468
19	Propyl acetate	0.32	3.12	0.480
20	Nitroethane	0.31	3.22	0.508
21	Heptylene	0.3	3.33	0.522
22	Nitromethane	0.28	3.58	0.554
23	Dioxane	0.28	3.58	0.554
24	Pentachloroethane	0.27	3.70	0.568
25	Ethylcyclopentane	0.26	3.85	0.586
26	Dimethylcyclohexane	0.24	4.16	0.620
27	Formalglycol	0.23	4.35	0.638
28	Dibutyl ether	0.22	4.55	0.658
29	Heptane	0.21	4.76	0.678
30	Methylcyclopentane	0.21	4.76	0.678
31	Vinyl butyrate	0.2	5.00	0.695
32	Furfural	0.19	5.26	0.720
33	1,1,2,2-Tetrachloroethane	0.19	5.26	0.720
34	Methylcyclohexane	0.19	5.26	0.720
35	Hexane	0.17	5.88	0.770
36	Hexylene	0.156	6.4	0.806
37	Pyridine	0.155	6.46	0.810
38	Tetrachloroethylene	0.15	6.66	0.824
39	Pentane	0.15	6.66	0.824
40	Cyclohexane	0.14	7.14	0.854
41	Ethyl acetate	0.13	7.68	0.885

Table 10. (*Continued*)

Number	Substance	A	$1/A$	$\text{Log}(1/A)$
42	Cyclopentane	0.11	9.10	0.960
43	Methyl propyl ketone	0.106	9.44	0.975
44	Toluene	0.097	10.30	1.012
45	Methyl methacrylate	0.091	11.00	1.042
46	Dimethyl ketone	0.088	11.35	1.055
47	Methyl ethyl ketone	0.082	12.20	1.086
48	Vinyl propionate	0.073	13.70	1.137
49	1,1,2-Trichloroethane	0.07	14.30	1.156
50	Methyl acetate	0.07	14.30	1.156
51	Propyl chloride	0.067	14.90	1.173
52	Bromoethylene	0.066	15.15	1.180
53	Carbon tetrachloride	0.065	15.40	1.188
54	Propyl bromide	0.063	15.80	1.195
55	1,1,1-Trichloroethane	0.06	16.70	1.223
56	Methyl acrylate	0.059	16.94	1.229
57	Trichloroethylene	0.058	17.23	1.237
58	Amylene (mixture)	0.058	17.23	1.237
59	Vinyl acetate	0.055	18.20	1.260
60	Diethyl ether	0.052	19.20	1.284
61	Divinylacetylene	0.05	20.00	1.300
62	1,3-Butadiene	0.03–0.05	33.0–20.0	1.518–1.300
63	1,2-Dichloroethane	0.046	21.70	1.336
64	1,2-Dichloroethylene	0.045	22.20	1.346
65	Benzene	0.043	23.20	1.366
66	1,2-Dichloropropane	0.04	25.00	1.398
67	Chloroethyl	0.04	25.00	1.398
68	Ethyl bromide	0.039	25.60	1.408
69	Thiofuran	0.036	27.80	1.444
70	1,1-Dichloroethane	0.033	30.16	1.482
71	Dimethyl ether	0.024	41.60	1.619
72	Methylene chloride	0.02	50.00	1.700
73	Chloroform	0.019	52.60	1.721
74	Methyl bromide	0.018	55.50	1.744
75	Monovinylacetylene	0.016	62.50	1.796
76	1,1-Dichloroethylene	0.015	66.60	1.824
77	Butyraldehyde	0.012	83.40	1.920
78	Propionaldehyde	0.01	100.0	2.00
79	Acetaldehyde	0.008	125.0	2.097
80	Vinyl chloride	0.0075	133.2	2.124
81	Chlorobutadiene	0.006	166.6	2.222
82	Methyl iodide	0.004	250.0	2.398
83	Methacrylonitrile	0.0042	238.0	2.378
84	Acrylonitrile	0.0013	770.0	2.890

values. It can be seen from the table that the real risk, as regards narcosis for mice, in the series of substances presented increases from no. 1 to no. 84, the last member being 694 times as hazardous as the first one.

The substances listed in the table may be divided into three real hazard categories as far as narcosis in mice is concerned: slight hazard, from propylbenzene to methyl propyl ketone (1–43); moderate hazard, from toluene to butyralidehyde (44–77); and high hazard, from propionaldehyde to acrylonitrile (78–84). This rating is highly tentative but convenient; the first member of each subsequent category presents a hazard 10 times greater than the first member of the preceding category; also, the integral part of any log $(1/A)$ value in one category differs by unity from that in the next category.

A similar scale, but based on lethal concentration and minimal lethal concentration data for mice with 2-hr exposure collected in the *Handbook of Toxicology* (Spector, 1956), is presented in Table 11. Another scale of real hazard was prepared using data from Table 10 on threshold concentrations for unconditioned reflex activity of rabbits with 40-min exposure (Table 12). The data of Tables 11 and 12, like those of Table 10, make it possible to classify substances as more hazardous and less hazardous with respect to death of mice and threshold action on rabbits.

It appears important to compare the real hazards as assessed by different criteria and on animals of different species. Accordingly, Tables 11 and 12 each include a column giving the numbers of substances from Table 10.

Table 11.   A Scale of the Real Hazards Presented by Freely Evaporating Substances (*Criterion:* death of white mice)

Number	Substance	A	$1/A$	Log$(1/A)$	Number in Table 10
1	Pentachloroethane	1	1	0	24
2	1,1,2,2-Tetrachloroethane	0.9	1.11	0.045	33
3	Ethylcyclohexane	0.51	1.96	0.292	10
4	1,2-Dichloroethane	0.4–0.52	2.5–1.92	0.398–0.284	63
5	1,1,2-Trichloroethane	0.42	2.38	0.376	49
6	Dimethylcyclohexane	0.27–0.32	3.7 –3.13	0.568–0.496	26
7	Methylcyclohexane	0.22–0.27	4.55–3.7	0.658–0.568	34
8	Cyclohexane	0.17–0.2	5.88–5.0	0.77–0.699	40
9	1,1,1-Trichloroethane	0.087	11.5	1.060	55
10	Carbon tetrachloride	0.077	13.0	1.114	53
11	Methylene chloride	0.071	14.1	1.150	70
12	Dichloromethane	0.03	33.3	1.523	72
13	Chloroform	0.026	38.5	1.586	73

Table 12. A Scale of the Real Hazards Presented by Freely Evaporating Substances
(*Criterion:* threshold action on unconditioned reflex activity in rabbits)

Number	Substance	A	$1/A$	Log($1/A$)	Number in Table 10
1	Cyclohexanone	0.455	2.2	0.342	
2	Butanol	0.2	5.0	0.700	2
3	Ethanol	0.052	19.2	1.284	7
4	Propanol	0.047	21.3	1.328	6
5	Xylidine (meta)	0.0364	27.5	1.440	
6	Toluidine (ortho)	0.0305	32.8	1.516	
7	Methanol	0.029	34.4	1.536	3
8	Styrene	0.029	34.4	1.536	12
9	Vinyl butyrate	0.02	50.0	1.700	31
10	1-Nitropropane	0.014	71.4	1.854	5
11	Aniline	0.0136	73.5	1.866	
12	Octane	0.0135	74.0	1.870	14
13	Methyl propyl ketone	0.0134	74.6	1.873	43
14	Methylaniline	0.0129	77.5	1.890	
15	Nitromethane	0.011	91.0	0.960	22
16	Furfural	0.0096	104.0	2.017	32
17	Methylpyridine	0.0086	117	2.068	
18	2-Nitropropane	0.008	125	2.097	11
19	Nitroethane	0.008	125	2.097	20
20	Ethyl acetate	0.0067	149	2.173	41
21	Xylene	0.0067	150	2.176	
22	Pyridine	0.0062	161	2.207	37
23	Methyl ethyl ketone	0.0062	161	2.207	47
24	Diethyl ether	0.0056	179	2.252	60
25	Toluene	0.0055	183	2.262	44
26	Vinyl propionate	0.005	200	2.300	48
27	Dimethyl ketone	0.0028	357	2.552	46
28	Benzene	0.0024	420	2.623	65
29	Butylamine	0.0024	420	2.623	
30	Carbon tetrachloride	0.002	500	2.700	53
31	Trichloroethylene	0.0016	625	2.796	57
32	1,2-Dichloroethane	0.0013	770	2.887	63
33	Chlorobenzene	0.0012	805	2.906	
34	Chloroform	0.001	1000	3.000	73
35	Vinyl acetate	0.0006	1668	3.222	59
36	1,1-Dichloroethylene	0.0004	2660	3.425	76
37	Dimethylamine	0.00013	7640	3.883	
38	Butyraldehyde	0.0001	10 000	4.000	77
39	Methylamine	0.00007	14 000	4.146	
40	Monochlorotrifluoroethylene	0.000004	256 000	5.408	
41	Formaldehyde	0.000002	526 000	5.720	

It will be seen from these columns that the real hazards, in terms of death of mice and conditioned reflex activity in rabbits, do not always agree with those in respect to narcosis in mice. To ascertain the degree of agreement, correlation coefficients were computed and were found to be .77 for the correlation between narcotic and lethal action data for mice and .94 for that between narcotic action data for mice and threshold action data for rabbits. Therefore there does exist an overall correlation between the hazards associated with the different toxic effects studied.

The departures from close correlation may be due in part to experimental errors involved in the determination of effective concentrations. In particular, this is indirectly indicated by the much lower correlation coefficient between narcosis and mortality data for mice (.77) than between narcosis data for mice and threshold action data for rabbits (.94). Indeed, whereas the narcotic and threshold action data were obtained in one laboratory, those on mortality in mice came from several sources. The principal reason for incomplete agreement, however, appears to be differences in the mechanisms by which the various selected effects develop. This may be illustrated by the following example.

Narcosis is of course a much less rigorous criterion than death and, other things being equal, usually occurs at a lower inspired concentration (e.g., when nonelectrolytic action results first in narcosis and then in death). Sometimes, however, narcotic concentrations are higher, and very much so, than lethal ones, as was strikingly demonstrated by Golubev (1957) for vinyl esters: the narcotic concentrations of these esters were also absolutely lethal, whereas lethal concentrations did not cause narcosis. These effects evidently develop by different mechanisms in such cases.

It may be concluded from the foregoing discussion that the thermodynamic activity and, consequently, the two-phase toxicity or the real hazard can serve as comparative criteria of the danger presented by freely evaporating substances only for a given kind of effect produced by such substances under identical conditions. Such a conclusion was to be expected. Obviously there cannot be a universal criterion of hazard (or of toxicity) for chemicals in view of the diversity in type and mechanism of their toxic actions.

On the other hand, a scale similar to those presented in Tables 10, 11, and 12 may be found useful for comparative assessment of toxicities when a particular effect is used as the toxicity criterion.

6. SOME IMPLICATIONS OF THE THERMODYNAMIC APPROACH TO
    THE STUDY OF THE ABSORPTION AND FATE OF SUBSTANCES IN
    THE BODY (POSSIBLE APPLICATIONS OF THE ACTIVITY CONCEPT
    IN BIOLOGY)

6.1. Range of Action; Thermodynamic Capacity of Biophases; Role of
      Activity in the Passage of Substances from External Phases to Biophases

The range of biological action of a substance may be defined as the range of its
activities (or fictitious activities), limited by two extreme (i.e., maximal and
minimal) selected effects.* One example of such effects is the action on
unconditioned reflexes at one extreme, and death with 2-hr exposure at the
other; another example is narcosis and death; and so on. A clearer idea of the
biological action range may be had from Tables 10, 11, and 12. Thus pentachloroethane causes narcosis in mice at an activity of 0.27 (Table 10) and
kills mice at an activity of about unity (Table 11). Ethylcyclohexane produces
the same effects at activities of 0.44 and 0.51, respectively. Pentachloroethane
has, therefore, a much wider range for mice than does ethylcyclohexane,
at least insofar as the selected effects are concerned.

Similarly, diethyl ether is effective at $A = 0.052$ (Table 10) and $A = 0.0056$
(Table 12), while vinyl propionate is effective at 0.073 and 0.005, respectively.
The former has a broader range as judged from tests on mice and on rabbits.

On the other hand, as shown by Tables 10 and 11, 1,1,2,2-tetrachloroethane
($A = 0.19$ and 0.9, respectively) and 1,1,2-trichloroethane ($A = 0.07$ and 0.42)
have approximately the same range for mice, although the latter compound
may be expected to have a somewhat wider range than the former if a
stricter criterion is applied, say death with 1-hr rather than 2-hr exposure.
Then 1,1,2-trichloroethane may be effective, and 1,1,2,2-tetrachloroethane
ineffective.

In pharmacology the therapeutic range of a drug is defined by its doses
from minimal effective to minimal toxic or, in the case of respirable substances, by the respective concentrations. Above, the action range was
defined in terms of thermodynamic activity. The difference between the
action ranges as defined by concentrations and by activities is apparent from
Table 13, which is based on data contained in Tables 8 and 9.

In Table 13 the biological action range is given by $(C_{narc} - C_{thr})$ or
$(A_{narc} - A_{thr})$ for the first group of substances and by $(C_{leth} - C_{narc})$ or
$(A_{leth} - A_{narc})$ for the second. When expressed in terms of concentration, the

---

* Strictly speaking, this range should be defined as the range of activities extending from minimal
threshold to lethal.

Table 13. Comparison of Ranges of Substance Action as Expressed in Terms of Effective Concentrations (mg/liter) and of Activities

Range: threshold effect on unconditioned reflexes in rabbits, narcosis in mice

Substance	Threshold for Rabbits[a]		Narcosis in Mice[a]		Difference	
	C_{thr}	A_{thr}	C_{narc}	A_{narc}	$C_{narc} - C_{thr}$	$A_{narc} - A_{thr}$
Dimethyl ketone	1.6	0.0028	50	0.088	48.4	0.085
Methyl ethyl ketone	1.9	0.0062	25	0.082	23.1	0.076
Methyl propyl ketone	1.9	0.0134	15	0.106	13.1	0.093

Range: narcosis in mice, death of mice

Substance	Narcosis in Mice		Death in Mice[a]		Difference	
	C_{narc}	A_{narc}	C_{leth}	A_{leth}	$C_{leth} - C_{narc}$	$A_{leth} - A_{narc}$
Cyclohexane	50	0.14	65	0.185	15	0.045
Methylcyclohexane	35	0.19	45	0.245	10	0.055
Dimethylcyclohexane	22.5	0.24	27.5	0.295	5	0.055

[a] C_{thr} = threshold concentration, A_{thr} = activity for threshold action, C_{narc} = narcotic concentration, A_{narc} = activity for narcotic action, C_{leth} = lethal concentration, A_{leth} = activity for lethal action.

range decreases with increasing molecular size for both groups. When stated in terms of activity, however, it remains approximately the same for either group.

A pharmacologist seeking to know the extent of permissible deviations from the mean dose (concentration) and the range of usable doses (concentrations) compares the doses (concentrations) in a range-finding test. In a homologous series the action range will then decrease with growing molecular size in accordance with decreasing saturated vapor pressure, solubility, and so on.

In some cases a biological action range defined in terms of activity offers certain advantages. An important advantage may be associated with the fact that the activity of a substance having the nonelectrolytic type of action characterizes that substance in the phase responsible for its action, so that the action range may yield information about changes in the state of the biophase or of the substance and about the binding and interactions of the substance on passing from one biological effect to another. Moreover, activity provides a more accurate and convenient description of the toxic action range from the standpoint of industrial toxicology. Thus, if two substances have the same action range in terms of activity, that is, if their activities change by the same magnitude in going from one selected effect to some other selected effect, it follows that, when either of these two substances has produced one such effect, the other selected effect should occur after the same time interval with both these substances, other things being equal.

Take, for example, methyl- and dimethylcyclohexane. As defined by activities, their narcosis—death ranges are the same. In terms of concentrations the range of the former is twice that of the latter. However, the time elapsing between the lower effect level (narcosis) and the additional evaporation of 10 mg/liter of methylcyclohexane and of 5 mg/liter of dimethylcyclohexane, required to attain lethal concentrations, will be the same for both substances. Therefore, as far as the true hazard is concerned, the toxic action ranges of these two substances are the same for the effects selected.

The example just given clearly indicates two possible approaches to defining the action range. If one is concerned with dosage, it is more convenient to use an absolute quantity such as dose or concentration, as is usually done in practice. If, on the other hand, one is concerned with industrial conditions, a relative quantity such as thermodynamic activity may be used to greater advantage.

A parallel may be drawn between the action range of a substance and the capacity of the biophases responsible for its action. Indeed, the wider the action range, the wider is the range of activities and, consequently, the more of the substance that can be contained in the biophases in the thermodynamic sense. This capacity may be termed the thermodynamic capacity of the effective biophase in respect to the substance concerned. Since the true thermodynamic activity can be determined only for substances with the nonelectrolytic type of action in a state of distribution equilibrium, the same applies to the thermodynamic capacity also. The numerical value of this capacity defined by the difference between activities will then characterize the substance at the site of its action.

As for substances having the specific type of action, the thermodynamic capacity will not be a thermodynamic capacity proper, for it will have been determined from fictitious activities. These fictitious activities, however, will fully retain their role as indicators of the true industrial hazards from freely evaporating substances. Accordingly, the fictitious thermodynamic capacity will give an indication of the likelihood and speed of change from one effect to another. It will differ from the true thermodynamic capacity only in that it will not be indicative of the state of the substance at the site of attack.

It seems pertinent to discuss briefly the activity and the action range in relation to the solubility. Generally, since the activities required to produce equal effects increase, whereas the solubilities decrease, in a homologous series, these two quantities are inversely related. The thermodynamic capacity and solubility, however, are not related either directly or inversely, at least apparently. When two substances having the same action range have different solubilities, this means that different absolute quantities of these substances are required to attain the same effect: a larger amount of the more readily soluble substance will be necessary. This is a consequence of the rapid augmentation of activity upon only a slight increase in the concentration of the substance in a medium where it is sparingly soluble and, conversely, of the slow rise in activity upon a considerable increase in the concentration in a medium where the substance is readily soluble.

The foregoing makes clear the relationship between the insecticidal potencies of substances applied in different phases. Thus Burtt (1945) found a solution of phenol in paraffin oil to be appreciably more toxic for sheep ticks than an aqueous solution of phenol at the same concentration. Since phenol is much more readily soluble in water, its thermodynamic activity in oil is much higher than in water at the same concentration. In accordance with the law of distribution, the rate of passage of phenol from the solution into the tick's body was the greater the higher its activity in the solution. At the same time, solutions of phenol in paraffin oil and water which were in equilibrium were found to have the same toxic effect on the ticks. This is understandable since their activities were the same, although their concentrations were very different.

The example just given shows that, when an effective substance is to be applied to a biological object in different phases, inquiry should first be made as to its activity in these phases.

The foregoing considerations also explain the finding of Ivens (1952) that some hydrocarbons are not toxic in air but are very toxic in liquids, as well as the examples given by Rich and Horsfall (1952) and Hadaway and Barlow (1958) to show that the toxicity of an insecticide depends on the solvent.

Hurst (1943, 1945), in discussing the role of insect cuticles in contact with insecticides, pointed out that insecticide potency often depends on cuticle permeability. The question arises as to what should be understood by "permeability" in this case. Cuticles (which are varied) appear to have different solubilities for different substances. If the solubility is low, the substance, having entered the cuticle in a small amount and with difficulty, shows considerable activity and, accordingly, readily passes on to inner phases. In this case the substance finds it most difficult to gain entry into the cuticle from the environment. If the solubility is high, the substance easily penetrates the cuticle from the outside, but it will encounter difficulty in passing into inner phases so long as it has not accumulated in a sufficient amount to develop a high thermodynamic activity in the cuticle. These relationships should be taken into account in discussing the role of cuticles or other intermediary membranes in the passage of foreign substances into living organisms.

6.2. Metabolism of Foreign Compounds

Except when chemically and toxicologically very active groupings are released, the metabolic transformation of nonelectrolytes results in products less toxic than the original compounds (Lazarev, 1938; Williams, 1959). At the same time more polar, that is, more water-soluble, compounds are formed. These two facts can be readily linked by the concept of activity.

When a more water-soluble substance forms, its activity in the body water is appreciably lower than that of the original compound. This makes it easy for the substance to accumulate in the aqueous phase and difficult in other phases where its activity is relatively high. Its accumulation in the aqueous phase, where its activity is relatively low, prevents its penetration into other biophases, thereby taking it farther from the sites of action and nearer to the routes of excretion. Hence its toxicity diminishes.

This may be illustrated by the following example. The esters of vinyl alcohols and fatty acids are rapidly and completely saponified in the body with the formation of acetaldehyde and various acids (Filov, 1959b). The changes in activity during that process are indicated in Table 14.

Table 14. Solubilities and Thermodynamic Activities of Some
Vinyl Esters and Their Metabolites in Water

Substance	Solubility (weight %)	Activity
Vinyl acetate	~2.5	
Vinyl propionate	~0.9	May be large
Vinyl butyrate	~0.3	
Acetaldehyde	∞	In practice cannot
Carboxylic acids or their salts	∞	be large

6.3. The Relationship of Physicochemical Properties, Toxic Concentrations, and Activities to the Positions of Substances in the Homologous Series

The biological potencies of nonelectrolytes are usually compared by measuring their external concentrations under the conditions of their equilibrium distribution between the external medium and the organism. A number of correlations were revealed when such equilibrium concentrations were studied in relation to physicochemical properties (Lazarev, 1944). These are correlations between the magnitudes of biological action of members of a homologous series and their solubilities, surface activities, saturated vapor pressures, partition coefficients, and so on.

In a homologous series such physicochemical properties show roughly parallel or, to be precise, symbatic changes, as can be clearly seen when the magnitudes of the properties are expressed in logarithmic form (Figure 8). Even a cursory look at this figure is enough to see that the variations in these properties are governed by the same law. No additional proof is required from the mathematical point of view. A close examination of the physical essence of the properties involved will reveal this law to hold good from the physical viewpoint as well. This is the law of distribution between heterogeneous phases.

Indeed, we see that the solubility is related to the distribution of the substance between the pure solid, liquid, or gaseous phase and the saturated solution. The saturated vapor pressure corresponds to the distribution between the pure solid or liquid phase and its vapors. The partition coefficient between any immiscible phases speaks for itself. The surface activity reflects the distribution between the bulk of the liquid and its surface. Finally, the equilibrium toxic concentration corresponds to the distribution between the external medium and the organism.

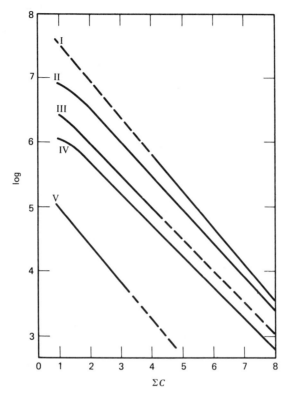

Figure 8. Variation in log values of some properties in homologous series. I, solubility (mole/liter × 10^{-6}); II, toxic concentrations for **B. typhosus** (mole/liter × 10^{-6}); III, concentrations reducing the surface tension of water to 50 dynes/cm (mole/liter × 10^{-6}); IV, vapor pressure at 25°C (mm Hg × 10^{4}); V, partition coefficient between water and cottonseed oil (× 10^{3}). Data for alcohols. (After Ferguson, 1939.)

The distribution law is characterized by the partition (distribution) coefficient. This coefficient has a definite value in each particular case and completely defines the state of equilibrium.

Thermodynamics gives the following expression for the partition coefficient:

$$\log K = -\frac{\Delta\mu}{RT}$$

where $\Delta\mu$ is the change in chemical potential attending the equilibrium transition of 1 mole of substance between the two phases, and T is the absolute temperature.

The distribution law thus has a logarithmic nature. This accounts for the logarithmic dependence of distributive properties in a homologous series. The thermodynamic meaning of this logarithmic dependence is that in the homologous series for each particular distributive property (solubility, vapor pressure, etc.) there is a constant increment in the chemical potential difference between the standard states in the two phases for each successive member of the series. This follows directly from the above formula, for when the temperature is constant log K is proportional to $\Delta\mu$.

All this has a direct bearing on the thermodynamic activity which characterizes the biological effects of nonelectrolytes. The logarithmic course of the thermodynamic activities required for equal effects (see Figures 5 and 7) is likewise accounted for by the distribution law. It should be stressed that, when members of a series of nonelectrolytes show proportional changes in log activities, this points to the nonelectrolytic type of action by these members. If one or more members of the series depart strongly from the linear logarithmic relationship shown by other members, this indicates that they have a different type of action, that is, tend to act specifically.

A linear relation similar to the ones depicted in Figure 7 is sometimes seen in a series of specifically acting substances as well. In our view this suggests that all members of the series have the same mode of action. Indeed, when log activities in a series change in a uniform manner, such changes are due solely to changes in physicochemical distributive properties, other things being equal; these "other things" include a common mechanism of action.

6.4. The Role of Ferguson's Principle in the Problem of Interaction between Foreign Substances and the Organism

Ferguson's idea of considering the biological action of foreign substances in thermodynamic terms, that is, on the basis of their chemical potentials and activities, did not introduce any new concept into the study of the mechanism of nonelectrolytic action. It did, however, make it possible to unite several physicochemical theories of narcosis and to describe their phase distribution essence in strict physical terms. A corollary to such description was clarification of the fact that, although the physicochemical properties which are associated with distribution relationships do not determine the mechanism of nonelectrolytic action directly, they do determine the transport of substances to the sites of their action.

As regards the mechanism of action, it is related to other physicochemical properties which appear to depend on the spatial structures of the molecules involved, on the distributions of their electromagnetic fields, and so on.

Although the thermodynamic conceptions cannot per se explain the intimate mechanism of molecular interaction underlying any action of substances in general and the nonelectrolytic action in particular, any future molecular theory of the biological action of substances will have to be amenable to a thermodynamic description.

In a more direct way the thermodynamic approach makes it possible to reach conclusions regarding the direction in which substances are moving and the conditions necessary for their equilibrium distribution both between the environment and the organism and within the organism itself; moreover, it may be useful for judging the possibility and pathways of metabolic transformations by particular compounds.

4

KINETIC ASPECTS OF THE ABSORPTION AND FATE OF POISONS IN THE BODY

1. GENERAL CONSIDERATIONS RELATING TO THE ABSORPTION, TRANSFORMATION, AND ELIMINATION OF POISONS

1.1. Absorption

Under conditions of occupational exposure, toxic substances can gain entry into the human body through the respiratory tract, the skin, and the gastro-intestinal tract. The most important of these three routes is the first because any toxic substance can exist in the form of gas, vapor, or aerosol, and it is often extremely difficult to afford adequate respiratory protection to workers from substances in such states of aggregation or to design a technological process that would completely preclude their release to the ambient air. Indeed, statistics shows that occupational poisoning is very frequently caused by poisons in the gaseous or vaporous state.

Absorption through the Respiratory Tract

The penetration of toxic substances by way of the respiratory tract depends on the state of aggregation of the poison, on its physicochemical properties, and, to a large measure, on its fate in the body. The conditions determining the true hazard of poisoning from volatile industrial poisons are discussed in Chapter 3.

Gases and Vapors. Gaseous or vaporous substances which undergo no changes in the body, or whose biotransformation is slow compared to their absorption, pass into the blood mainly by way of the alveoli and are distributed throughout the body by the bloodstream. Of certain importance also in their penetration are other parts of the respiratory tract whose role in this process is the greater the higher the water solubility of the substance (Gadas-kina, 1949).

The absorption of stable substances into the blood and tissues can be des-

94

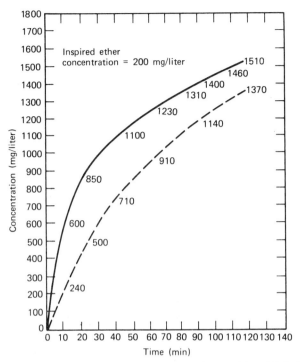

Figure 9. Concentration-time curves for ethyl ether in the arterial (solid line) and venous (dashed line) blood of a dog inhaling ether vapors. (From Lazarev, 1938.)

cribed to a first approximation by an exponential expression (this is discussed in detail later). A substance depends for its absorption on its dynamic distribution, in which the blood acts as an intermediate phase in receiving the substance from the inspired air and giving it off to tissues which vary in their affinity for the substance concerned and in their blood supply. This leads to a characteristic pattern of absorption for a slowly reacting substance whose concentration in the arterial blood at first rises much more steeply than in the venous blood. With the course of time, as the tissue concentration of a given substance progressively rises and approaches equilibrium with the arterial blood concentration, the difference between the arterial and venous concentrations gradually decreases (Figure 9). A direct result of this is a progressive rise in the expired concentration, which in the limit tends to the inspired concentration, that is, to a steady state. This relationship is illustrated by the curve of Figure 10, constructed from data on halothane inhalation by human subjects in a study (Sechzer et al., 1963) where the inspired concentration (C_0) of halothane was held constant and the C_{exp}/C_0 ratio was determined by

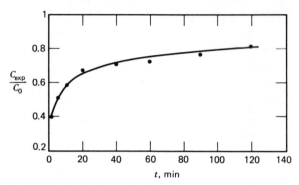

Figure 10.   Ratio of end-expired and inspired halothane concentrations. See text for explanation. (From Sechzer et al., 1963.)

measuring the expired concentration (C_{exp}). This ratio may vary from 0 to 1; it is unity when a steady state has been reached.

A similar absorption pattern is seen in the case of a gaseous substance whose rate of biotransformation is comparable to that of absorption. The picture here is, however, more complicated because of the more or less prominent role played by processes of breakdown in addition to those of absorption and distribution.

The situation is different with rapidly metabolizable substances. Some of these are broken down on moist mucosal surfaces and enter the bloodstream as metabolites. An important part in their absorption may be played by the upper air passages. As shown by Gadaskina (1937), the degree of retention of such substances within these passages depends on their solubility: the more soluble the substance, the more of it will be absorbed through the upper air passages, and vice versa.

A rapidly metabolizable substance fails to saturate the body, and this is reflected in the retention of its vapors, which does not change with time. This constancy was shown, in particular, by Filov (1959b) in a study on the metabolic fate of esters of vinyl alcohol and fatty acids. As shown schematically in Figure 11, the difference between the inspired and expired concentrations of vinyl esters is constant, that is, the amount retained does not change with time; these esters cannot be recovered in the expired air after the cessation of inhalation because all of the retained amount is immediately transformed.

In the process of biotransformation, rapidly metabolizable substances may give rise to reasonably stable metabolites, which in turn accumulate in the blood and tissues. This is illustrated by Figure 12, which reproduces data from an experiment on the retention and transformation of methyl acetate in rabbits (Filov, 1961b). Methyl acetate does not accumulate in the body: when

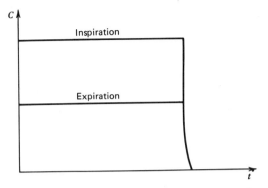

Figure 11. Inspired and expired ester concentrations. The area between the concentration lines corresponds to the amount of ester retained in the body. C, ester concentration; t, time.

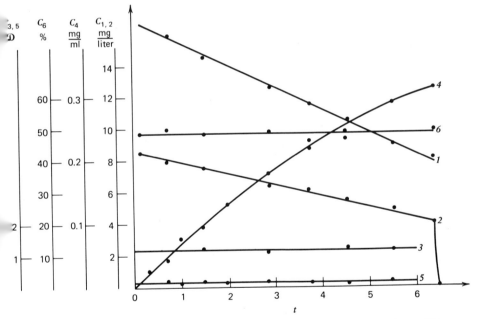

Figure 12. Results of an experiment on the inhalation of methyl acetate vapors by a rabbit; t, time in hours. *1*, Inspired methyl acetate concentration; *2*, expired methyl acetate concentration; *3*, blood level of esters (in optical density units); *4*, blood concentration of methanol; *5*, blood level of formaldehyde (in optical density units); *6*, percent retention of methyl acetate vapors (as calculated from data on *1* and *2*.)

its vapors are inhaled, the blood level of the esters does not increase; accordingly, the degree of retention of its vapors remains constant. At the same time the blood concentration of its slowly transformed metabolite, methanol, is rising. The next metabolite, formaldehyde, does not accumulate either because of its rapid transformation.

A rather interesting quantity is the percentage retention of gaseous substances on inhalation. Percentage retention remains constant for rapidly metabolizable compounds and progressively decreases for those which are transformed slowly. This difference in retention may form the basis of a method for estimating the persistence of substances in the body. The percentage retention of a substance should be determined on an individual basis because of its great variation between individuals. Thus the retention of trichloromethylchloroformate in the respiratory tract of rabbits was found to vary from 63 to 93% from one animal to another (Gadaskina, 1937). Such variations have as their basis the physiological and biochemical variability between individuals.

Particulate Matter. The retention of inhaled particulates (aerosols) occurs throughout the respiratory tract, from the nasal cavities downward. Amounts retained vary from one area of the tract to another, depending mainly on the physical properties of particles, primarily their size. The percentage of particles retained is lower the smaller their size. As the size increases, more and more particles tend to be retained in the upper airways because larger and heavier particles settle more readily on mucous membranes, especially where the air passages are curved. Particles about 1μ in size settle mainly in the alveoli, while those over 5μ tend to deposit in the upper airways, notably in the nasal cavities.

The site and degree of retention also depend on the density, shape, hygroscopicity, and electric charge of the particles, as well as on the breathing frequency and inspiratory capacity. As the number of particles retained in the upper respiratory tract increases, the possibility of further retention diminishes.

The fate of retained particles depends on several factors such as retention site, particle size, and the physicochemical properties of the substance concerned. The most important of these properties is solubility.

Unless the particles retained in the upper air passages, that is, primarily larger particles, are readily soluble, they are removed mainly by the action of the cilia of the ciliated epithelium lining the air passages. The speed of upward movement of mucus in the human trachea is 3 to 4 cm/min. Removal is facilitated by coughing.

The dust which has gained access to the alveoli is retained there for a considerable period of time, thus favoring its dissolution and also its direct passage into the blood. This explains why finely dispersed particulates are more toxic than coarsely dispersed ones.

Clearly, the more easily soluble a substance, the more of it will pass into the blood. The solubility of a substance on mucous membranes of the respiratory tract is usually much higher than its solubility in water. Quartz dust, for example, which is virtually insoluble in water, is partially soluble in alveoli. Such an increase in solubility is brought about by the action of biochemical mechanisms which are still poorly understood.

A high solubility of dust in water and on mucosal surfaces may have either a beneficial or a detrimental effect. The dust of low-toxic substances acts mainly as a mechanical irritant on the tissues, so that high solubility favors its rapid removal from the respiratory tract. In contrast, the easily soluble dust of a highly toxic substance is conducive to poisoning.

Various aspects of particulate matter penetration into the body and of resulting intoxications are discussed, for example, by Navrotsky (1963) and Katsnelson (1976).

Absorption through the Skin

The skin is permeable to gases, liquids, and solids, most of which are non-electrolytes. As a rule, the intact skin is impermeable to electrolytes. Exceptions are heavy metals and their salts, which are absorbed into the blood through the skin barrier to a small extent.

The ability of a substance to penetrate the skin depends mainly on its lipid and water solubilities (Lazarev et al., 1931, 1933). Lipid-soluble substances are capable of moving through the fatty layers of the skin, but their further absorption will be hindered if their hydrophobic properties prevent their dissolution in the blood. Skin absorption is also affected by such factors as temperature, contact surface area, and duration of contact.

In order for a substance to produce a toxic effect, it must penetrate through the skin in an effective toxic dose. The accumulation of such a dose may be prevented by processes of biotransformation and excretion.

In experimental studies of skin absorption it must be remembered that the skin of laboratory animals is usually more permeable than human skin and that the ratio of body surface area to body volume in small animals is different from that in large ones; these facts should be taken into account when transferring animal data to man.

Absorption through the Gastrointestinal Tract

Toxic substances may be ingested with swallowed dust, tobacco smoke, food, and so on. Some substances, especially if lipid soluble, can pass into the blood from the oral cavity, thus avoiding the liver and entering the systemic circulation directly.

Gastric absorption depends on the nature and quantity of gastric contents. Gastric secretions may considerably alter a poison and increase its solubility. Intestinal secretions may similarly affect substances that have not been changed or absorbed earlier. Poisons may also be transformed by intestinal bacteria. For example, aromatic nitro compounds are reduced by bacteria to amines (Bray et al., 1953).

After their absorption from the stomach and intestine, substances first enter the liver, where many poisons undergo various transformations. These are mainly directed toward detoxication, but more dangerous compounds may sometimes result. One example is the well-known lethal synthesis. Another example is the oxidation of β-naphthylamine to 2-amino-1-naphthol, which, though less toxic than the parent compound, has marked carcinogenic properties (Boyland, 1959). Some compounds are absorbed into lymphatic pathways and bypass the liver.

1.2. Distribution

The vast majority of industrially used organic poisons are nonelectrolytes. The basic principles underlying the distribution of a nonelectrolyte between the blood and various tissues are fairly simple. As it is absorbed into the blood, a nonelectrolyte is carried to all organs and tissues, where it is retained to varying degrees. During this initial stage of distribution, the absorption of a substance into tissues (or organs) depends mainly on the blood supply of the tissue (or organ): the greater the blood supply, the more of the substance will accumulate there. This first stage may therefore be referred to as one of dynamic distribution determined by the intensity of blood supply.

With the passage of time, however, the distribution becomes more and more influenced by the sorptive properties of the tissues themselves. The substance is gradually redistributed and accumulates predominantly in tissues whose affinity for that particular substance is greatest. The final distribution may be called static: it marks the attainment of equilibrium distribution of the substance among all body tissues and organs. In such a state the substance is distributed between the blood and tissues in accordance with the tissue/blood partition (distribution) coefficient.

This is of course a most general, idealized description of the distribution process. The distribution of each particular substance may be influenced by a number of other factors, primarily by biotransformations. If the process of metabolism is very rapid, the concept of static distribution becomes meaningless.

The absorption of stable metabolites into tissues is likewise determined by their tissue/blood partition coefficients.

As regards inorganic poisons and various electrolytes, their distribution usually follows other patterns, related to the physicochemical mechanisms of their interaction with the biological structures of tissues. An electrolyte dissociates in the body into cations and anions, whose fate is always different; the distribution of electrolytes is thus the distribution of their ions.

The most characteristic feature of the distribution of inorganic substances is nonuniformity. A typical example is lead. The bulk of lead is concentrated in the bones, but some is found in the liver and kidneys. Lead is detectable in bones for months after intake. This exemplifies the possibility of the formation of long-lasting depots of inorganic compounds in the body.

Inorganic compounds of arsenic and cyanide compounds when introduced directly into the bloodstream disappear completely from the blood within seconds or minutes, being, as it were, dipped out by tissues from the blood. The tissue/blood partition coefficient, which so conveniently characterizes the distribution of organic compounds, becomes meaningless in this case.

The above examples (many more could be given) show that the distribution of inorganic compounds is markedly different from that of organic compounds.

1.3. Transformation

When absorbed into the body, most poisons undergo transformations which vary in degree, depending on the poison, and may affect all or part of its molecules. The untransformed molecules are eliminated unchanged.

The number of substances that are entirely eliminated in their original form is small. Examples are lower aliphatic hydrocarbons and, expecially, inert gases from the zero group of the periodic table.

Many compounds are metabolized completely, some of them being broken down to the end products, CO_2 and H_2O. Examples of completely metabolizable compounds are many esters of fatty acids and of aliphatic alcohols.

The most common case appears to be partial breakdown, wherein a portion of the compound is eliminated in the unchanged state. The ratio between the amount eliminated unchanged and the amount transformed to one degree or another depends on the inspired concentration of the toxic compound or on the dose of it that has entered the body in one way or another.

The type of biotransformation is largely determined by the physicochemical properties of the substance, but other factors may also be of importance, including route of entry, diet, and species.

Transformations occur in various tissues and organs, including the blood, depending on the structure of the poison. The most important organ in this respect is of course the liver.

Metabolic products are usually less toxic than the original substance, that is, the transformations of poisons are directed toward their detoxication. There are exceptions to this general rule, as already indicated.

It is significant that most metabolites are more polar and, consequently, more soluble in water than the original compounds (Lazarev and Staritsina, 1935), thus facilitating their renal excretion. The structural changes leading to this constitute one of the most important detoxication mechanisms.

Poisons are altered in the body through biochemical reactions, the four main types of reaction being oxidation, reduction, hydrolysis, and synthesis. The reactions of oxidation, reduction, and hydrolysis are many and varied; but, in general, compounds of similar structure are oxidized, reduced, or hydrolyzed in a similar manner. The synthetic reactions, or conjugation (binding) processes, are much less varied. In the process of metabolism, one type of transformation is often succeeded by another. Thus benzene is oxidized to phenol, which conjugates with glucuronic acid or sulfate and is eliminated in a conjugated form. Synthetic reactions are frequently the final, if not the only, phase of transformation. All phases of biotransformation usually involve various enzymes. Some of these are inherent in the organism, lack narrow specificity, and catalyze many similar transformations. Others, known as induced enzymes, may form *de novo* in the course of particular transformations.

In the most general schematic form the biotransformation of toxic substances may be represented as follows:

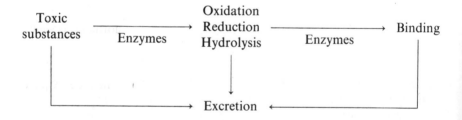

1.4. Elimination

Industrial poisons and their metabolites are cleared from the body by various channels, mainly through the lungs, the kidneys, and the intestine. Volatile substances, which are of special concern in industrial toxicology, are largely eliminated in the expired air. This applies in particular to many volatile organic solvents with low solubility coefficients. As a rule the expired air contains unchanged substances, either alone or together with their nearest volatile metabolites. In rare cases nonvolatile compounds give rise to volatile ones in the process of metabolism. These, too, are eliminated mainly through the lungs.

Compounds which are readily soluble in water are excreted chiefly through the kidneys. As already mentioned, most biotransformations give rise to substances with increased solubility, which facilitates their excretion in the urine.

The gastrointestinal tract is a far less important route of elimination. In fact it is of practical importance only for salts of heavy metals. Sweat, saliva, milk, and other body fluids may also participate to some extent in the elimination of certain substances.

Not infrequently, toxic compounds and their metabolites are concurrently eliminated through several routes, some one of which is of particular significance. One example is ethyl alcohol, the bulk of which undergoes transformation and about 10% of which is eliminated unchanged, predominantly in the expired air, but also in the urine and, in small amounts, in the feces, saliva, sweat, and milk.

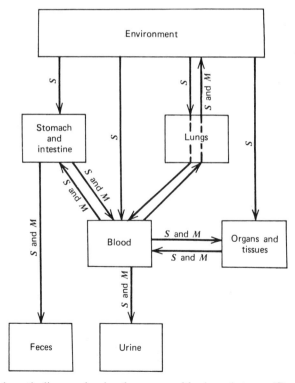

Figure 13. Schematic diagram showing the passage of foreign substances (S) and their metabolites (M) through the body.

The process of elimination by any route can be described to a first approximation by an exponential expression, which is discussed in detail in Sections 3.1 and 4.

1.5. General Scheme of Substance Passage through the Body

The routes of entry of poisons into the body, the main directions of their possible movement there, and the route by which they and/or their metabolites are eliminated are shown diagrammatically in Figure 13. In addition to the portals of entry most common for industrial poisons, there are shown the parenteral routes that, though uncommon in practice, are often used in toxicological experiments.

Naturally, different compounds have different movement patterns and fates in the body. Also, each particular compound or group of compounds has its characteristic route of entry. In most cases the distribution of substances in the body is intimately associated with their metabolism.

2. MODELING: SCOPE AND PURPOSE

Important tools in the study of the movement and metabolism of toxic substances are models which permit vivid representation and detailed interpretation of the processes under consideration.

Broadly speaking, a model is a physical or theoreticomathematical analogue of a process, usually simpler than the process itself and, in any case, susceptible to analysis. Although a model, like any analogue, is inferior to the phenomenon which it is designed to simulate, it facilitates analysis of that phenomenon. By making the model more and more complex, one can approximate the phenomenon as closely as one wishes. Very close approximation is usually unnecessary, however, because it would eliminate the basic idea behind modeling, which is to simplify analysis by excluding less relevant factors from consideration. The purpose of modeling is to assure the simplest possible analysis of the phenomenon under study. This purpose can be served by different kinds of models. According to Krüger-Thiemer (1964), pharmacokinetics, toxicokinetics, and related disciplines make use of three groups of models: graphic, mathematical, and real (physical). This subdivision is somewhat artificial but useful.

An example of a graphic model is the diagram shown in Figure 13; other examples will be given later in this chapter.

Any mathematical expressions describing a process of substance movement or metamorphosis in the body may be regarded as a mathematical model. When one is concerned with a fairly general process or when the system designed to simulate the organism is simple (e.g., consists of one or two homogeneous parts) and the process occurring in the system is subject to constraints, a mathematical model is relatively simple and usually consists of exponential equations with a small number of parameters. Such equations are not difficult to solve with the aid of a simple calculating machine —or even without it. As we advance to more complicated situations (e.g., as the system or process is made more complex in order to approximate it to reality), more complicated mathematical models must be used whose solution may require an electronic computer. The subject of mathematical modeling is treated in a systematic way by Rashevsky (1961) and, with special reference to problems of industrial toxicology, by Piotrowski (1971).

Real (physical) models comprise various kinds of physical elements whose laws of operation are known beforehand. Such a model may consist, for example, of liquid-filled vessels linked in a particular way. It is customary, however, to use capacitors, resistors, transistors, and other components interconnected to form an electrical network where current simulates the flow of substance in a living system.

The most generally applicable are mathematical models, but they are not explicit enough. Graphic models are too general; also, a graphic model usually requires a mathematical description, so that a combined model results. Mathematical description is necessary for many physical models as well. On the other hand, a complex mathematical model may be inapplicable in practice because the researcher does not know how to solve it or its solution is too laborious. In such cases recourse must be had to a high-speed digital or analogue computer. One example of a combined (physical-mathematical) model is the model designed to demonstrate the effect of protein binding and of ionization on the distribution and the kinetics of elimination of substances, described by Krüger-Thiemer et al. (1964).

Electronic simulation is very widely used because it enables simple analogies to be drawn between the main characteristics of the substance-organism system, on the one hand, and certain electrical characteristics, on the other. The flow of substance is simulated by electric current, as already mentioned. The volumes of biological compartments are represented by capacitors; the concentrations of substances by voltages; the rate constants characterizing the transferences of substances between, or their loss from, the compartments, by resistances; and so on. Electronic circuits are easy to assemble, they are compact, and all the processes occur in them at high speeds and can be followed on an oscilloscope screen.

The more or less complex networks made up of such components to simulate various real processes, such as the passage of a substance through the body, are known as analogue machines, analogue computers, or just analogues. An analogue computer, in addition to its use as an analogue of a living system, can serve to perform continuous computations from the equation embodied in it. However, the true value of analogue models for pharmacokinetics and toxicokinetics consists not so much in the solution of equations describing variable processes as in the simulation of processes for which equations are too difficult to derive or impossible to solve. Analogue computer simulation may give valuable indications as to which parameters of the simulated system are most important and what should be measured experimentally.

Complex kinetic equations are more amenable to solution on digital computers. These, unlike analogue machines, cannot simulate the physical processes occurring in a living system, but they can solve equations describing, to any desired degree of accuracy, the behavior of substances in any system, however complicated it may be.

To construct a mathematical model adequately describing the behavior of a substance in such a sophisticated system as the living organism, the latter must be mentally simplified by separating it into parts, or compartments. Thus it may be assumed that the blood plasma and the major organs and tissues of the body are all homogeneous and isotropic. Then the organism may be regarded as a system consisting of a finite number of compartments, each compartment having defined physicochemical properties and being distinct from any other. Separation into compartments may be done at the cellular level rather than at the level of organs or tissues. Such simplification will obviously be a closer approximation to reality, but the number of compartments will increase greatly. Similar compartmentalization is conceivable at the subcellular or any other level.

The distribution of a substance among the individual compartments of a system consisting of n compartments lends itself to mathematical calculation. The calculation will be the simpler the smaller the n. The most general compartmental system is the one which imposes no constraints on the exchange of the substance between the compartments (or, more broadly, on such exchange of its metabolites formed in all or some of the compartments). A model of this kind is shown schematically in Figure 14.

The movement of substance in this model is describable by nth-order differential equations which are extremely difficult to derive, let alone solve. In some cases, however, an n-compartment system can be greatly simplified. This is possible, for example, when some of the compartments are not involved in substance exchange, a situation that has many broad analogies in biology. Two simplified models of this kind were described in detail by Sheppard and Householder (1951). One of them (mammillary model) is shown in Figure 15, and the other (catenary) in Figure 16.

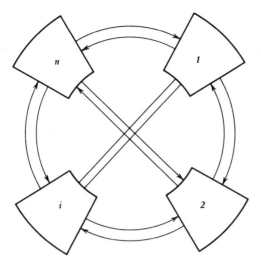

Figure 14. Model of an unconstrained system consisting of n compartments, where substances can move from any compartment to any other. Here, and in two subsequent figures, *1*, *2*, *i*, and *n* designate compartment numbers from *1* to *n*. (After Sheppard and Householder, 1951.)

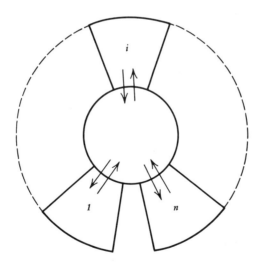

Figure 15. Model of a system consisting of n compartments, one of which is centrally located and communicates with all peripheral comparements (mammillary model). (After Sheppard and Householder, 1951.)

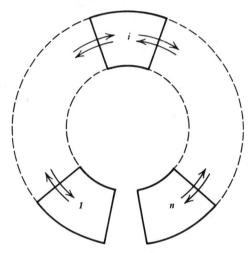

Figure 16. Model of a system consisting of n compartments which communicate chainwise (catenary model). (After Sheppard and Householder, 1951.)

The central compartment of the mammillary model may represent the plasma, while the peripheral compartments may represent the cells; the exchange of substance between the cells can occur only through the plasma. This model may be found convenient in the study of distribution processes. The catenary model may be of interest in metabolic studies. The above authors presented, for each of these models, a mathematical description of the distribution kinetics between the compartments and discussed in detail the kinetic features of the central and peripheral compartments. The proposed mathematical expressions are, however, of limited practical use because of their complexity and of the uncertainty of the models.

The kinetics of distributive processes in n-compartment systems is discussed by Filov (1967) and Atkins (1969).

Results of kinetic studies are expressible by mathematical equations in a compact form and, at the same time, with sufficient completeness. Although a mathematical equation is derived from experimental data which are always more or less limited, it can provide a concept of the whole process under study, as well as of the magnitudes of its parameters of interest (e.g., the blood concentration of a substance) at any instant of time.

Alternatively, an equation for a process can be constructed from theoretical considerations and then tested against experimental data and made more precise if necessary. If one is concerned with a fairly general problem of principle, there is often no need to fit experimental data to a proposed equation: the form of the equation and the functional relationship embodied in it, coupled with a consideration of a few particular cases, may prove to be quite sufficient.

Mathematical models of kinetic relationships can serve a variety of purposes. A mathematical model, as already indicated, may sum up the results of a study by clearly formulating the relationship discovered. Or it may serve as a hypothesis requiring validation or a hypothesis pointing out a new line of research. On the other hand, a mathematically flawless model (or, in a more explicit manner, its physical analogue) may help one to discard an inconsistent concept, however attractive it may seem. Indeed, it often happens that an author is so convinced of the validity of his theoretical propositions that he may mistake the desired for the real. The criterion of truth in such a situation can be a mathematical model (or any other suitable model) which works in a fairly objective way and is devoid of any emotions or bias.

A kinetic model that describes the behavior of a substance in the body makes it possible to obtain qualitatively new information on the biological fate and mode of action of that substance. It may form a basis for the control of the process of substance elimination from the body. Furthermore, mathematical relationships, if firmly established, make it possible to dispense with much of the time-consuming and detailed experimental work involved in the study of particular substances. When an adequate equation is available, such work can be reduced to a few experiments to determine the main constants. By substituting these constants into the equation, one can see the whole process under study.

The mathematical description of the kinetics of substance behavior in the body places the study of kinetic problems on a quantitative basis. That any quantitative method has advantages over its qualitative counterpart does not need any special proof. Nevertheless it seems appropriate to quote here the following words of Kelvin:

I often say that when you can measure what you are speaking about, and express it in numbers, you know something about it, but when you cannot express it in numbers, your knowledge is of a meager and unsatisfactory kind; it may be the beginning of knowledge, but you have scarcely, in your thoughts, advanced to the stage of science whatever the matter may be (quoted from Nelson, 1964).

The subsequent sections of this chapter describe some of the simpler and, at the same time, more widely used mathematical models for the absorption (with or without biotransformation), distribution, and elimination of substances, either in unchanged form or as metabolites. For some of the models examples will be given to indicate their possible practical applications. Particular attention will be devoted to the derivation of models and to methods for the calculation of kinetic parameters that characterize the movement of substances through the body.

3. ELEMENTS OF MATHEMATICAL MODELING; MODELS FOR ABSORPTION

3.1. Basic Equations and Their Graphic Interpretation

Kinetic Constants

Taking cognizance of the general principles underlying the free absorption of substances into the body from the environment, outlined in Section 1 of this chapter, we are now in a position to derive the simplest mathematical model for absorption which will be valid for any route of entry. Let us consider a system where a substance is assumed to be present in the external medium in a practically constant concentration despite its continued absorption into the living organism placed in that medium. This assumption, which is certainly valid when the concentration is specifically held constant, will be also valid if the medium has a much larger volume than the organism. This is often the case in industrial practice (e.g., the volume of a factory workroom or of some other enclosed workplace, as compared to that of the persons present there). As a first approximation, the organism may be regarded as a certain homogeneous system into which the substance penetrates by a process of diffusion and where it is perfectly mixed and accumulates to a certain limit. It should be further assumed that the substance undergoes slow or no change in the body. The latter assumption will simplify our task; moreover, it is valid for a wide range of substances encountered in practice (hydrocarbons, ethers, etc.). The mixing of the substance is accomplished by the bloodstream.

The most arbitrary of the above assumptions is that the organism is homogeneous; this assumption should introduce most of the error in the calculations to be made using the mathematical model which we will now proceed to construct.

Absorption begins when the organism is introduced into the medium, where the substance is present in a concentration C_0. The limit for absorption is given by the product λC_0, where λ is the partition coefficient of the substance between the organism and the medium. This will be the blood/air partition coefficient if the substance is absorbed into the blood from inhalation. For many substances the latter coefficient may be replaced, for practical purposes, by the water/air solubility coefficient, which can be readily determined experimentally. The greater the difference between the maximum possible concentration in the body (λC_0) and the actual concentration (C) at a time t, the more intensive is the absorption (this follows from the diffusion nature of the process). This can be stated mathematically as

$$\frac{dC}{dt} \propto (\lambda C_0 - C)$$

which means that the increment in concentration dC for every infinitesimal time interval dt is proportional to the difference between the maximum possible and the actual concentrations of the substance. Introducing a proportionality constant k, we can write the above expression as a differential equation for absorption:

$$\frac{dC}{dt} = k(\lambda C_0 - C) \tag{1}$$

To solve this equation, we separate the variables dC and dt:

$$\frac{dC}{k(\lambda C_0 - C)} = dt$$

and integrate:

$$\frac{1}{k} \int \frac{dC}{\lambda C_0 - C} \int = dt$$

$$\int \frac{d(\lambda C_0 - C)}{\lambda C_0 - C} = -k \int dt$$

$$\ln(\lambda C_0 - C) = -kt + a$$

where a is the constant of integration.
Taking the antilogarithm, we have

$$\lambda C_0 - C = A \cdot e^{-kt}$$

A being the constant of integration. Hence $C = \lambda C_0 - A \cdot e^{-kt}$. The constant A is found from the initial condition that, at $t = 0$, $C = 0$. (This means that the substance is absent from the organism at the time when the latter is introduced into the medium, and it is convenient to take this time as zero.) Then $A = \lambda C_0$, and

$$C = \lambda C_0(1 - e^{-kt}) \tag{2}$$

Equation 2 is the simplest mathematical model of the process by which a substance is absorbed into the body unchanged. This is an exponential equation with the constant k, which in this case is called the rate constant for absorption. The processes described by exponential expressions like (2) are first order. The processes governed by diffusion are always first order.

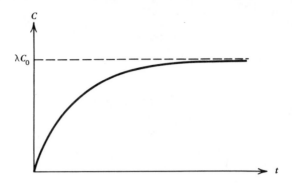

Figure 17.   Kinetic curve describing the absorption of substance in a biological system by a first-order process.

A graphic model corresponding to the mathematical model just derived is shown in Figure 17. Although of limited use, such models describe more or less adequately the absorption of many substances into the blood and other body fluids, especially when the observation period is relatively short, as well as, more crudely, into the body as a whole. One example is shown in Figure 9, where the absorption of ethyl ether into the venous blood of a dog is described by an exponential curve for an observation period of 2 hr. Other examples are given in the next section. The practical significance of the model is discussed by Tolokontsev (1959, 1960c) and Liublina (1964).

As regards the elimination of substances, the simplest model is the one describing the elimination of a substance by some one route, for example, in the expired air or in the urine, or its loss by way of metabolism. In the most common situation the decrease in the amount of the substance is proportional to its concentration:

$$\frac{dC}{dt} \propto -C \quad \text{or} \quad \frac{dC}{dt} = -\kappa C \tag{3}$$

where κ is the proportionality constant, and the minus sign before C shows that the concentration declines with time. Integration yields

$$\int \frac{dC}{C} = -\kappa \int dt$$

$$\ln C = -\kappa t + a$$

which, on taking the antilogarithm, gives $C = A \cdot e^{-\kappa t}$.

The constant A is found from the initial condition that, at $t = 0$, $C = C_0$

(This means that the maximal concentration C_0 occurred at the time when elimination started.) Then $A = C_0$, and

$$C = C_0 \cdot e^{-\kappa t} \tag{4}$$

This is the simplest mathematical model of the process by which a substance is eliminated from the body. It is an exponential equation with the constant κ called the rate constant for elimination. The elimination process is first order.

In (1) to (4) the amount of substance D may be substituted for the concentration C. It is often convenient to deal with amounts when applying the elimination equation for practical purposes; then

$$D = D_0 \cdot e^{-\kappa t} \tag{5}$$

This is not so with the equation for absorption because the partition coefficient λ is defined in terms of concentrations.

The model for elimination, (4) and (5), can often describe satisfactorily an actual excretory or metabolic process (e.g., Bray and White, 1966; Filov, 1967) and so may find many practical uses. A graphic interpretation of this model is presented in Figure 18.

Another graphic interpretation of the model is worth mentioning. By putting (4) in its logarithmic form, we have

$$\log C = \log C_0 - \frac{\kappa}{2.3} t \tag{6}$$

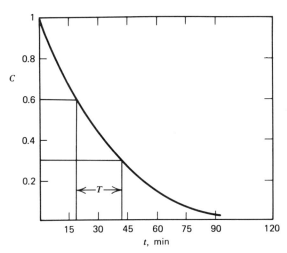

Figure 18. Kinetics of butyl acetate hydrolysis in human blood. T is the half-life of butyl acetate. (See p. 115 for a discussion of half-life.)

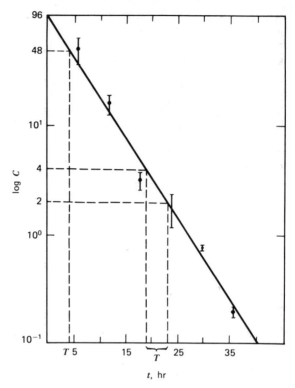

Figure 19.   Decline of benzene concentration in the epididymal fat of rats ($T = 4.2$ hr). (After Mironis, 1970.)

which is an equation of a straight line relating log C and t. If experimental points lie on a straight line, they are described by (6) and (4) and consequently obey first-order kinetics. It is convenient to construct such graphs on semi-logarithmic paper so that the values of C, rather than their logarithms, can be plotted against time to describe the relationship log $C = f(t)$.*

Such a graph, describing the disappearance of benzene from a biological substrate by one route, is presented in Figure 19. A graph like this is of practical use for the estimation of a number of kinetic parameters, primarily the elimination constant κ. Moreover, it allows one to judge the nature of the elimination process. Indeed, if the experimental points lie on a straight line, as shown, for example, in Figure 19, the process of excretion (or metabolism) obeys first-order kinetics and so can be described by (6) and, consequently,

---

* It reads: the logarithm of concentration is a function of time. This is a shortened and generalized form of writing various equations —(4) in this case.

(4). If the points do not lie on a straight line, the elimination occurs by a process more complex than exponential. Thus the disappearance of a substance may be described by the sum of two or more independent exponentials. A biexponential plot describing the loss of carbon disulfide from subcutaneous fat is shown in Figure 28 on p. 145, where more complex elimination processes are also discussed.

It follows from (1) to (6) that the time courses of absorption and elimination are governed by the constants k and κ, respectively. When the numerical values of these constants are known, the concentration of the substance in the system can be readily calculated for any instant of time. In the case of elimination, it will be necessary to know only the initial concentration of the substance, which may be determined experimentally or just given. In the case of absorption, it will be necessary to know, in addition, an approximate value of λ.

As can be seen from (2) and (4), the constants k and κ are expressed as reciprocals of time. Thus, in (4), the cofactor $e^{-\kappa t}$ must be a dimensionless quantity, which is possible only if the exponent is dimensionless. Accordingly, since t is measured in units of time (sec, min, hr, etc.), κ must be measured in reciprocal times (1/sec, 1/min, 1/hr, etc.).

The physical meanings of these constants are as follows: κ shows what fraction of the substance present in the biological system is eliminated per unit time, while k indicates what fraction of the maximum possible amount of the substance that can be absorbed into the system is actually absorbed per unit time.

Constants Characterizing Half-Completion of a Process

The constants k and κ are closely related to the constants called the elimination half-life and the saturation half-life. Since the elimination half-life is of particular importance in toxicology, we will discuss it at some length, bearing in mind that everything that concerns this constant essentially applies to the saturation half-life as well.

The terms "elimination half life," "biological half-life," and "half-life" (or "half-life period") are all used to mean the time required for half the amount of a substance present in a biological system to be eliminated or to disappear. The processes or pathways by which the elimination occurs are immaterial. Thus it may occur by one or more pathways and may or may not involve degradation or binding of the substance. This is a purely physiological concept which characterizes the system "organism-substance."

Denoting the elimination half-life by T and using (4), we can write

$$\frac{C_0}{2} = C_0 \cdot e^{-\kappa T}$$

and

$$e^{-\kappa T} = \tfrac{1}{2}$$

or, in logarithmic form, $\kappa T = \ln 2 = 0.693$, which clearly shows the numerical relation between the elimination rate constant and the half-life; thus

$$\kappa = \frac{0.693}{T}$$

and

$$T = \frac{0.693}{\kappa} \qquad (7)$$

The value of T can be easily found graphically, for example from elimination data plotted on semilogarithmic scales, exemplified in Figure 19. It is also possible to find T from a concentration versus time plot, as shown in Figure 18. Straight-line plots are, however, preferable, since they permit inter- and extrapolation and give greater accuracy in graphic manipulations.

If the substance is eliminated by an exponential process, T can also be determined by calculation from the formula

$$T = \ln\left(\frac{t_2 - t_1}{\ln C_1 - \ln C_2}\right) \qquad (8)$$

where C_1 and C_2 are the blood concentrations at times t_1 and t_2.

It is of interest that 29% of the substance is eliminated for $0.5T$, 75% for $2T$, 87.5% for $3T$, and 93.8% for $4T$. Here are two numerical examples involving T.

EXAMPLE 1.   What fraction of the original amount of a given substance remains in the body after a time equal to $9T$?

$$C = C_0 \cdot e^{-\kappa \cdot 9T}; \qquad \frac{C}{C_0} = -\frac{1}{e^{\kappa T \cdot 9}} = \frac{1}{e^{\ln 2 \cdot 9}} = \frac{1}{2^9} = \frac{1}{512}$$

Answer: $C \approx 0.002$ of C_0.

EXAMPLE 2.   How much of the substance will be contained in the body after 50 hr if $T = 14.3$ hr?

$$\frac{50}{14.3} = 3.5; \qquad \frac{C}{C_0} = \frac{1}{2^{3.5}} = \frac{1}{11.3}$$

Answer: $C \approx 9\%$ of C_0.

For a more detailed discussion of the concept of half-life reference may be made, for example, to the papers by Garrett and Alway (1964) and Wilbrandt

(1964). The latter paper also describes methods for calculating the half-lives of substances from urinary or blood level data.

The constants k and κ, as well as the half-life T, are of course subject to biological variation, as are any other biological characteristics.

The Apparent Volume of Distribution

Another parameter characterizing the behavior of a foreign substance in the body is the apparent volume of distribution.* This quantity is often used, mainly outside the USSR, in studies concerned with the kinetics of distributive processes. The volume of distribution is the fictitious volume that would be occupied by a given substance in a state of homogeneous distribution equilibrium in the body:

$$V = \frac{W}{C} \tag{9}$$

where W is the amount of the substance in the body in units of weight, and C is its concentration in the tissue through which the distribution volume is defined. If, for example, W is in milligrams and C in milligrams per milliliter of blood plasma, V will be in milliliters as defined from plasma concentration. A V calculated from plasma concentration data will differ from one calculated from concentration data for another tissue, say muscular. The volumes of distribution determined from blood and plasma concentrations will differ if the concentrations themselves are different.

The concept of a volume of distribution allows one to obviate the difficulties associated with the presence of different quantities of substance in different tissues at equilibrium. In other words, it makes it possible to exclude from consideration the partition coefficients of substance between different tissues (λ_i). This is an important advantage because such coefficients are often difficult, if not impossible, to determine, for it is not known in which tissues the substance is distributed. The distribution volume characterizes the ability of a substance to penetrate into tissues, to combine with biological components, and to be stored in various regions of the body.

It is not difficult to determine V if an intravenously administered substance attains equilibrium in a matter of minutes. Therefore, a few minutes after the intravenous injection of a known dose, the blood concentration of the substance should be determined several times at regular intervals, and a plot of concentration against time constructed in semilogarithmic coordinates, similar to the plot shown in Figure 19. A straight-line plot will indicate that an

---

* Hereafter the word "apparent" is omitted.

equilibrium was reached. Extrapolating the plot to the y axis will allow one to find the value of C_0 and to calculate V from the formula

$$V = \frac{\text{dose}}{C_0}$$

Another method for calculating V requires the determination of the amount of substance in the urine and in the plasma, but dispenses with the need for rapid establishment of equilibrium (it is applicable only to substances whose sole or main route of elimination is urine):

$$V = \frac{W - M_t}{C_t}$$

where W is the amount of administered substance, M_t is the amount excreted in urine to time t, and C_t is the concentration in plasma at time t. The numerator thus gives the amount of substance in the body at time t.

Here is an example of calculation by this formula. Suppose that the plasma concentration of a substance is 0.06 mg/ml at t hours after its intravenous injection in a dose of 2 g. By that time 0.62 g of the substance has been excreted in the urine. Therefore

$$V = \frac{2000 - 620}{0.06} = 23{,}000 \text{ ml}$$

The percent volume of distribution can be calculated by the formula

$$V\% = \frac{V}{V_{\text{body}}} \cdot 100 \tag{10}$$

where V_{body} is the total body volume, which in most cases is numerically equal to the body weight in grams. There is little variation in $V\%$ from one individual to another within a species.

Substituting the value for V from (9) into (10), we arrive at a relationship very useful for certain calculations:

$$V\% \cdot V_{\text{body}} = \frac{W}{C} \cdot 100$$

A knowledge of V sometimes allows one to draw immediate conclusions of practical importance. Thus, according to Milne (1964), the volume of distribution of many substances in an adult human being is about 14 liters, which is approximately equal to the extracellular fluid volume. The distribution volume of some substances penetrating inside body cells is about 42 liters, that is, equal to the total body water in the average human being. Milne used the "volume of distribution" concept to discuss practical aspects of the potentiation of urinary excretion of poisons. (This question is also dealt with in Section 5.4.)

References to the literature concerned with the volume of distribution are given by Filov (1967, 1973). Methods for the calculation of V and possible errors involved in its evaluation are discussed by Riegelman et al. (1968).

The half-life of a substance excreted in urine is related to its distribution volume by the equation

$$T = \ln 2 \cdot \frac{V}{C} \tag{11}$$

where C is the plasma clearance, as calculated from the formula

$$C = \frac{C_u \cdot v}{C_{pl}}$$

in which C_{pl} and C_u are the plasma and urine concentrations, respectively, of the substance, and v is the volume of urine excreted per minute.

In conclusion, here is an example of calculations of the constants k, κ, and λ from experimental data. Figure 20 shows the results of an experiment on the saturation and desaturation of the omentum with benzene in rats inhaling benzene vapors in a concentration of 3 mg/liter (Mironos, 1970). These results are sufficient to calculate the constants.

For the calculations two concentrations were chosen, C_t and C_{2t}, corresponding to times t and $2t$. Applying (2), we have

$$C_t = \lambda C_0 (1 - e^{-kt})$$

and

$$C_{2t} = \lambda C_0 (1 - e^{-k2t})$$

The parentheses in the latter expression contain the difference of squares, which can be written as

$$C_{2t} = \lambda C_0 (1 - e^{-kt})(1 + e^{-kt})$$

Dividing C_{2t} by C_t, we get

$$\frac{C_{2t}}{C_t} = 1 + e^{-kt}$$

and

$$e^{-kt} = \frac{C_{2t} - C_t}{C_t}$$

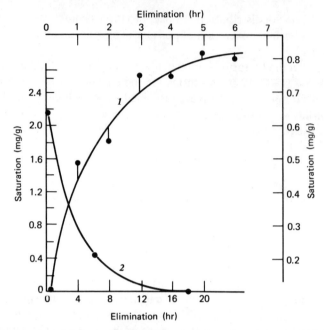

Figure 20. Experimental curves describing the saturation of rat omentum with benzene (*1*) and its elimination from the omentum (*2*). Each point is the average of three determinations in different rats.

Taking the logarithms gives

$$-kt = \ln\left(\frac{C_{2t} - C_t}{C_t}\right)$$

whence

$$k = \frac{1}{t} \cdot \ln\left(\frac{C_t}{C_{2t} - C_t}\right) \tag{12}$$

This expression is sufficient for calculating k. For convenience, a t of 1 hr was chosen, as shown in Figure 20. Then $C_t = 440\ \mu g/g$, $C_{2t} = 595\ \mu g/g$, and k can be readily calculated:

$$k = \frac{1}{1} \cdot \ln\left(\frac{440}{595 - 440}\right) = \ln 2.84 = 1.04\ hr^{-1}$$

Similarly, to calculate λ, we substitute the value of k from (12) into the equation $C_t = \lambda C_0(1 - e^{-kt})$, and after transformations we find an expression convenient for calculating λ:

$$C_t = \lambda C_0 \left\{ 1 - \exp\left[-t \times \frac{1}{t} \ln\left(\frac{C_t}{C_{2t} - C_t} \right) \right] \right\}$$

$$= \lambda C_0 \left\{ 1 - \exp\left[\ln\left(\frac{C_{2t} - C_t}{C_t} \right) \right] \right\}$$

$$= \lambda C_0 \left(1 - \frac{C_{2t} - C_t}{C_t} \right) = \frac{\lambda C_0(2C_t - C_{2t})}{C_t}$$

whence

$$\lambda = \frac{C_t^2}{C_0(2C_t - C_{2t})} \tag{13}$$

Supposing that the C_t in micrograms per gram is approximately equal to the C_t in milligrams per liter, and substituting the concrete values into (13), we find

$$\lambda = \frac{440 \times 440}{3 \times (880 - 595)} \approx 230$$

To calculate κ, we transform (4) so that

$$\kappa = -\frac{1}{t} \ln\left(\frac{C}{C_0} \right) \tag{14}$$

In our case $C_0 = 2150 \ \mu g/g$, and we take a t equal to 5 hr, so $C = 600 \ \mu g/g$. Hence

$$\kappa = -0.2 \cdot \ln 0.28 \approx 0.26 \ hr^{-1}$$

It should be noted that this is not the simplest method for calculating κ. It would be simpler to turn curve 2 in Figure 20 into a straight line by constructing a plot in semilogarithmic coordinates and to calculate the constant as described on p. 114. As for k, it has been calculated in the simplest way.

In this section we have considered the simpler methods of calculating some kinetic parameters. These methods are far from being always applicable in practice. In the subsequent sections more complicated methods are described, and their scopes of application are indicated.

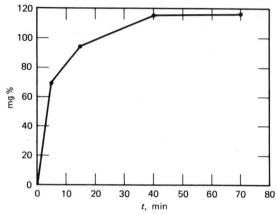

Figure 21.   Saturation of the cerebrospinal fluid with ether in a dog. (From Fedorov, 1963.)

3.2.   Absorption of Inert Gases into Tissues; a Complete Equation for Absorption

Here further examples will be given to illustrate the absorption of reasonably inert gases. Figure 21 shows the time course of diethyl ether absorption into the cerebrospinal fluid of a dog inhaling ether vapors. The experimental points connected by straight lines fit an exponential curve sufficiently well for the entire process to be describable by (2). Figure 22 compares an experimental curve describing the saturation of rat omentum with benzene during the inhalation of its vapors in a concentration of 3 mg/liter (dotted line) and a theoretical exponential curve for this process (solid line). These curves are practically identical, thus confirming the validity of model (2) in this case. This method is used to judge how closely experimental data fit theoretical kinetic concepts. Figure 10 shows that an exponential equation can also be used to describe the absorption of halothane into the human body.*

Although we have been trying to demonstrate (in particular, by giving the above examples) the practical value of (1) and (2) for absorption studies, we must not forget their limitations. For one thing, these first-order kinetic equations were derived on the assumption that the organism can be regarded as a one-compartment system rather than the multicompartment system which it actually is. For another, absorption from inhalation is affected by a number of physiological parameters such as alveolar ventilation; residual volume; thickness and permeability of the alveolar-capillary membrane; rate of pulmonary blood flow; cardiac output; total blood volume; pul-

---

* This process can probably be described more accurately by the sum of several exponentials.

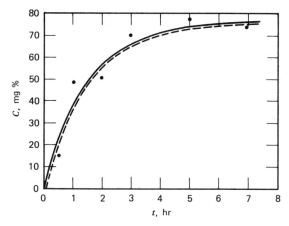

Figure 22. Comparison of experimental and theoretical curves for the saturation of rat omentum with benzene. See text for explanation. (After Mironos, 1970.)

monary tissue mass; partition coefficients between air and pulmonary tissue, between air and blood, and between blood and various tissues; and volume, blood supply, and diffusion parameters of particular tissues.

All these parameters are incorporated into the absorption rate constant k. If they vary during absorption, so does the value of k, and the absorption will be governed by a relationship more complex than exponential. Moreover, physiological parameters such as cardiac output vary within a species from one individual to another. These variations make k variable even if the experiments are identical but use different animals.

Attempts have been made to describe the absorption process more precisely by taking into consideration the basic physiological parameters. One of the early attempts was made by Y. Henderson and H. Haggard, whose model is discussed by Lazarev in his *General Principles of Industrial Toxicology* (1938). A number of other models were reviewed by Filov (1967). Here we will describe what we believe to be one of the best models, which takes account of the more important physiological parameters. The model is given below in its final form, without derivation, reproducing only the constraints imposed by the authors on the system representing the organism (Paton and Speden, 1965).

The first assumption is that the substance is almost instantaneously diffused from the alveolar space to lung capillaries. Furthermore, we assume that there are no pulmonary vascular shunts and that the perfusion-ventilation relations are constant throughout the lungs. In addition, we suppose that the capacity of the lung tissue itself for the absorbed substance is negligibly small.

Turning to the transfer of the substance from the blood to tissues, we assume that the substance is rapidly diffused and that there are no vascular shunts in the body. We also suppose that pulmonary ventilation is a continuous process and that all physiological parameters remain unchanged. The organism is regarded as consisting of a finite number of compartments.

With these assumptions it is possible to write a differential equation describing the arterial concentration of the substance (C) as a function of the inspired concentration (C_0) and of the following physiological parameters: alveolar ventilation (M), lung volume (V_l), cardiac output (F), concentrations of the substance in particular tissues $(C_1, C_2,$ etc.) and in the venous blood (C_v), volume of these tissues $(V_1, V_2,$ etc.), blood flow through the tissues $(f_1, f_2,$ etc.), and the partition coefficients between the blood and air (λ) and between the blood and the various tissues $(\lambda_1, \lambda_2,$ etc.). This equation has the form

$$\frac{dC}{dt} = \frac{M}{V_l}(\lambda C_0 - C) + \frac{\lambda F}{V_l}(C_v - C) \tag{15}$$

Equations describing changes in particular tissues will have the form:

$$\frac{dC_i}{dt} = \frac{f_i}{\lambda_i V_i}(\lambda_i C - C_i) \tag{16}$$

where the subscript i is the number of tissue concerned (1 or 2 or 3, etc.).

Concentration in the venous blood will be defined by the relation

$$C_v = \frac{f_1 C_1}{F\lambda_1} + \frac{f_2 C_2}{F\lambda_2} + \frac{f_3 C_3}{F\lambda_3} + \cdots \tag{17}$$

Equations 15 to 17 describe the process of absorption more accurately than (1) but are much more difficult to apply in practice. Whereas it is very easy to integrate (1) and to convert it to form (2), which is not difficult to solve, the solution of (15) to (17) requires the use of a digital or, preferably, an analogue computer. The principles of operation and possible applications of analogue computers in toxicokinetic studies are discussed, for example, by Filov (1967).

Analogue computer simulation has shown, in particular, that if the substance being inhaled is readily soluble in an aqueous phase, the approach to steady-state concentration is slow and that the main physiological parameter limiting this process is pulmonary ventilation. If the solubility is moderate, the limiting parameter is cardiac output. Analogue computers make it possible to compare the effects of partition coefficients and other parameters on the absorption of a substance into different tissues of the organism.

3.3.   A Model for the Absorption of a Gaseous Substance Which Is Inhaled Periodically

When a person is occupationally exposed to a gaseous substance, this substance is absorbed into the body during the working hours and eliminated from the body during the hours off work. If exposure periods regularly alternate with periods free from exposure, the whole cycle can be described by simple mathematical methods. If the substance is eliminated at a slow rate and over a period much longer than the period of absorption, a model for the process of saturation and desaturation of body tissues may be represented in graphic form as shown in Figure 23.

For a more detailed mathematical description of the process (Filov, 1969), certain limitations have to be imposed. The main limitation will be introduced by the assumption that the absorption and elimination are first-order processes. Moreover, our consideration will be confined to substances which are eliminated unchanged at a far faster rate than the rate of their transformation in the body. It is also possible to consider metabolizable substances, provided that their elimination is interpreted as representing the sum of excretory and metabolic processes; such interpretation is permissible only as a certain approximation. Finally, the organism will be considered to be a one-compartment system.

With these assumptions the absorption of a substance into body tissues previously free from that substance can be described by (2):

$$C_1 = \lambda C_0 (1 - e^{-kt}),$$

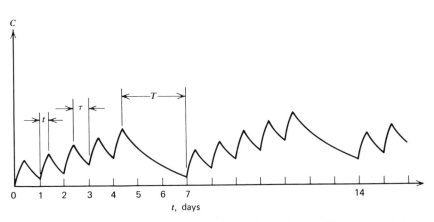

Figure 23.   The time course of saturation and desaturation of tissues with a gaseous substance under conditions of a 5-day work week. See text for details.

where C_0 is the inspired concentration and C_1 is the concentration in the tissues at a time t; elimination can be described by (4): $C = C_1 \cdot e^{-\kappa t}$.

Consider now a situation corresponding to our task: periods of occupational exposure (t) to a substance whose environmental concentration remains constant (C_0) regularly alternate with exposure-free periods (τ) during which the substance is eliminated only.

During the first workday, the substance will be absorbed to a level C_1 over a working time t. Thereafter it will undergo elimination, and its concentration will decline to the level $C_1 \cdot e^{-\kappa \tau}$ over the period of time τ that will have elapsed by the beginning of the next workday. Absorption will then resume, so that by the end of the second workday the concentration will be

$$C_2 = C_1 \cdot e^{-\kappa \tau} + (\lambda C_0 - C_1 \cdot e^{-\kappa \tau})(1 - e^{-kt}) \qquad (18)$$

The first term in this equation is the concentration remaining from the first workday at the beginning of the second, while the second term corresponds to the exponential relationship for absorption, taking into account the initial level of the substance, $C_1 \cdot e^{-\kappa \tau}$. [Clearly, if practically all of the substance has been eliminated during the exposure-free period τ, the term $C_1 \cdot e^{-\kappa \tau}$ will be equal to zero, so that (18) will reduce to (2).]

Multiplying and rearranging terms in (18) enables us to reduce it to the form

$$C_2 = \lambda C_0 (1 - e^{-kt}) \left[1 + e^{-(kt + \kappa \tau)} \right]$$

By the beginning of the third workday the concentration will decline to $C_2 \cdot e^{-\kappa \tau}$, to rise again during that day to the level

$$C_3 = C_2 \cdot e^{-\kappa \tau} + (\lambda C_0 - C_2 \cdot e^{-\kappa \tau})(1 - e^{-kt})$$
$$= \lambda C_0 (1 - e^{-kt}) \left[1 + e^{-(kt + \kappa \tau)} + e^{-2(kt + \kappa \tau)} \right]$$

Proceeding in this way, we will observe a regular pattern which can be represented by a formula giving the concentration in tissues after any nth workday, provided that the situation (i.e., the environmental concentration and the exposure and exposure-free periods) remains unchanged:

$$C_n^{\max} = \frac{\lambda C_0 (1 - e^{-kt}) \left[1 - e^{-n(kt + \kappa \tau)} \right]}{1 - e^{-(kt + \kappa \tau)}} \qquad (19)*$$

By the beginning of the next workday the concentration will be

$$C_n^{\min} = C_n^{\max} \cdot e^{-\kappa \tau} \qquad (20)$$

* This mathematical model is very similar to those describing the kinetics of drugs during their periodic parenteral administration (see Filov, 1967).

If we let n tend to infinity in (19), we will get the maximum possible concentration value under the given conditions:

$$C_{n \to \infty}^{\max} = \lambda C_0 \frac{1 - e^{-kt}}{1 - e^{-(kt + \kappa\tau)}} \tag{21}$$

This concentration will always be lower than the one developing in the case of continuous inhalation without exposure-free periods (i.e., when $\tau = 0$ and $C = \lambda C_0$), because the denominator in (21) is always greater than the numerator. This mathematical inference is of course fully consistent with the simple logical inference that a smaller amount of substance can accumulate in the body with discontinuous than with continuous daily exposure. The magnitude of the limit of absorption will depend on the values of t, τ, k, and κ.

Let us consider now a more practical situation where exposure by inhalation occurs during the working week only, so that account must be taken not only of daily exposure-free periods but also of the longer-lasting weekend periods. Denote the weekend duration by T, with $T > \tau$.

Suppose that the working cycle consists of a days. By applying the same reasoning as above in deriving (19), we can arrive at a formula for the concentration of substance in body tissues by the end of the mth working cycle (mth working week):

$$C_m^{\max} = \frac{\lambda C_0(1 - e^{-kt})[1 - e^{-a(kt + \kappa\tau)}]}{1 - e^{-(kt + \kappa\tau)}}$$

$$\cdot \frac{1 - \exp\{-m[akt + (a - 1)\kappa\tau + \kappa T]\}}{1 - \exp\{-[akt + (a - 1)\kappa\tau + \kappa T]\}} \tag{22}$$

By the end of the weekend period T, that is, by the start of the next $(m + 1)$ working week, the concentration will be

$$C_m^{\min} = C_m^{\max} \cdot e^{-\kappa T} \tag{23}$$

The concentration by the end of any workday p belonging to the $(m + 1)$ week will be given by the equation

$$C_{am + p}^{\max} = \frac{\lambda C_0(1 - e^{-kt})[1 - e^{-p(kt + \kappa\tau)}]}{1 - e^{-(kt + \kappa\tau)}} + C_m^{\min} \cdot e^{-pkt} \cdot e^{-(p - 1)\kappa\tau} \tag{24}$$

where $0 \leq p \leq a$.

If $p = a$, that is, for the end of a working week, (24) will convert to (22). The latter will in turn reduce to (19) if we suppose that all exposure-free periods are equal (i.e., $T = \tau$ and $am = n$).

Equations 19, 22, and 24 are mathematical models for the absorption of gaseous substances. Clearly, these equations are of limited use. They were derived on the assumption that the variation in working conditions is strictly periodic. Such an ideal situation can be produced only in experiment. In real life there will always be deviations from the ideal, and the greater the deviations the less applicable will be the models.

The partition coefficient λ, the absorption constant k, and the elimination constant κ must be known in order for the above equations to be used in practice. Values of these constants for a limited range of substances are available in the literature; for most substances, however, they are unknown and must be determined in special experiments.

Let us illustrate the application of these equations by considering two substances, chloroform and ethanol, the constants for which were known or were calculated from experimental data obtained by Tolokontsev (1960a).

Suppose that the workday period t is 8.4 hr, the off-work period $\tau = 15.6$ hr, and the number of workdays n is 5 days. The constants for chloroform are as follows: $\lambda = 10.3$, $k \approx \kappa \approx 0.08$ min^{-1}.

The concentration of chloroform in tissues by the end of the working week will be given by (19):

$$C_{5\text{th day}}^{\max}$$

$$= 10.3 \times C_0 \frac{[1 - \exp(-0.08 \times 8.4 \times 60)]\{1 - \exp[-5(0.08 \times 8.4 \times 60 + 0.08 \times 15.6 \times 60)]\}}{1 - \exp[-(0.08 \times 8.4 \times 60 + 0.08 \times 15.6 \times 60)]} \approx 10.3 \times C_0$$

The concentration by the end of any other working day will also be $10.3 \times C_0$. This means that, when chloroform is inhaled in the concentration C_0, an equilibrium saturation of the tissues is attained every working day.

The elimination of chloroform will be given by (20):

$$C^{\min} = 10.3 \times C_0 \cdot \exp(-0.08 \times 15.6 \times 60) \approx 0$$

This means that chloroform does not cumulate. Each day the body is saturated with chloroform vapors and then completely cleared of chloroform. This result fully agrees with the conclusion reached in an experimental study by Morris et al. (1951).

The constants for ethanol are as follows: $\lambda = 2000$ and $k \approx \kappa \approx 0.0007$ min^{-1}. Therefore

$$C_{5\text{th day}}^{\max} = 2000 \times C_0$$

$$\cdot \frac{[1 - \exp(-0.0007 \times 8.4 \times 60)]\{1 - \exp[-5(0.352 + 0.655)]\}}{1 - e^{-1.007}}$$

$$= 2000 \times C_0 \times 0.47 = 940 \times C_0$$

From (22) we find that the concentration of ethanol will be $942 \times C_0$ by the end of the second week, $944 \times C_0$ by the end of the third week, and so on, that is, the tissue content of the alcohol will progressively increase, though very slowly. The body will not be completely free from it even after a weekend $(T = 63.6)$:

$$C^{min} = 940 \times C_0 \cdot \exp(-0.0007 \times 63.6 \times 60)$$

$$= 940 \times C_0 \times 0.032 = 30 \times C_0$$

Direct measurements showed similar behavior of ethyl alcohol in the blood of human beings inhaling its vapors (Lester and Greenberg, 1951).

The mathematical models just described can be used in a variety of situations, in particular for the interpretation of animal experiments and in model biological systems, provided that the conditions specified in the second paragraph of this section (p. 125) are observed.

Here is an example to show how one of those models (19) can be applied to the results of an animal experiment. In one of our experiments (Mironos, 1970) rats were regularly exposed to benzene vapors, and their fat was examined for benzene content at various times during and after exposure to clarify the role of fatty tissues in benzene deposition. By applying the procedures described in Section 3.1, we first calculated the main kinetic parameters characterizing rat fatty tissues (the omentum and epididymis) as benzene depots. For the omentum, λ was found to be 230; k, 1.04 hr^{-1}; and κ, 0.26 hr^{-1} (the calculations are described on pp. 119–121; those were the highest k and κ values). For the epididymal fat, $\lambda = 270$, $k = 0.28$ hr^{-1}, and $\kappa = 0.1$ hr^{-1} (the lowest k and κ values) (Filov and Mironos, 1967).

The above values are sufficient to calculate benzene contents in the omental and epididymal fats of rats for any exposure regimen. Using (19) and (20), we performed calculations for daily 6-hr exposures to benzene vapors in a concentration of 3 mg/liter—the same regimen as had been used by Mironos in her laborious experiments of many days' duration. The calculations are given in Table 15.

As can be seen from the table, the maximum possible amount of benzene had been absorbed into the omentum as early as on day 1 of exposure. Later, somewhere between days 1 and 10, the benzene concentration reached its peak in the epididymal fat. This shows that neither the omentum nor the epididymis can act as a significant benzene depot in rats. This theoretical conclusion is in complete agreement with the conclusion reached from the long-continued experiments. Mathematical methods similar to the one described here have an advantage over experimental methods not only in that they can produce results readily and rapidly, but also in that these results have predictive value enabling the researcher to follow the time course of the process under study.

Table 15. Benzene Concentrations in Omental and Epididymal Fat of Rats in the Course of 20 Days of Daily 6-Hr Exposures (C_0 = 3 mg/liter; C in mg/kg)

Fat	Concentration	Exposure Day		
		1	10	20
Omental	C^{max}	690	690	690
	C^{min}	6.2	6.2	6.2
Epididymal	C^{max}	660	680	680
	C^{min}	92	95	95

3.4. Absorption of Metabolizable Substances

The absorption of a substance undergoing more or less rapid biotransformations would be expected to follow a more complicated pattern than the absorption of inert substances that remain unchanged (see Section 3.1). Let us consider this process (Filov, 1964a). The system will be essentially the same as before: a medium containing a substance in a constant concentration C_0 and a living system (assumed to be single-compartment for simplicity) into which the substance is absorbed from the medium. However, in addition to being absorbed, the substance is broken down at a rate that depends on the characteristics of the living system and the nature of the substance.

Most breakdown processes involving xenobiotics that are present in the body in relatively small quantities are well describable by first-order kinetic equations, their rates being proportional to the amount or concentration of particular substances in the medium concerned. Therefore we can write a differential equation which differs from (1) only in having one additional term:

$$\frac{dC}{dt} = k(\lambda C_0 - C) - \kappa C \qquad (25)$$

The left-hand side of this equation gives the instantaneous velocity of absorption into the organism, while the right-hand side gives the components of that velocity which depend on absorption (the first term) and degradation (the second term). The designations are as follows: C_0 is constant external concentration of the substance, C is internal concentration of the substance at time t, λ is partition coefficient of the substance between the external medium and the living system, k is rate constant for absorption, and κ is rate constant for degradation. To solve this equation we rearrange the right-hand side:

$$\frac{dC}{dt} = k\lambda C_0 - (k + \kappa)C$$

separate the variables of integration:

$$\frac{dC}{(k + \kappa)C - k\lambda C_0} = -dt$$

and integrate:

$$\frac{1}{k + \kappa} \int \frac{d[(k + \kappa)C - k\lambda C_0]}{(k + \kappa)C - k\lambda C_0} = -\int dt$$

$$\ln (k + \kappa)C - k\lambda C_0 = -(k + \kappa)t + a$$

a being the constant of integration. Hence

$$(k + \kappa)C - k\lambda C_0 = Ae^{-(k+\kappa)t}$$

where A is the same constant after the taking of antilogarithms.

The constant A can be found from the initial condition that $C = 0$ when $t = 0$; consequently $A = -k\lambda C_0$. Hence the final form of the equation describing the concentration of a substance which is freely absorbed into and undergoes biotransformation in a biological system is as follows:

$$C = \frac{k\lambda C_0}{k + \kappa} [1 - e^{-(k+\kappa)t}] \tag{26}$$

It follows from this equation that the substance, even if it undergoes degradation, still continues to accumulate in the living system under the conditions specified (i.e., when its circumambient external concentration remains constant and it freely penetrates into the living system from the environment). Apart from the external concentration and the partition coefficient, the limit of absorption depends on the ratio between the absorption and degradation constants, as can be seen when $t \rightarrow \infty$.

Absorption in this case proceeds by an exponential process whose rate constant is equal to the sum of the absorption and degradation constants. In other words, the saturation of the living system with a reactive substance occurs more rapidly than its saturation with an unreactive substance having otherwise identical physicochemical properties (this is shown in graphic form in Figure 24).

The inferences to be drawn from (26) for reactive substances may be illustrated by considering three specific cases.

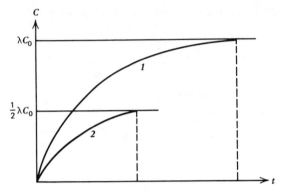

Figure 24. Graphic representation of relationships governing the absorption of unreactive (*1*) and reactive (*2*) ($k = \kappa$) substances having equal λs and the same C_0.

1. Absorption is much more rapid than degradation, that is, $k \gg \kappa$. Then κ can be neglected, so that

$$C = \lambda C_0(1 - e^{-kt})$$

This is of course (2), as was to be expected.

2. The rate constants for absorption and degradation are equal ($k = \kappa$). Then, substituting k for κ, we have

$$C = \tfrac{1}{2}\lambda C_0(1 - e^{-2kt})$$

Letting t go to ∞, we get the limit to which the concentration will tend: $C \to \tfrac{1}{2}\lambda C_0$. This limit is half that for an unreactive substance having the same λ and C_0, but it will take only half as long to attain this limit for a reactive substance, as can be readily seen from Figure 24.

3. Degradation occurs at a much faster rate than absorption, that is, $k \ll \kappa$. Then

$$C = \frac{k\lambda C_0}{\kappa}(1 - e^{-\kappa t})$$

When $t \to \infty$, $C \to (k/\kappa)\lambda C_0$. This means that, although accrual of the substance occurs, its upper limit will be low, and the lower the smaller is k compared to κ; this limit tends to zero.

Physically, the absorption of a substance whose degradation rate constant is much greater than its absorption rate constant may be visualized as follows. A certain, if only a very small, amount of the substance must of course be absorbed before its breakdown can begin. The rate of degradation, which is measured in terms of the number of molecules broken down per unit time, is the faster the higher the total content of the substance. At a certain concentration the rate of degradation becomes equal to that of absorption, indicating that a steady-state concentration of the substance has been reached.

After this theoretical consideration of absorption kinetics for metabolizable substances, it is appropriate to turn to experimental data. A number of our studies (Filov, 1961a, 1961b, 1964b) were concerned with the fate of acetic esters in the body. These esters were shown to undergo degradation, and the degradation rates of some of them were estimated in model experiments. No esters were detectable in the blood of rabbits inhaling ester vapors in moderate concentrations, despite their retention in the body. Esters were found to be present, however, in the blood of rats on the inhalation of massive concentrations. This confirmed the theoretical prediction.

To apply (26) to particular metabolizable substances, the constants λ, k, and κ of these substances must of course be known. The blood/air partition coefficients of many substances are close to their water/air partition coefficients (Lazarev, 1938); these have been determined for a number of esters (Filov, 1957a). Filov (1961a) also presented experimentally determined degradation constants (κ) for some esters. The constants for methyl, ethyl, and butyl acetates are given in Table 16.

As for k, information about this constant appears to be scarce and confined to unreactive substances and to those whose reactive capacity is negligibly small (see, e.g., Tolokontsev, 1960c). Values of k for biotransformable compounds are probably unobtainable without recourse to (26). We calculated k values for the three above-mentioned esters from the results of one of our experimental studies (Filov, 1964b). These results are summarized in Table 17.

The data of Table 17, together with those given in Table 16, are quite sufficient to calculate the values of k and, therefore, to be able to follow the process of ester absorption into the blood of each rat. Clearly, these calculations are approximate because we use the water/air rather than the blood/air partition coefficient and, especially, because the values of κ are averages and so

Table 16.   Values of λ and κ for Some Esters

Constant	Ester		
	Methyl Acetate	Ethyl Acetate	Butyl Acetate
λ at 37°C	138	97.4	44.4
κ for blood of white mice (min^{-1})	0.005	0.01	0.06

Table 17.   Time of Falling on One Side and Narcotic Concentrations of Esters in the Blood of Rats Exposed to an Atmosphere of Saturated Ester Vapors

Ester:	Methyl Acetate				Ethyl Acetate				Butyl Acetate			
Saturation concentration at 20° (mg/liter):	690				72.8				14			
Test number:	1	2	3	4	1	2	3	4	1	2	3	4
Time taken by rats to fall on one side (min):	20	15	15	12	20	15	12	12	40	15	20	15
Narcotic concentration in blood (mg %):	72	61	72	102	28	24	27	21	19	22	13	20

are only rough guides to the esterase activity in the blood of individual animals. Indeed, it has been shown that this activity may vary up to about two-fold between individuals of the same species (Filov, 1963b).

Here is the calculation for Test 1 with methyl acetate. In this case $\lambda = 138$, $\kappa = 0.005$ min^{-1}, $C_0 = 690$ mg/liter, $t = 20$ min, and $C = 720$ mg/liter. By substituting these figures into (26), which describes the kinetics of reactive substances in a biological system (in the rat blood in this case), the value of k can be found and the concentration of the ester calculated for any time. Hence we have

$$720 = \frac{k \times 138 \times 690}{k + 0.005} \{1 - \exp[-(k + 0.005) \times 20]\}$$

After several arithmetic operations this can be written as

$$e^{-20k} = 1.097 - 4.16 \times 10^{-5} \times \frac{1}{k}$$

and can be solved by one of the methods available for the approximate solution of such equations. We used the method in which two plots are constructed [for $X = e^{-20k}$ and $X = 1.097 - 4.16 \times 10^{-5} \times (1/k)$] and the value of k is found at the point of intersection of these plots; in this case $k = 0.00037$ min^{-1}. The values of k calculated in this way for all the tests are shown in Table 18.

The example just given illustrates one possible application of (26) for practical purposes.

Table 18.   Rate Constants for the Absorption of Some Esters into the Blood of White Rats

Ester:	Methyl acetate			
Test number:	1	2	3	4
$k(\text{min}^{-1})$:	3.7×10^{-4}	4.3×10^{-4}	5×10^{-4}	9.2×10^{-4}
Average:	5.5×10^{-4}			
Ester:	Ethyl acetate			
Test number:	1	2	3	4
$k(\text{min}^{-1})$:	2.2×10^{-3}	2.4×10^{-3}	3.8×10^{-3}	2.9×10^{-3}
Average:	2.8×10^{-3}			
Ester:	Butyl acetate			
Test number:	1	2	3	4
$k(\text{min}^{-1})$:	2.8×10^{-2}	4.8×10^{-2}	2.2×10^{-2}	4.2×10^{-2}
Average:	3.5×10^{-2}			

3.5.   Absorption of a Known Dose

How will the content of a substance in the blood vary when a known dose of the substance is gradually absorbed and eliminated simultaneously? This question often arises in considering the absorption of a known dose from the gastrointestinal tract or by some other route. Let D be the known dose being absorbed into the blood by an exponential process, which, as already mentioned, is what actually happens in most cases. Elimination from the blood is also supposed to be a first-order process. Designate the constants of these two processes by k and κ, respectively.

In this case, the curve describing the variation in the content of a substance in the blood will obviously be the resultant of the curves for absorption and elimination. Such a curve, together with its two component curves, is shown in Figure 25. Let us now derive a mathematical model for the total process.

Absorption (curve 1) is described by

$$y_1 = D(1 - e^{-kt}) \tag{27}$$

and elimination (curve 2), by (5):

$$y_2 = D \cdot e^{-\kappa t}$$

The find the overall law governing the variation in the blood content of a substance we have to consider infinitesimal variations in the ordinate y

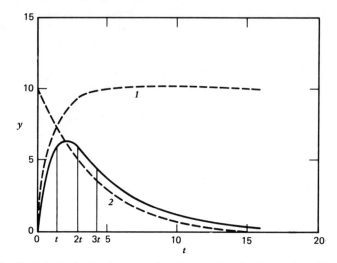

Figure 25. Variation in the blood content of a substance given in a known dose D in the course of its concomitant absorption and excretion by a first-order process. The graph has been plotted for $D = 10, k = 1$, and $\kappa = 0.25$. See text for explanation.

caused by absorption and elimination in an infinitesimal time interval. In other words, we have to differentiate (27) and (5) and to add up the derivatives:

$$y_1: \qquad \frac{dy_1}{dt} = Dke^{-kt}$$

and

$$y_2: \qquad \frac{dy_2}{dt} = -D\kappa e^{-\kappa t} = -\kappa y_2$$

The derivative of the resultant function y

$$\frac{dy}{dt} = \frac{dy_1}{dt} + \frac{dy_2}{dt} = Dke^{-kt} - \kappa y_2 \qquad (28)$$

Since absorption and elimination occur simultaneously, their separation, as above, is artificial. Actually there is a single process y which coincides with y_1 and y_2 when dt is infinitesimal. This allows one to simplify (28):

$$\frac{dy}{dt} = Dke^{-kt} - \kappa y \qquad (29)$$

The integral of (29) will be the required function, $y = f(t)$. We now proceed to solve (29) by the method of variation of constants, as described by Dost (1953). Suppose that its solution exists in the form

$$y = C_1 e^{-\kappa t} + C_2 e^{-kt} \tag{30}$$

which will be valid if C_1 and C_2 are so defined as to satisfy condition (29). Accordingly, we differentiate (30):

$$\frac{dy}{dt} = -C_1 \kappa e^{-\kappa t} - C_2 k e^{-kt} \tag{31}$$

and substitute (31) and (30) into (29):

$$-C_1 \kappa e^{-\kappa t} - C_2 k e^{-kt} = Dk e^{-kt} - C_1 \kappa e^{-\kappa t} - C_2 \kappa e^{-kt}$$

or

$$(Dk + C_2 k - C_2 \kappa)e^{-kt} = 0$$

For finite t's the exponential function is not equal to 0; therefore

$$Dk + C_2 k - C_2 \kappa = 0$$

whence

$$C_2 = \frac{Dk}{\kappa - k}$$

Substituting this value of C_2 into (30), we have

$$y = C_1 e^{-\kappa t} + \frac{Dk}{\kappa - k} e^{-kt}$$

whence the value of C_1 can be found from the obvious initial condition that $y = 0$ when $t = 0$:

$$C_1 = -\frac{Dk}{\kappa - k}$$

The final form of the function describing the behavior of a substance in a one-compartment biological system into which a known dose D of that substance is absorbed exponentially and then eliminated, also by an exponential process, is

$$y = \frac{Dk}{\kappa - k}(e^{-kt} - e^{-\kappa t}) \tag{32}$$

This model is the mathematical form of the resultant curve, shown in Figure 25. It can be seen from this curve that the content of the substance in the blood attains its maximum value at a time t_{max}. The determination of this time may be of interest, in particular, from a purely practical point of view. It is not difficult to find t_{max} from (32) if we recall that the derivative of a function at an extremum (at the maximum in our case) is zero. Accordingly, we differentiate and equate the derivative to zero:

$$\frac{dy}{dt} = -\frac{Dk^2}{\kappa - k} e^{-kt} + \frac{Dk\kappa}{\kappa - k} e^{-\kappa t} = 0$$

whence

$$ke^{-kt} = \kappa e^{-\kappa t} \qquad \text{at } t = t_{max}$$

Now, by simple mathematical transformations, primarily by taking logarithms to base e, we come to the expression for t_{max}:

$$t_{max} = \frac{1}{k - \kappa} \ln\left(\frac{k}{\kappa}\right) \tag{33}$$

Substituting the value of t_{max} into (32), we find y_{max}, or the magnitude of the highest rise in the blood content of the substance. This operation of substituting (33) into (32) likewise requires some simple transformations which we omit. The result is

$$y_{max} = D\left(\frac{k}{\kappa}\right)^{\kappa/(\kappa - k)}$$

Examples showing that the concentration of a substance in the blood obeys (32) are common in pharmacological literature, where the description of the kinetic behavior of a known dose of a drug is of prime concern. In toxicology the above relationship is primarily encountered in experimental studies where a known amount of poison is introduced into the stomachs of animals. Results of one such study are presented in Figure 26, which shows that cyclohexylamine, administered into the stomach of a rabbit, rapidly appears in the blood, where it attains considerable concentration concurrently with its accumulation in the urine; subsequently the blood is seen to be cleared of the poison, whose urinary concentration continues to rise steadily; the blood concentration of the amine varies in accordance with (32).

Methods for calculating the constants k and κ from (32) are discussed in Section 5.1.

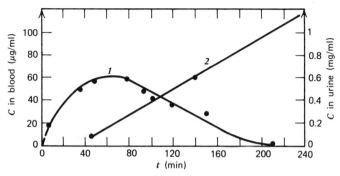

Figure 26.   Results of an experiment with cyclohexylamine ingestion by a rabbit and subsequent determination of the poison in the blood (*1*) and the urine (*2*). (From Filov, 1968.)

3.6.   Penetration from Blood Plasma into Other Tissues

Let us consider a specific case where a substance penetrates from blood plasma into cerebrospinal fluid (CSF) (Mayer et al., 1959). Here the substance must pass across the blood-brain barrier, or a certain lipoprotein membrane, before it can enter the CSF. It will then accumulate in the CSF phase until a steady state is reached. Let C_{pl} be the concentration of substance in plasma dialysate (for simplicity, C_{pl} is supposed to be constant) and C_{CSF} its concentration in the CSF.

If the absorption is by a process of diffusion, that is, obeys first-order kinetics, we may write the differential equation as

$$\frac{d(C_{pl} - C_{CSF})}{dt} = -k(C_{pl} - C_{CSF}) \tag{34}$$

where k is a permeability constant that is a measure of the rate at which the substance enters the CSF and that depends entirely on the properties of the substance and of the membrane.

After transformations, this equation can be solved for k:

$$k = -\frac{1}{t} \ln\left(\frac{C_{pl} - C_{CSF}}{C_{pl}}\right) \tag{35}$$

It follows from (35) that a plot of $\log(C_{pl} - C_{CSF})/C_{pl}$ against time should be a straight line.

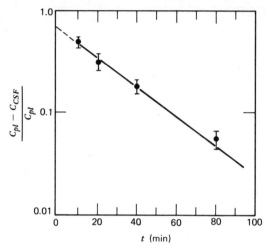

Figure 27. The penetration of acetanilide into cerebrospinal fluid. See text for details. (After Mayer et al., 1959.)

Mayer and co-workers tested a number of drugs and found a linear relationship to hold in all cases. Figure 27 shows the plot obtained for acetanilide (N-acetylaniline); straight lines had of course different slopes for different substances.

The linearity of the plots proves that absorption from plasma into CSF is indeed first order, that is, occurs by a process of diffusion. The values of k calculated from experimental data are sufficient for describing the kinetics of this process.

4. ELIMINATION

In Section 3.1 we presented mathematical models for the elimination (or, rather, disappearance) of substance from the body, based on the assumption that this process is first order and occurs by some one route. Here we will discuss models for more complex cases, giving a more accurate description of what actually happens, for example, when elimination is by more than one route, or when the living organism cannot be regarded as a one-compartment system. But first let us consider a rather common case of exponential elimination by urinary excretion, that is, by only one route, a process described by (5), discussed on p. 113. We will thus continue our consideration of the simplest and also the most important method of elimination.

4.1.   Elimination in the Urine

Suppose that a foreign substance has been absorbed into the body in a total amount D_0 and is being excreted in the urine in accordance with (5). Then, at every instant of time, D_0 may be considered as comprising the amount of substance still present in the body (D) plus the amount already excreted in the urine (E): $D_0 = D + E$ and $E = D_0 - D$. But, according to (5), $D = D_0 e^{-\kappa t}$, or

$$E = D_0(1 - e^{-\kappa t}) \tag{36}$$

The accrual of excreted substance in the urine is thus an exponential process.* A graphic representation of the decline in the amount of substance in the body and its accrual in the urine will, as might be expected, give symmetrical curves similar to those shown in Figures 17 and 18. The sum of D and E will always be equal to D_0.

The velocity of urinary excretion (V) can be found in the ordinary way, by differentiating (36):

$$V = \frac{dE}{dt} = D_0 \cdot \kappa \cdot e^{-\kappa t} \tag{37}$$

Alternatively, V could be obtained from (5); the expression for V would then differ from (37) only by the minus sign, indicating the loss of substance from the body, in contrast to (37), which indicates its accrual in the urine. As can be seen from (37), the excretion velocity shows an exponential decrease with time. The maximum velocity is the initial one, V_0, corresponding to zero time:

$$V_0 = D_0 \kappa \tag{38}$$

Accordingly, (37) can be rewritten as

$$V = V_0 \cdot e^{-\kappa t} \tag{39}$$

The total amount of substance excreted in urine (E_∞) can be found by integrating (39)† from zero to infinity:

$$E_\infty = V_0 \int_0^\infty e^{-\kappa t}\, dt = -\left.\frac{V_0}{\kappa}\right|_0^\infty e^{-\kappa t} = \frac{V_0}{\kappa} \tag{40}$$

---

* Without taking account of the increase in urine volume.
† Indeed, since $dE = V\, dt$, as can be seen from (37).

Equations 38 and 40 are identical, that is, $E_\infty = D_0$, as could have been inferred a priori, since it was stipulated that the substance is to be eliminated by urinary excretion only.

In this way it is possible to calculate the amount of substance excreted in the urine in any time interval, say from t_1 till t_2 :

$$B_{1,2} = \int_{t_1}^{t_2} V\, dt = V_0 \int_{t_1}^{t_2} e^{-\kappa t}\, dt = -\frac{V_0}{\kappa}\bigg|_{t_1}^{t_2} e^{-\kappa t} = \frac{V_0}{\kappa}(e^{-\kappa t_1} - e^{-\kappa t_2}) \quad (41)$$

The above calculations are of interest per se. The mathematical procedures used are simple, even elementary, while the results, expressed by (36) to (41), are evidently of practical utility. One should only bear in mind the ideality of the situation just considered, that is, the assumptions that the elimination is by one route, that there is no metabolism, and so on.

4.2.   Elimination by Two or More Independent Routes

It often happens that a foreign substance is cleared from the body by several independent routes, being eliminated in the urine, in the expired air, by way of metabolism, and so on. Here we will consider the simplest, but fairly common, case of elimination by two independent routes, which can then be generalized to include three or more such routes.

If A is the amount of a substance in the body and B and E are the amounts eliminated by the two routes at rates κ_1 and κ_2, respectively, the process may be represented schematically as follows

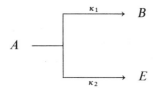

The differential equation for elimination includes two parameters:

$$-\frac{dA}{dt} = \kappa_1 A + \kappa_2 A = (\kappa_1 + \kappa_2)A \quad (42)$$

Integration and other operations already performed in deriving (40) lead to

$$A = A_0 \cdot e^{-(\kappa_1 + \kappa_2)t} \quad (43)$$

where A_0 is the initial content of substance in the body.

Model 43 is the same as model 5* except that the elimination rate constant κ is the sum of the elimination rate constants by two independent routes $(\kappa_1 + \kappa_2)$.

The velocity of elimination (V) by each route depends on the respective elimination rate constant and the amount of substance in the body. Thus, for route B, $V_B = \kappa_1 A$. Substituting the value for A from (43), we have

$$V_B = \kappa_1 \cdot A_0 \cdot e^{-(\kappa_1 + \kappa_2)t} \tag{44}$$

The initial elimination velocity V_0 can be obtained from (44) on condition that $t = 0$:

$$V_{0,B} = \kappa_1 \cdot A_0 \tag{45}$$

Therefore (44) can be written as

$$V_B = V_{0,B} \cdot e^{-(\kappa_1 + \kappa_2)t}$$

Integrating the latter equation from zero to infinity will allow us to find the total amount of substance eliminated by route B [all the operations will be similar to those used in deriving (40)]:

$$B_\infty = \frac{V_{0,E}}{\kappa_1 + \kappa_2}$$

Accordingly, for route E,

$$E_\infty = \frac{V_{0,E}}{\kappa_1 + \kappa_2}$$

Dividing one of the two last expressions by the other and taking cognizance of (44) and (45) for route B and of the analogous equations for route E, we get important proportions:

$$\frac{B_\infty}{E_\infty} = \frac{V_{0,B}}{V_{0,E}} = \frac{V_B}{V_E} = \frac{\kappa_1}{\kappa_2} \tag{46}$$

Therefore the amounts of a substance eliminated by the different routes are proportional to the velocities of elimination by the respective routes and to the respective elimination constants.

---

* Or as (4) if A (amount) is replaced by C (concentration).

4.3. Complex Elimination

So far we have been concerned with the elimination of substance from a living organism that can be regarded as a one-compartment system. In such situations the process of elimination can be described by a simple exponential equation which gives a straight line when plotted in semilogarithmic coordinates (see Section 3.1). In some cases such a line is well fitted by experimental data, thus indicating that the simple exponential model adequately describes the elimination process under study. Such close fits are, however, rare, occurring mostly in studies concerned with the clearance of an individual tissue, as exemplified in Figure 19. As regards the organism as a whole, a simple exponential expression is usually inadequate, especially when the experimental information is extensive and accurate. Then the data points cannot be fitted to a straight line, even approximately, on semilogarithmic scales. However, in many cases it is found possible to draw through the points not one but two or more straight lines. The resultant elimination curve is then a composite of two or more curves, each describing elimination as a first-order process.

Figure 28 shows, in semilogarithmic coordinates, experimental data on the elimination of carbon disulfide from the subcutaneous fat of rats after a long-term exposure to vapors of that compound. It can be seen from the figure that the two straight lines fit the experimental points rather well. Each of the lines is an individual exponential, and their sum gives a complex elimination curve. The experimental data presented are sufficient for the determination of the numerical characteristics of the exponentials. The y intercept obtained by extrapolating each line will give the log C_0 and, hence, the value of C_0. In our example $C_{0,1} = 8.66$ and $C_{0,2} = 0.052$. Next, we have to find the elimination rate constants κ_1 and κ_2. The simplest way to do this is to determine the elimination half-life T and to calculate κ from (7). The half-life T can be readily found graphically, as shown, for example, in Figure 19. In our case $T_1 = 1.5$ hr and $T_2 = 19.75$ hr. Accordingly, $\kappa_1 = 0.46$ hr^{-1} and $\kappa_2 = 0.035$ hr^{-1}. Therefore the full equation for the elimination of carbon disulfide from rat subcutaneous fat is

$$C = C_{0,1}e^{-\kappa_1 t} + C_{0,2}e^{-\kappa_2 t} = 8.66e^{-0.46t} + 0.052e^{-0.035t} \quad (47)$$

This equation suggests that carbon disulfide occurs in two different states in the subcutaneous fat as far as the degree of its binding is concerned: a more labile and a less labile. The less labile carbon disulfide is eliminated over a longer period of time.

An example of a three-exponential curve is the curve for the elimination of diethyl ether in expired air in human beings (Onchi and Asao, 1961). This experimental curve is shown in Figure 29. Using the procedure described

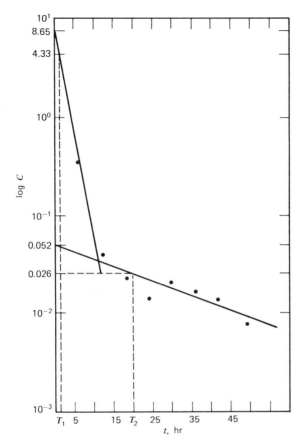

Figure 28. Decline of carbon disulfide concentration in the subcutaneous fat of rats. $T_1 = 1.5\,\text{hr}$; $T_2 = 19.8\,\text{hr}$. (After Mironos, 1970.)

above, it is possible to resolve the curve, in semilogarithmic coordinates, into three straight lines and to calculate the numberical value of each elimination parameter. The overall equation for ether elimination is

$$C = 3.47e^{-0.326t} + 1.61e^{-0.075t} + 1.13e^{-0.005t} \tag{48}$$

Bolanowska et al. (1967) presented equations for the elimination of lead from various tissues in rats. In particular, the fall in the blood level of lead was described by the equation

$$C = 18e^{-0.8t} + 4e^{-0.037t} + 1.1e^{-0.0067t} + 0.16e^{-0.0006t} \tag{49}$$

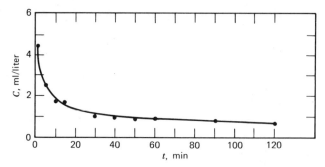

Figure 29.   Elimination of ether in expired air in human beings. (From Onchi and Asao, 1961.)

These and similar equations emphasize the multiphasic nature of the bio-logical objects from which the substances under study undergo elimination. The word "multiphasic" should be understood not only literally, that is, to mean, for instance, distinct tissues with sharply different physicochemical properties, but also in the sense that a given substance may be bound to differing degrees to different components of one and the same tissue. One example of such interpretation is provided by (47) for the biexponential elimination of carbon disulfide from subcutaneous fat. As regards the four-exponential Equation 49, it describes, according to Bolanowska et al., the disposal of lead from such tissues as blood, muscle, skin, and bone, in the decreasing order of disposal rate.

It would seem appropriate to point out here some of the errors to be avoided, or rather allowed for, when constructing empirical equations of experimental curves and interpreting such equations. Thus, although the two exponentials in Figure 28 are rather different from each other (such big differences always facilitate the task), the flatter line could well have been drawn flatter or, on the contrary, steeper. The implications of this are all the greater because every data point obtained from experiments of this kind is itself subject to considerable error, due not so much to assay and sampling errors as to the biological variability of the test material.

A certain degree of arbitrariness is shown in constructing exponential straight lines in the following cases: when the number of data points is small or when these points are widely scattered,* when the exponentials making up the elimination curve have similar slopes, and when the transition zones near the junction of straight lines are so large as to blur the straight-line pattern.

---

* Errors in this case stem from the considerable errors involved in the points themselves and so cannot be disposed of by resorting to special methods such as a least squares fit.

For this reason it seems hardly justified to calculate the numerical values of the parameters in such great detail as, for instance, in (48). It would have been sufficient to have given only one digit after the decimal point for the coefficients and one or two significant figures for the elimination constants.

In certain cases only the qualitative result may be shown. Thus one may merely state that the elimination curve is three-exponential; such a statement may be sufficient and at the same time quite reliable. On the other hand, a seemingly precise description of exponentials may be based on very unreliable data.

In Sections 4.1, 4.2, and 4.3 situations were discussed where a steady state of diffusion of the substance between all body parts was presumed to have been attained by the beginning of elimination (or, at any rate, by the time when consideration of the elimination process was started). This condition is fulfilled in practice in a number of situations, but mainly in the case in which the study of elimination is started when absorption has been in progress long enough for a steady state to be reached and in the case of substances which are rapidly and homogeneously distributed in their characteristic distribution volumes without being selectively absorbed into particular organs or tissues (nondepositing substances). In the section which follows account is taken of substance distribution as well.

4.4. Elimination of a Substance Undergoing Distribution in the Body

Consider the following system. A substance present in a compartment A is eliminated into a compartment E by an exponential process with a rate constant κ and is simultaneously absorbed into a compartment B, whence it can again pass into A. The rate constants for absorption into and elimination from B are k_1 and k_2, respectively, while the processes themselves occur at velocities proportional to the concentrations of the substance. A graphic model for this system is fairly simple:

$$A \underset{k_2}{\overset{k_1}{\rightleftarrows}} B$$

$$\kappa \downarrow$$

$$E$$

Physically, this model in the most common case includes the blood (A), the urine (E), and the organ or tissue (B) where the substance accumulates. There may be several B compartments [k being different for different compartments (r)], but here only one will be considered for simplicity.

If A, B, and E are understood to mean the concentrations of the substance in the respective compartments of the model, a system of differential equations can be written describing the behavior of the substance in the model in accordance with first-order kinetics:

$$
\left.
\begin{aligned}
\frac{dA}{dt} &= -(k_1 + \kappa)A + k_2 B \\[2mm]
\frac{dB}{dt} &= -k_1 A - k_2 B \\[2mm]
\frac{dE}{dt} &= \kappa A
\end{aligned}
\right\}
\tag{50}
$$

To find the integral forms of the equations describing the variation of substance content in the different compartments of the model, we have to solve system 50. First we differentiate the first equation:

$$
\frac{d^2 A}{dt^2} = -(k_1 + \kappa)\frac{dA}{dt} + \frac{dB}{dt}
$$

Substituting the value for dB/dt into this equation from the second equation of (50) and transferring everything to the left-hand side, we get

$$
\frac{d^2 A}{dt^2} + (k_1 + \kappa)\frac{dA}{dt} - k_1 k_2 A + k_2^2 B = 0
$$

Substituting into this equation the value for $k_2 B$ from the first equation of (50), we have

$$
\frac{d^2 A}{dt^2} + (k_1 + k_2 + \kappa)\frac{dA}{dt} + k_2 \kappa A = 0
$$

or

$$
\frac{d^2 A}{dt^2} + \alpha\frac{dA}{dt} + \beta A = 0
$$

where $\alpha = k_1 + k_2 + \kappa$ and $\beta = k_2 \kappa$.

In its general form the integral of this equation is

$$
A = c_1 e^{r_1 t} + c_2 e^{r_2 t}
\tag{51}
$$

where c_1 and c_2 are the constants of integration, and

$$
r_{1,2} = \frac{-\alpha \pm \sqrt{(\alpha^2 - 4\beta)}}{2}
\tag{52}
$$

The next step is to find the values of c_1 and c_2. To do this we substitute A from (51) into the first equation of system 50:

$$r_1 c_1 e^{r_1 t} + r_2 c_2 e^{r_2 t} = -(k_1 + \kappa)(c_1 e^{r_1 t} + c_2 e^{r_2 t}) + k_2 B$$

Multiplying, rearranging terms, and expressing in respect to B, we get

$$B = \frac{r_1 + k_1 + \kappa}{k_2} c_1 e^{r_1 t} + \frac{r_2 + k_1 + \kappa}{k_2} c_2 e^{r_2 t} \tag{53}$$

Now we have to set the initial conditions on which the concrete values of c_1 and c_2 will depend. Let us take the simplest case, in which the substance is instantaneously introduced into A. Then $A = A_0$ and $B = 0$ at $t = 0$. Substituting these conditions into (51) and (53), we have

$$A_0 = c_1 + c_2$$

and

$$\frac{r_1 + k_1 + \kappa}{k_2} c_1 + \frac{r_2 + k_1 + \kappa}{k_2} c_2 = 0$$

By simple substitution we now calculate the values of c_1 and c_2 from the above equations:

$$c_1 = -\frac{r_2 + k_1 + \kappa}{r_1 - r_2} A_0$$

$$c_2 = \frac{r_1 + k_1 + \kappa}{r_1 - r_2} A_0 \tag{54}$$

Thus we have obtained relationships describing variations in concentration in the A and B compartments, respectively. In the former case the relationship is (51) after the substitution of (52) and (54), and in the latter case it is (53) with the same substitutions.

The third equation in system 50 describes the elimination velocity V_E. Substituting the value for A from (51) into this equation, we get an equation for elimination velocity:

$$\frac{dE}{dt} V_E = \kappa c_1 e^{r_1 t} + \kappa c_2 e^{r_2 t} \tag{55}$$

It can be seen from (55) that elimination is described in this case by a curve which is the sum of two exponentials. If we considered a more heterogeneous system consisting of several differing B compartments, (55) would be more complex. In the case of two B compartments, for example, it would be three-exponential.

Here is a numerical example taken from Piotrowski (1963). Suppose that we are concerned with the elimination by urinary excretion of a substance which tends to be absorbed into some one organ or tissue. Let $A_0 = 1000$ mg (the amount introduced into the blood). The excretory process will be governed by the rate constants of its individual phases: k_1, k_2, and κ. Let these constants be equal to 0.2 day^{-1}, 0.02 day^{-1}, and 0.1 day^{-1}, respectively. We calculate the values of the constants from (52) and (54) and substitute them into (55): the calculation gives $r_1 = -0.313$, $r_2 = -0.0064$, $c_1 = 958$, and $c_2 = 42$, and the equation for urinary excretion velocity is as follows:

$$V_E = 95.8 \times e^{-0.313t} + 4.2 \times e^{-0.0064t} \text{ mg/day}$$

On semilogarithmic scales a plot of this equation will be a broken line consisting of two straight lines (as a first approximation), similar to the one shown in Figure 28. Another concrete example illustrating the use of this model concerned nitrobenzene (Piotrowski, 1966).

The situation considered above is a particular case of a much more general situation where a substance is absorbed over a period of time, rather than being instantaneously introduced into the blood. A graphic model for this situation is as follows:

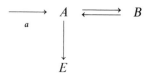

where a is the law governing the absorption of substance into the blood from the environment or from the gastrointestinal tract. Analysis of this general situation is more complex than the one presented above, although the steps are the same. Piotrowski (1965) made such an analysis for the case of continuous absorption of substance from inspired air. For this purpose he solved system 50, in which the first equation was modified. This modified equation includes the rate constant for absorption into compartment A and has the form

$$\frac{dA}{dt} = a - (k_1 + \kappa)A + k_2 B$$

4.5.   Elimination of Metabolite

Let us consider the simplest case, in which a substance A is metabolized and a metabolite M is eliminated from the body by one route, for example, in the urine (E). Here, as in most other cases, both metabolism and elimination obey first-order kinetics. The model for our system is $A \overset{k}{\to} M \overset{\kappa}{\to} E$, where k

and κ are the rate constants for metabolism and metabolite excretion, respectively.

In this case there are two consecutive processes. The first of them is governed by relationship 5. The rate of the second process is the sum of the rates of metabolite loss and metabolite formation from the precursor A. The entire model is describable by the following system of equations:

$$-\frac{dA}{dt} = kA$$
$$\frac{dM}{dt} = kA - \kappa M$$
$$(56)$$

The first step in solving this system is the substitution of the integral form of the first equation (5) into the second equation:

$$\frac{dM}{dt} = kA_0 e^{-kt} - \kappa M$$

or

$$\frac{dM}{dt} + \kappa M = kA_0 e^{-kt}$$

Integration of this differential equation (the details of integration are omitted) gives $M = k/(\kappa - k)A_0 e^{-kt} + ce^{-\kappa t}$, where c is the constant of integration. As usual, c is found from the initial conditions, which, in this case, are taken to be that the metabolite was initially ($t = 0$) absent from the system ($M = 0$). Then $c = k/(\kappa - k)A_0$.

The final form of the mathematical model for metabolite excretion is

$$M = \frac{kA_0}{\kappa - k}(e^{-kt} - e^{-\kappa t}) \qquad (57)$$

Evidently the amount of metabolite excreted into the urine (E) at each instant of time will be $E = A_0 - (A + M)$, account being taken, of course, of the stoichiometry of metabolism. Figure 30 (Piotrowski, 1963) shows plots of variation in A, M, and E for $A_0 = 1000$ mg, $k = 0.7$ hr^{-1}, and $\kappa = 0.1$ hr^{-1}. The rate of metabolite excretion is, as always, the derivative of the amount of metabolite in the urine with respect to time and is proportional to M: $V_E = dE/dt = \kappa M$. Substituting the value for M from (57), we have

$$V_E = \frac{k\kappa}{\kappa - k} A_0(e^{-kt} - e^{-\kappa t}) \qquad (58)$$

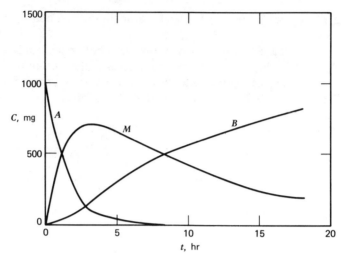

Figure 30.   Curves describing the concentrations of a substance (A) and its metabolite (M) in the blood and the excretion of the metabolite in the urine (E). (After Piotrowski, 1963.)

As can be inferred from (58) and Figure 30, the process of metabolite excretion is characterized by, in addition to the elimination constant κ, a certain instant of time when the elimination velocity is maximal. This time (t_{max}) can be found in the ordinary way, by equating to zero the derivative of a function, in this case the time derivative of velocity:

$$\frac{dV_E}{dt} = \frac{k\kappa}{\kappa - k} A_0(\kappa e^{\kappa t_{max}} - ke^{-kt_{max}}) = 0$$

The latter equation is fulfilled only if the expression in parentheses vanishes, or $\kappa e^{-\kappa t_{max}} = ke^{-kt_{max}}$. Hence, after taking the logarithm, we have

$$t_{max} = \frac{2.3}{\kappa - k} \log\left(\frac{\kappa}{k}\right) \tag{59}$$

In the example given above and shown in Figure 30 $t_{max} = 3.2$ hr.

Substitution of the value for t_{max} into (57) will give the value of M_{max}. Such substitution involves a number of simple algebraic operations which are omitted here. As the result we can arrive at the expression

$$M_{max} = A_0\left(\frac{\kappa}{k}\right)^{\kappa/(k-\kappa)} \tag{60}$$

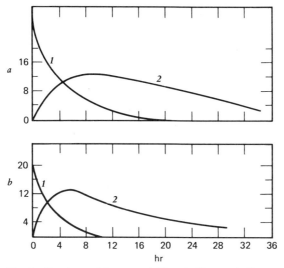

Figure 31. Blood levels of unchanged 2-propanol (*1*) and of its metabolite acetone (*2*) following the administration of 2-propanol to dogs (*a*) (*n* = 5) and rats (*b*) (*n* = 6). (After Abshagen and Rietbrock, 1969.)

It would seem interesting to consider the particular cases of (58) in which $k \gg \kappa$ and $\kappa \gg k$ in order to determine the parameters affecting the elimination process when one rate constant is much greater than the other. We leave this opportunity to those who are interested in such analysis.

A good example of all the relationships given above is provided by Abshagen and Rietbrock (1969) in a study on dogs and rats administered 2-propanol, which is completely converted to acetone, the latter being eliminated. The results are shown in Figure 31. The values of A_0, t_{max}, and M_{max} can be determined graphically. Formulas 57 to 60 enable one to calculate the values of k and κ. These values are given in Table 19.

Table 19.   Values of Kinetic Parameters in Experiments with 2-Propanol

Test Objects	A_0 (mM/liter)	t_{max} (hr)	M_{max} (mM/liter)	k (hr^{-1})	κ (hr^{-1})
Dogs	23.4	9.15	11.6	0.18	0.06
Rats	22.3	5.02	12.7	0.40	0.08

Source. Abshagen and Rietbrock (1969).

A rather common case is the elimination of unchanged substance along with its metabolite. If the elimination of both occurs by the same route, say by urinary excretion, the model of this system may be represented as follows:

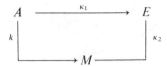

where κ_1 and κ_2 are the rate constants for the excretion of unchanged substance and metabolite, respectively. The system of differential equations for this model is

$$-\frac{dA}{dt} = (k + \kappa_1)A$$

$$\frac{dM}{dt} = kA - \kappa_2 M$$

(61)

This system does not appear to be much more complex than (56), and its solution involves the same operations. The result, however, will be more complex, for it will reflect a more complicated case.

There are also other problems whose solutions may be of importance for various practical situations but would considerably enlarge the size of this chapter. Thus we have not discussed the case of consecutive transformations of a substance to several metabolites with their subsequent elimination, or the case of parallel conversions of the precursor to various metabolites with different fates, or such cases as the elimination of unchanged substance and of its metabolites by different routes. The principles underlying the solutions of all such problems will, however, remain the same as in the situations described above. In conclusion, mention may be made of two studies concerned with problems of this kind. Dominguez (1950) considered the formal kinetics of elimination of both metabolizable and inert substances not only during the steady state of distribution but also before such a state. Wagner and Nelson (1964) considered a number of kinetic problems involving zero-order processes of substance movement through a biological system.

4.6. General Considerations Concerning the Formation and Elimination of Metabolites and the Elimination of the Parent Substance Itself

An extraneous compound is cleared from the body through processes of excretion and metabolism. A metabolite may be excreted, or it may undergo transformation and then be excreted in the form of additional metabolites. Parallel formation of several metabolites may also occur. All this may be represented by consecutive and parallel processes which in most cases obey first-order kinetics (as is assumed to be the case here). The following theoretical account of the fate of a certain foreign substance A in the body is taken from the paper by Cummings et al. (1967). We begin our consideration with the instant of time ($t = 0$) when A has reached a steady state in all compartments of its distribution in the body.

The substance A is considered to undergo elimination by being excreted unchanged with the rate constant κ and by the simultaneous formation of metabolites M_1, M_2, ... with the rate constants k_1, k_2, ..., respectively. The overall rate constant for the disappearance of A from the body is K:

$$K = \kappa + k_1 + k_2 + \cdots \tag{62}$$

The metabolites are assumed to undergo no further transformation and to be instantaneously equilibrated within the compartments of their distribution. Their elimination rate constants are $\kappa_1, \kappa_2, \ldots$. This may be represented schematically as follows:

$$
\begin{array}{llll}
 & \xrightarrow{k_1} M_1 & \xrightarrow{\kappa_1} & B_1 \\
 & \xrightarrow{k_2} M_2 & \xrightarrow{\kappa_2} & B_2 \\
A \xrightarrow{\kappa} & \xrightarrow{k_i} M_3 & \xrightarrow{\kappa_i} & B_i \\
 & \xrightarrow{\kappa} & & A_B
\end{array}
$$

This system may be characterized by a set of equations which are given here without derivation, since all the necessary steps have been presented in the preceding sections. Our consideration concerns only one metabolite, but it may be extended to cover any number of metabolites by substituting the appropriate rate constants. In these equations A_0 is the amount of the substance in the body at zero time, A_t is its amount in the body at time t, A_B is its amount excreted unchanged to time t, M is the amount of metabolite formed to time t, M_t is the amount of metabolite in the body at time t, and B is the amount of metabolite excreted to time t. Then,

$$A_0 = A_t + A_B + M \quad \text{and} \quad M = M_t + B$$

Since $dA_t/dt = -KA_t$,

$$A_t = A_0 e^{-Kt} \tag{63}$$

Also, since $dA_B/dt = \kappa A_t = \kappa A_0 e^{-Kt}$, we have

$$A_B = \frac{\kappa A_0}{K}(1 - e^{-Kt}) \tag{64}$$

Similarly, since $dM/dt = kA_0^{-Kt}$, we get

$$M = \frac{kA_0}{K}(1 - e^{-Kt}) \tag{65}$$

The rate of change in the amount of the metabolite in the body is equal to its rate of formation minus its rate of excretion, so that

$$\frac{dM_t}{dt} = kA_0 e^{-Kt} - \kappa_1 M_t$$

Integrating this equation with the condition that, at $t = 0$, $M_t = 0$, we get

$$M_t = \frac{kA_0}{\kappa_1 - K}(e^{-Kt} - e^{-\kappa_1 t}) \tag{66}$$

Then

$$\frac{dB}{dt} = \kappa_1 M_t = \frac{k\kappa_1 A_0}{\kappa_1 - K}(e^{-Kt} - e^{-\kappa_1 t})$$

Hence

$$B = \frac{kA_0}{K(\kappa_1 - K)}\left[\kappa_1(1 - e^{-Kt}) - K(1 - e^{-\kappa_1 t})\right] \tag{67}$$

Equations 63 to 67 fully describe the kinetics of the appearance of metabolites in the body, as well as the kinetics of the disappearance of both the substance and its metabolites from the body.

Metabolite Kinetics

Let us discuss in more detail the kinetics of metabolite formation and behavior in the body. Under the conditions specified, the metabolite is absent from the body at $t = 0$, but, as can be seen from (65), it is formed in increasing amounts to approach asymptotically a value of $(k/K)A_0$. The amount of metabolite in the body, however, depends not only on its formation but also on its excretion; the main parameter of the latter process is the constant κ_1. The overall kinetics of metabolite in the body is described by (66).

The rate of change in the amount of metabolite in the body can be obtained by subtracting the rate of metabolite excretion from the rate of metabolite formation or by differentiating (66):

$$\frac{dM_t}{dt} = \frac{dM}{dt} - \frac{dB}{dt} = \frac{kA_0}{\kappa_1 - K}(\kappa_1 e^{-\kappa_1 t} - Ke^{-Kt}) \tag{68}$$

This equation shows that the amount of metabolite in the body will increase while $dM/dt > dB/dt$, will reach its maximum value when $dM/dt = dB/dt$, and will decrease when $dM/dt < dB/dt$. Of particular interest is the maximum value of M_t, attained when $dM_t/dt = 0$. The latter condition is fulfilled when the quantity in the parentheses in (68) vanishes. Then the time when the maximum amount of metabolite is achieved will be

$$t_{max} = \frac{1}{\kappa_1 - K} \ln\left(\frac{\kappa_1}{K}\right) \tag{69}$$

The value of $M_{t,max}$ can be obtained by inserting (69) into (66):

$$M_{t,max} = \frac{kA_0}{\kappa_1 - K}\left[\left(\frac{K}{\kappa_1}\right)^{K/(\kappa_1 - K)} - \left(\frac{K}{\kappa_1}\right)^{\kappa_1/(\kappa_1 - K)}\right] \tag{70}$$

Table 20 shows the values of $M_{t,max}$ and t_{max}, calculated from (69) and (70) as a function of κ_1 at fixed K and k, which makes it possible to estimate the effect of κ_1 on the amount of metabolite attained in the body and the time of its attainment. It can be seen from the table that, when κ_1 is small, there is considerable accrual of the metabolite in the body. When κ_1 is large, accrual of the metabolite still occurs, but to a small extent.

Table 20. Relationship between the Rate Constant for Metabolite Excretion, $M_{t_{max}}$, and t_{max} at $K = 0.3$ Hr^{-1}, $k = 0.1$ Hr^{-1}, and $A_0 = 1$

κ_1 (hr^{-1})	$M_{t_{max}}/A_0$	t_{max} (hr)	t_{max}/T
0	0.33	∞	∞
0.05	0.23	7.16	3.10
0.10	0.19	5.50	2.38
0.50	0.09	2.55	1.10
1.00	0.06	1.72	0.74
1.50	0.04	1.34	0.58
3.0	0.03	0.85	0.37

Source. Cummings et al. (1967).

The last column of Table 20 shows the ratio of t_{max} to the half-life of the substance in the body ($T = \ln 2/\kappa_1$). This ratio is a function of κ_1/k only, whereas t_{max} depends, in addition, on the absolute values of κ_1 and K, as can be seen from (69). This can be readily shown:

$$\frac{t_{max}}{T} = \frac{\ln(\kappa_1/K) \cdot \kappa_1/K}{\ln 2[(\kappa_1/K) - 1]} \tag{71}$$

Cummings and Martin (1963) advanced theoretical considerations suggesting that the value of κ_1 cannot exceed 3 hr^{-1} and will probably not exceed 1 hr^{-1}. The half-life of most foreign substances does not exceed 7 hr. When $T = 7$ hr, $K = 0.1$ hr^{-1}, so that κ_1/K will not exceed 30, a more probable figure being 10.

Excretion Rate of the Substance and Its Metabolites

Taking logarithms of the differential form of (64), which describes the excretion of unchanged substance, we have

$$\ln\left(\frac{dA_B}{dt}\right) = \ln(\kappa A_0) - Kt \tag{72}$$

This is an equation for the straight line obtained by plotting the log rate of substance excretion against time. The line has an intercept on the $\ln(dA_B/dt)$ axis equal to $\ln(\kappa A_0)$ and has a slope equal to $-K$.

Equations similar in form to (72) may also be obtained for the metabolites, provided that t is sufficiently large. To do this, the differential form of (67) should be considered. When κ_1 is greater than K, the term $e^{-\kappa_1 t}$ can be neglected, and this equation, in its logarithmic form, will reduce to

$$\ln\left(\frac{dB}{dt}\right) = \ln\left(\frac{k\kappa_1 A_0}{\kappa_1 - K}\right) - Kt \tag{73}$$

When $\kappa_1 < K$, then

$$\ln\left(\frac{dB}{dt}\right) = \ln\left(\frac{k\kappa_1 A_0}{K - \kappa_1}\right) - \kappa_1 t \tag{74}$$

The rate of excretion of metabolite, always in parallel with the amount of metabolite in the body, will increase beginning with $t = 0$, to attain a maximum value at a time t_{max}, given by (69). It will thereafter decline, and the decrease of the log rate with time will eventually become linear. A graphic representation of these relationships is given in Figure 32. The linear portions of the curves are described by (73) and (74). The slope of the curve is equal to $-K$ when $\kappa_1 > K$, and to $-\kappa_1$ when $K > \kappa_1$. When κ_1 and K are very different in magnitude, a linear plot will be obtained after a relatively short

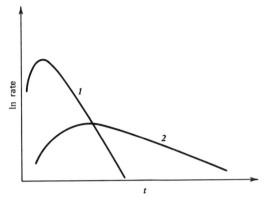

Figure 32. A plot of the log rate of metabolite excretion against time. $K = 0.3$ hr^{-1}; $k = 0.15$ hr^{-1}. 1, $\kappa_1 > K$ ($\kappa_1 = 1$ hr^{-1}); 2, $\kappa_1 < K$ ($\kappa_1 = 0.1$ hr^{-1}). (After Cummings et al., 1967.)

time; when κ_1 and K are nearly equal, the plot will become linear after a long time. When κ_1 is equal to K, (66) and (67) are not usable in the forms given and alternative expressions have to be obtained. For example, the differential form of (67) may be written as

$$\frac{dB}{dt} = \frac{k\kappa_1 A_0}{\kappa_1 - K} e^{-Kt}[1 - e^{(K - \kappa_1)t}]$$

On expansion of $[1 - e^{(K - \kappa_1)t}]$ and division by $-(K - \kappa_1)$ we have

$$\frac{dB}{dt} = k\kappa_1 A_0 e^{-Kt}\left[t + \frac{K - \kappa_1}{21} t^2 + \frac{(K - \kappa_1)^2}{31} t^3 + \cdots\right]$$

which, when $\kappa_1 = K$, reduces to

$$\frac{dB}{dt} = KkA_0 te^{-Kt}$$

Writing the last equation in its logarithmic form, we get

$$\ln\left(\frac{dB}{dt}\right) = \ln(KkA_0) + \ln t - Kt$$

or

$$\ln\left(\frac{1}{t} \cdot \frac{dB}{dt}\right) = \ln(KkA_0) - Kt \tag{75}$$

Therefore, when $\kappa_1 = K$, a plot of $\ln[(1/t)(dB/dt)]$, rather than of $\ln(dB/dt)$, against time should be constructed to obtain a straight line with a slope equal to $-K$. Similarly, (66) and (67) must be replaced by

$$M_t = kA_0 t e^{-Kt} \quad \text{and} \quad B = \frac{kA_0}{K}(1 - e^{-Kt} - Kt e^{-Kt})$$

respectively.

The above procedures for the construction of linear plots make it possible to calculate values of K from experimental data and so are of practical use. This method of data treatment, known as the "rate" method, was introduced by Swintosky (1957). Since then, it has been developed further and has also been applied, as shown above, to the elimination of unchanged substance and its metabolites. In practice, the amounts of substance (ΔA_B) or of metabolite (ΔB) excreted in a series of equal time intervals (Δt) are first determined, the excretion rates dA_B/dt or dB/dt are replaced, as a first approximation, by $\Delta A_B/\Delta t$ or $\Delta B/\Delta t$, and a straight-line plot is obtained by plotting their logarithms against time.

It may happen that a metabolite or an unchanged substance cannot be determined separately; in such cases it is possible to estimate only the overall elimination rate $d(A_B + B)/dt$, which is the sum of the rates of excretion for all metabolites and for the unchanged substance:

$$\frac{d(A_B + B)}{dt} = \frac{dA_B}{dt} + \sum_1^i \frac{dB_i}{dt}$$

$$= A_0\left[\kappa e^{-Kt} + \sum_1^i \frac{k_i \kappa_i}{\kappa_i - K}(e^{-Kt} - e^{-\kappa_i t})\right]$$

Then, provided that all the κ_i are greater than K and that t is large, this equation can be written in a form suitable for the graphical determination of K:

$$\ln\left[\frac{d(A_B + B)}{dt}\right] = \ln\left[A_0\left(\kappa + \sum_1^i \frac{k_i \kappa_i}{\kappa_i - K}\right)\right] - Kt \tag{76}$$

Treatment of Excretion Data by the "Sigma-Minus" Method

An alternative procedure for determining K, which has been used more extensively than the "rate" method, is the "sigma-minus" method, first described by Bray et al. (1951).

When applied to the excretion of unchanged substance, this method consists of plotting $\ln(A_{B_\infty} - A_B)$ against time, where $(A_{B_\infty} - A_B)$ is the difference between the sum (sigma) of the amounts of substance ultimately excreted

$(A_{B\infty})$ and the cumulative amount of substance excreted to a time t. Mathematically, the method is based on (64), which may be rewritten as

$$(A_{B\infty} - A_B) = \frac{\kappa A_0}{K} e^{-Kt}$$

and, in the logarithmic form, as

$$\ln(A_{B\infty} - A_B) = \ln\left(\frac{\kappa A_0}{K}\right) - Kt \qquad (77)$$

Equation 77 is thus identical in form to (72), the straight line having a slope equal to $-K$.

The application of the sigma-minus method to the excretion of metabolites is more complex, but, as in the rate method, equations of the same form as (77) can be derived. If the total amount of excreted metabolite is B_∞, then, since $M = M_t + B$, we have $(B_\infty - B) = B_\infty - M + M_t$; substituting the values for $(B_\infty - M)$ from (65) and (67), we have $(B_\infty - B) = (kA_0/K)e^{-Kt} + M_t$. Substituting now the values for M_t from (66), we get

$$(B_\infty - B) = \frac{kA_0}{K} e^{-Kt} + \frac{kA_0}{\kappa - K}(e^{-Kt} - e^{-\kappa_1 t})$$

When $\kappa_1 > K$ and t is large, the latter equation reduces to

$$(B_\infty - B) = \frac{\kappa_1 kA_0}{K(\kappa_1 - K)} e^{-Kt}$$

or, in the logarithmic form,

$$\ln(B_\infty - B) = \ln\left(\frac{\kappa_1 kA_0}{K(\kappa_1 - K)}\right) - Kt \qquad (78)$$

whence the value of K can be found.

Comparison of (72) and (77) and of (73) and (78) shows that, when t is large, the plots of excretion data which are obtained by the rate method and by the sigma-minus method are described by equations of the same type. The straight lines described by these equations have a slope equal to $-K$, but the intercepts of the "rate" plots differ from those of the "sigma-minus" plots by $\ln K$. These two methods were compared in detail by Martin (1967a), who also (Martin, 1967b) devised a combined method for the determination of excretion rate constants for metabolites.

Determination of the Excretion Rate Constants for Metabolites

The foregoing methods involve the assumption that the substance is absorbed instantaneously and is in a steady state in the body. If the substance is absorbed gradually, the above equations cannot be applied until after the absorption has ceased.

The combined method described below does not involve the assumption of complete absorption, but it is necessary to specify that absorption is relatively rapid and to assume that both the substance and its metabolites rapidly attain equilibrium distribution in the body. Also, the duration of the study must be much longer than the time required for complete absorption.

This "rate versus amount" method (Martin, 1967b) for the determination of κ_1 is based on the construction of a plot of dB/dt (rate) versus M_t (amount) and the determination of κ_1 from its slope. If substance elimination is a first-order process, κ_1 will be given by the slope of the straight line $dB/dt = \kappa_1 M_t$ passing through the origin.

The value of dB/dt can be calculated as in the rate method. To determine M_t, consider the proportion $M/A_B = k/\kappa = B_\infty/A_{B_\infty} = r$ [cf. (46)]. Since $M_t = M - B$, $M_t = rA_B - B$, and M_t can now be calculated for any time from data on the amounts of the substance and its metabolite excreted by that time and the total amounts of them ultimately excreted.

The experimental procedure for calculating κ_1 thus consists of collecting the same data which are required for the rate and the sigma-minus methods (both for the unchanged substance and metabolite) and of constructing a linear plot with a slope equal to κ_1.

4.7. Relationship between the Elimination of a Substance and the Decline of Its Biological Activity; Calculation of the Disappearance Rate Constant

Let us consider the most common case, in which the biological effect is determined by the substance itself rather than by its metabolites (Levy, 1964). In most cases the magnitude of the biological effect (I) is a linear function of the logarithm of the substance content in the body (A). This relationship is described by the following equation, widely used in pharmacology:

$$I = m \log A + i \tag{79}$$

where m and i are constants, m being the slope of the straight line obtained by plotting I against $\log A$, and i usually being negative.

If the body content of the substance decreases in accordance with first-order kinetics, as is usually the case, we have from (5)

$$\log A = \log A_0 - \frac{\kappa}{2.3} t \tag{80}$$

where A is the body content of the substance at time t, and A_0 is the body content at zero time.

Substituting now the value for $\log A$ from (70) into (80), we have

$$\frac{I - i}{m} = \frac{I_0 - i}{m} - \frac{\kappa}{2.3} t$$

which can be reduced to

$$I = I_0 - \frac{\kappa m}{2.3} t \tag{81}$$

Equation 81 is a zero-order equation, which shows that the biological activity declines linearly with time as the substance is eliminated exponentially from the body. Therefore, while the amount of the substance in the body declines exponentially, its biological effect decreases linearly, that is, at a constant rate. This theoretical conclusion, which needs experimental verification, is contrary to the frequently expressed view that the change in biological action with time parallels that of the concentration or content of the substance in the body.

It should be noted that indications of zero-order decrease in activity can be found in pharmacological literature. One example is the exponential decrease in the concentration of tubocurarine (muscle relaxant) in blood plasma and the linear decrease in grip strength observed in an animal experiment (Levy, 1964).

Let us consider now one possible method for the calculation of the disappearance rate constant κ (and, accordingly, the half-life) of a substance by determining the duration of its biological effect. To calculate this constant, a minimal body content of the substance is necessary to elicit a measurable biological effect; also, it is necessary that the substance be absorbed rapidly, for example intravenously (Levy and Nelson, 1965).

Now suppose that a dose D has been administered and that the substance will produce an effect during a time t, which is the time necessary to decrease the initial body content of the substance to d. From (80)

$$\log d = \log D - \frac{\kappa}{2.3} t$$

whence

$$t = \frac{2.3}{\kappa}(\log D - \log d)$$

The value of $(2.3/\kappa)\log d$ is constant; if we denote it by α, then

$$t = \frac{2.3}{\kappa}\log D - \alpha,$$

that is, $\log D$ is linearly related to t.

The value of κ can be calculated from the slope of the straight line obtained by plotting the duration of effect against the logarithm of the dose. By determining the value of α from the same plot, d can be found from the following equation: $\log d = \kappa\alpha/2.3$.

This method for the approximate calculation of κ may be found useful when for some reason it is not possible to determine the content of a substance in the blood or urine.

5. SOME METHODS FOR THE CALCULATION OF RATE CONSTANTS; FACTORS INFLUENCING THE ELIMINATION KINETICS

Sections 3 and 4 were concerned with the simpler or most often used methods for the calculation of kinetic characteristics. Since the most important characteristics are the rate constants for absorption, metabolism, and elimination, as well as the associated half-lives of these processes, here we briefly discuss some other methods for the calculation of these constants.

5.1. Calculation of the Rate Constants for Absorption and Elimination in the Case of Gradual Absorption of a Substance Administered in a Known Dose

The kinetics of substance behavior in this case is describable by the curves of Figure 25 and by (32), given in Section 3.5. In the method for the calculation of k and κ described here, three values of the function, y_1, y_2, and y_3, at times t, $2t$, and $3t$, are taken on the experimental curve $y = f(t)$ (see Figure 25) so that t is smaller than t_{max}. These data are sufficient for a simple calculation, as is shown in the following paragraphs.

First let us write (32) in a shorter form, designating $Dk/(\kappa - k)$ by A, e^{-kt} by x, and $e^{-\kappa t}$ by z; then $y_1 = A(x - z)$, $y_2 = A(x^2 - z^2)$, and $y_3 =$

$A(x^3 - z^3)$. Hence $y_2/y_1 = x + z$ and $y_3/y_1 = x^2 + xz + z^2$, so $(y_2/y_1)^2 = x^2 + 2xz + z^2$, whence $xz = y_2^2/y_1^2 - y_3/y_1$. Note the value of $(x - z)^2$:

$$(x - z)^2 = x^2 - 2xz + z^2 = \frac{y_3}{y_1} - 3xz = 4\frac{y_3}{y_1} - 3\frac{y_2^2}{y_1^2}$$

Thus we have a system of equations:

$$x + z = \frac{y_2}{y_1}$$

$$x - z = \sqrt{\left(4\frac{y_3}{y_1} - 3\frac{y_2^2}{y_1^2}\right)}$$

whence

$$x = \frac{1}{2}\left[\frac{y_2}{y_1} + \sqrt{\left(4\frac{y_3}{y_1} - 3\frac{y_2^2}{y_1^2}\right)}\right]$$

$$z = \frac{1}{2}\left[\frac{y_2}{y_1} - \sqrt{\left(4\frac{y_3}{y_1} - 3\frac{y_2^2}{y_1^2}\right)}\right]$$

We have

$$k = -\ln x = -2.3 \log x$$

and

$$\kappa = -\ln z = -2.3 \log z$$

Therefore, in order to find k and κ, the values of x and z must be calculated. This is possible only if y_1, y_2, and y_3 satisfy two conditions: (1) x and z are not complex numbers, and (2) z is positive. Condition 1 means that $4(y_3/y_1) - 3(y_2^2/y_1^2) \geq 0$, an expression which can be reduced to $(y_1 y_3)/y_2^2 \geq \frac{3}{4}$. Condition 2 means that $y_2/y_1 \geq \sqrt{[4(y_3/y_1) - 3(y_2^2/y_1^2)]}$, an expression which can be reduced to $(y_1 y_3)/y_2^2 \leq 1$.

Therefore the choice of points on the experimental curve for the calculation of k and κ by this method is limited by the condition

$$1 \geq \frac{y_1 y_3}{y_2^2} \geq \frac{3}{4} \tag{82}$$

This condition can always be observed. Calculations should be begun with the proper choice of time t so that condition 82 is fulfilled.

Dost and Medgyesi (1964) described a similar procedure for calculating k

and κ, but with a different choice of t: t, $2t$, and $4t$, rather than t, $2t$, and $3t$, which led to the condition

$$2 \geq \frac{y_2^3}{y_3 y_1^2} \geq 1$$

5.2. Calculation of the Rate Constants for Absorption, Metabolism, and Excretion from Urinary Excretion Data

Here we will indicate one possible method for the calculation of rate constants in a more complex case than the ones considered above, including Section 4.6. This method of calculation from data on the urinary excretion of a substance and its metabolite is applicable to the most general situation where a known amount of the substance is present in a compartment A of the body, whence it is absorbed with the rate constant k into the blood and other fluids (compartments) of distribution (B). In B the substance is metabolized with the rate constant k_1, and the metabolite (M) is excreted into the urine (E) with the rate constant κ_1. In addition, the substance can be excreted from B unchanged with the rate constant κ and undergo other transformations with the rate constant k_2. The overall process can be represented schematically as follows:

The loss of substance from B by all processes can be characterized by an overall rate constant K incorporating three first-order constants: $K = \kappa + k_1 + k_2$.

Such a method for calculating rate constants from urinary excretion data was developed by Wagner (1967), who also gave examples of detailed calculation. The method is not described here because it pertains more to the field of pharmacology and requires much space.

5.3. Computer-Assisted Calculation of Kinetic Constants

Wiegand and Sanders (1964) proposed a method for the simultaneous calculation of three parameters from blood concentration data—the rate constants for absorption and disappearance and the volume of distribution, with determination of standard errors to assess the accuracy. The calculations were programmed for a digital computer and can be made from data obtained on individual animals. The authors consider such individual determinations preferable because the values of the parameters can then be treated statistically to estimate their variances in a population of subjects.

5.4. Factors Determining the Elimination Kinetics and Affecting the Blood Concentrations of Substances

In the most general form the elimination of a substance is described by (4) or by the differential equation (3). The elimination process is fully defined by the constant κ, whose mathematical significance and physical meaning were discussed above. Here we will concentrate on the biological factors involved in this constant as its component parts.

Evidently, the more rapid the elimination, the greater is κ, that is, there exists a proportionality between the two. This is just what is expressed by (3) at a fixed value of the concentration C. It is also evident that κ is inversely proportional to the apparent volume of distribution V. Formally, this follows from (11) and (7). Logically, it is easy to conclude that, other things being equal, the greater the volume of the living organism in which the substance is distributed the slower its elimination, and vice versa.

The elimination of substances or, more broadly, their clearance from the organism occurs by various routes—through the kidneys and intestines; in the expired air, sweat, and milk; by way of metabolism; and so on. The relative importance of these routes varies from one substance to another, but the principal routes involve the kidneys, metabolism, and, for a number of industrially used low-molecular-weight compounds, the lungs. The overall elimination rate (let us designate it by v) may therefore be resolved into its component rates of elimination by the different routes, for example, in the urine (v_u), through the lungs (v_l), and by metabolism (v_m), so that $v = v_u + v_l + v_m$.

Moreover, the speed of elimination is proportional to the concentration of the substance in blood plasma—not to the total concentration, which is usually determined in quantitative studies of the blood, but to the concentration which is present in solution without being firmly bound to plasma proteins. A part of a foreign compound (different for different compounds) is often firmly bound in the plasma to certain proteins, mainly albumins. Without going into a discussion of the various aspects of protein binding, we will merely note that, if it is not very labile, such binding can be considered as a distribution of the substance in a body compartment, just like its distribution in the muscles, organs, and so on. If we designate by f the ratio of free concentration to total concentration, then, in view of the foregoing, we can write (3) in the form

$$-\frac{dC}{dt} = \frac{(v_u + v_l + v_m)f}{V} C \qquad (83)$$

where V is the apparent distribution volume, and the formal proportionality constant κ has been replaced by its composite biological equivalent.

Any factors that can alter the biological constants of (83) will also affect the rate of clearance of the foreign compound from the body. It must be re-emphasized here that, in view of the extreme complexity of the living organism, (83) is nothing more than an approximation. Nevertheless it is quite satisfactory as a first approximation and may be employed for practical purposes, say in searching for means of enhancing the excretion of poisons from the body.

The parameters of (83) depend on many factors, some of which will be mentioned now. But first it should be noted that "pure" elimination can be expected only in the absence of simultaneous processes of absorption and distribution, that is to say, in a steady state. If this condition is not fulfilled, (3) and consequently (83) are inapplicable.

Regarding the distribution volume V, it is to be noted that this quantity characterizes distribution only as a state, not as a process. It may be quite a satisfactory characteristic when the exchange of the substance between the tissues of distribution and the blood is rapid, that is, when a steady state may be considered to persist during elimination. When the substance is distributed, in addition, in body compartments from which its exit is very difficult, the concept of distribution volume is disturbed. One example of such a "deep" compartment is the bony tissue; the deep compartments are accessible to highly lipophilic or ionized molecules. The presence of deep compartments disturbs the exponential elimination of the substance and greatly prolongs the process of its disappearance from the body.

The quantity f in (83) is subject to the influence of many factors. It is characteristic of each compound binding to albumins, but is not a constant. The value of f depends mainly on the concentration of albumin and the concentration of substance in the blood. Its relationship to albumin is clear: the less albumin, the greater the value of f, that is, the less of the substance is in the blood in bound form. One would expect the result to be accelerated elimination of the substance. This is not always the case, however, because an increase in f (or, in other words, an increase in the plasma content of free substance) not only facilitates excretion but also makes it easier for the substance to pass to other compartments. This is equivalent to an increase in the effective volume of distribution, which results in a decreased excretion rate. For this reason the excretion rates of some substances may remain unchanged despite increased f.

The relationship of f to the concentration of substance is far from clear. It is a fact, however, that as the concentration increases, so does f, though to varying degrees for different substances. In this case, too, an increase in f may lead to increased V.

It should be added that the binding of substances to plasma proteins is unspecific. A substance may be competitively displaced from its binding sites by other substances, thus increasing the value of f. Effective displacing agents are metabolites. Thus metabolism by itself clears the blood of a foreign substance and, in addition, may affect this process in an indirect way, by increasing f.

Turning now to the expression for the overall elimination rate in (83), it may be noted that, if the foreign substance is disposed of by one process only, say by renal excretion, (83) will of course be greatly simplified since only the term v_u will remain. Clearly, any of the factors affecting the renal function may also alter the excretion rate. A highly important factor is renal disease. Renal excretion may also be blocked by a competitive excretory process. In the case of an acid or basic compound the speed of renal excretion is also influenced by the urine pH because the degree of ionization of a compound in the urine is pH-dependent—the excretion of acid compounds is speeded up, and that of basic compounds is slowed down. These and a number of other factors influencing the elimination of substances by renal excretion and some other routes are discussed in greater detail by Dettli and Spring (1968).

The elimination of volatile compounds in the expired air depends on the minute volume of respiration and the intensity of pulmonary blood flow. Therefore any factors that alter these two parameters (e.g., cardiovascular and respiratory diseases) also influence the rate of elimination.

The various factors influencing metabolic processes have been adequately described in the literature (e.g., Dettli and Spring, 1968; Kritsman and Konikova, 1968) and will not be discussed here.

All of the factors affecting the elimination kinetics of a substance also influence the content of the substance in the blood. Of particular importance here is the tissue distribution of the substance, on the one hand, and the elimination rate itself, on the other.

ADDENDUM: TOXICOKINETICS

The past decade has witnessed the rapid development of pharmacokinetics. Several monographs and monographic reviews have been published, a number of symposia and conferences have been held, and journals devoted especially to this relatively new field of study have appeared. We will mention here only three comparatively recent publications that sum up the results obtained, describe the state of the art, and outline prospects for the future; these are the review by Filov (1973); the proceedings of an international conference, edited by Teorell et al. (1974); and the monograph by Notari (1975).

By analogy with pharmacokinetics one can speak of toxicokinetics. The former concerns itself primarily with medicinal substances (drugs); the latter, with toxic chemical compounds (Filov, 1974). Except for the naturally occurring metabolites used as drugs, which should be regarded as falling within the province of biochemical kinetics, pharmacokinetics and toxicokinetics may be united in the framework of the kinetics of the passage of foreign substances (xenobiotics) through an organism. They are in effect the two sides of a single coin, and it is difficult to draw even an arbitrary demarcation line between them, since any drug can also act as a toxic agent.

Industrial toxicology deals chiefly with poisons that enter the body from the environment, predominantly by inhalation but also through the skin and by ingestion. Of special importance for the development of toxic effect is the process of poison absorption, which often extends over a long period. Accordingly, the toxicokinetics of industrial poisons concentrates largely on the absorption of poisons into the body. In drug therapy, on the other hand, a substance is administered by a particular route, so pharmacokinetics focuses on drug distribution, metabolism, and elimination. This suggests the possibility of differentiating between pharmacokinetics and toxicokinetics in terms of the emphasis they place, while at the same time indicating that they have much in common.

Toxicokinetics may be tentatively defined as the study of the time courses of the passage of poisons through the organism, including their absorption, distribution, metabolism, and elimination, as well as the study of the time courses of toxic effects. In the latter area (i.e., in the study of toxic effect–time relationships) there remains very much to be done, at least insofar as quantitative mathematical description is concerned.

The essentials of toxicokinetics were set forth in Chapter 4, where the discussion is centered on one-compartment and other simple models. A systematic account of various models with special reference to their applications in industrial toxicology can also be found in the already cited book of Piotrowski (1971). This author first defines the compartments, dividing them into two main groups—the rapid-exchange (more generally known as shallow) and the slow-exchange (deep) compartments—and then proceeds to a kinetic consideration of open models with one and two compartments, as well as metabolic models, and, finally, of more complex models, giving practical examples from studies on the toxicokinetics of mercury and lead.

This addendum is primarily concerned with the aspects of toxicokinetics that have been developed in the past few years or are receiving the attention of investigators. In addition, some topics omitted for various reasons from Chapter 4 (e.g., methods of toxicokinetics) will be touched upon here, as well as toxicokinetic studies that seem to present special interest. When a particularly important aspect of toxicokinetics has not been developed to a sufficient degree by toxicologists, the appropriate examples have been taken from pharmacological literature.

A1. METHODS OF TOXICOKINETICS

The methods employed in toxicokinetics may be subdivided into two groups: those used at the experimental stage and those utilized in the analysis of experimental findings or of theoretic concepts. The former group comprises methods for the quantitative assay of xenobiotics in biological substrates, while the latter includes compartmental analysis and techniques of mathematical modeling (Filov, 1976) and of analogue computer simulation.

The experimental stage in most toxicokinetic studies involves determining the concentrations of a given substance and/or of its metabolites at different times and in different biological media such as blood, plasma, urine, expired air, and tissues. Accordingly, toxicokinetics makes use of all the methods that are available for the determination of foreign substances in the body or in individual biological media. These include photometric and spectrophotometric analyses, polarography, various kinds of chromatography, fluorimetry, neutron activation analysis, tracer techniques, and atomic absorption spectrophotometry, as well as a number of other analytic tools permitting quantitative determinations of specific industrial poisons in biological substrates.

Whatever the method used, a most important requirement is sensitivity, since all foreign substances gaining access to the body—and, even more so, their metabolites—are in reality always present in relatively low concentrations (except for cases of forensic medical or other special interest). This requirement is best met by the various procedures utilizing radioactivity, and the kinetic behaviors of many poisons are studied by determining the radioactivity of biological specimens sampled at different times or of the organism as a whole after the administration of a labeled test substance. While highly sensitive and simple to use, these techniques have limitations due to the difficulty of interpreting the results, for it is hard to differentiate between the substance and its metabolites. Worthy of mention are the papers of Cohen (1970,

1971) giving details of radioactive isotope application in kinetic studies. Many stable isotopes can also be employed. Assays based on stable isotope techniques have been developed in the past few years because of the advent of more or less readily available instrumentation. The application of stable isotopes in kinetic studies of foreign substances is specifically discussed by Roncucci et al. (1976).

Great opportunities for mass spectrometry in this field are afforded by its use in conjunction with gas chromatography. This combination makes it possible to realize in practice the ability of the gas chromatograph to separate complex mixtures into individual components and to identify them virtually unequivocally on a mass spectrometer. This gas chromatographic-mass spectrometric method has the advantages of high sensitivity, accuracy, rapidity, and high reproducibility. Its applications to the determination of xenobiotics and their metabolites have been reviewed by Kozlov and Rudzit (1976). Another development has been the use of a gas chromatographic-mass spectrometric-computer system (Horning et al., 1975). Such a system integrates the methods of both groups mentioned at the beginning of this section and permits the researcher to obtain the end result without intermediate steps in a single experiment.

Methods for determining the more common organic and inorganic industrial poisons in various biological substrates have been described in detail by Gadaskina and Filov (1971) and Gadaskina et al. (1975).

Toxicokinetic methods of the second group have been described in sufficient detail in Chapter 4. Various aspects of electronic modeling and computer application for kinetic purposes have been reviewed by Filov (1973), and so here we will confine ourselves to mentioning the chapter entitled "Compartments" by Rescigno and Beck (1972), where all aspects of compartmental analysis are expounded in a systematic way, and the papers by Devissaguet and Le Verge (1975), Hattingberg (1973), and Rauws (1975), devoted to analogue computer applications for toxicokinetic and pharmacokinetic purposes. The first two of these three papers describe principles of analogue computer operation with special reference to kinetics, while the third considers in turn five examples of increasing complexity to show the opportunities offered by analogue computer simulation in toxicology.

A2.   NONLINEAR EFFECTS IN TOXICOKINETICS

In Chapter 4, where the basic toxicokinetic relationships are described, we have repeatedly emphasized that these relationships follow first-order kinetics. This implies that the rate of transfer and/or metabolism of a substance is proportional to the difference between its concentrations in the various compartments among which it is transferred. All kinetic constants, that is, transfer constants and half-lives, are indeed constant quantities that do not change with time or with variation in the experimental conditions [e.g., as the amount (dose) of the substance is altered]. In actual practice, however, the situation is more complicated, as anyone who has conducted toxicokinetic experiments is well aware. Kinetic parameters rarely remain constant. In most instances the experimenter observes their greater or lesser variations, but these may usually be neglected. Linear pharmacokinetics may be said to be a particular case of nonlinear pharmacokinetics wherein nonlinear effects are disregarded (or nonexistent). Graphically a nonlinear effect will appear as a nonlinear plot in semilogarithmic coordinates, in contrast to the graph shown, for example, in Figure 19 or in Figure 28.

The extent to which nonlinear effects are distributed may be judged from the paper of Wagner (1974), which presents in tabular form evidences for nonlinearities in the absorption, distribution, and metabolism of xenobiotics, in the renal excretion of unchanged substance and its metabolites, in the biliary excretion, and, finally, in the biologic action of xenobiotics.

The causes of such nonlinearities are many and varied and lie primarily in the living organism, with its great diversity of adaptive responses and powerful capacities for varying the functioning of organs and systems; or, in the language of pharmacokinetics, these nonlinearities are due to instability of the compartments. On the other hand, a nonlinearity may be related to the behavior of xenobiotics. In the case of absorption, for instance, nonlinear effects may be due to poor solubility of the substance, resulting in a low rate of its dissolution and, consequently, of its absorption. Among the major causes of deviations from linearity are the saturability of active absorption processes at high dose levels of xenobiotics; hemodynamic changes in the absorption site; variations in pH in the gastrointestinal tract that modify the fate of ionized compounds; and a more or less firm binding of part of the substance to the intestinal mucosa, tissues, blood proteins, and so on. Without mentioning the publications from which various evidences of nonlinearity were collected by Wagner (1974), most of which appeared before 1972, we will discuss a number of more recent studies, after considering at some length the quantitative expression of nonlinear effects and comparing them to linear ones.

A.2.1. Quantitation of Nonlinear Effects

One example of nonlinear processes is the kinetics of enzymatic metabolism when the metabolized substance is present in sufficiently high concentrations.

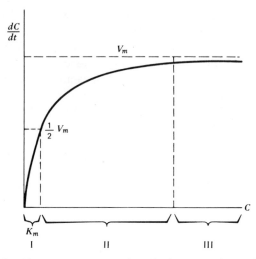

Figure A1. Relationship between concentration of substance and rate of its enzymic transformation. I, zone of first-order reaction; II, zone of mixed reaction; III, zone of zero-order reaction.

Nonlinearity in this case is due to the limited resources of the enzyme involved. The enzyme is progressively blocked by the substance as the concentration of the latter increases. The effect of concentration (C) on the rate of enzymatic transformation (dC/dt) is illustrated in Figure A1. At low concentrations the rate is proportional to the concentration. This is of course a first-order reaction for which all relationships described in Chapter 4 are valid. Here the proportionality factor is the constant for substance degradation and determines the slope of the linear relationship $dC/dt = kC$. In Figure A.2 straight lines 1 and 2 correspond to the degradation rate constants 2.2 and 0.55, respectively.

Actually, however, the increase in degradation rate tends to slow down as the concentration rises because the enzyme system becomes saturated and is no longer able to metabolize the substance completely. In this concentration range (zone II in Figure A1) the reaction is no longer first order but a mixed one. As the concentration increases further, the reaction rate becomes virtually constant and concentration-independent, attaining the maximum possible level. This rate is usually denoted by V_m ($dC/dt \rightarrow V_m$ as $C \rightarrow \infty$). Once it is attained, the reaction becomes a zero-order one so that a definite amount of substance is transformed per unit of time irrespective of the concentration.

These relationships, which are discussed here in very general terms, underlie the quantitative theory of enzymatic reactions; its basic equation is the

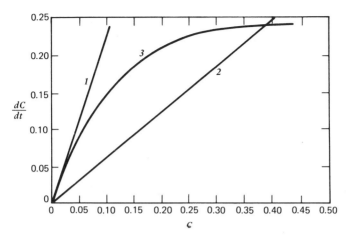

Figure A2. Comparison of linear and nonlinear toxicokinetics. The linear processes (*1* and *2*) have *k* constants equal to 2.2 and 0.55, respectively; the nonlinear process (*3*) has parameters $V_m = 0.22$ and $K_m = 0.1$.

equation of Michaelis and Menten (originators of the theory):

$$\frac{dC/dt}{V_m} = \frac{C}{K_m + C} \tag{A1}$$

The constant K_m is the Michaelis constant. It can be seen from Figure A1 that the value of K_m is given by the substance concentration at which the reaction rate is half its maximal value. This can be readily inferred from (A1). Details of the Michaelis-Menten nonlinear theory can be found in biochemistry texts (e.g., Lehninger, 1972).

Clearly, (A1) can be applied to enzymatic conversions of any industrial poisons. It will also be valid for nonenzymatic processes when the deviation from linearity is caused by saturation phenomena. An example is the saturation of tubular secretion in the kidneys when the concentration of the substance in the blood is high and it is excreted in the urine.

Linear and nonlinear kinetics are compared in Figure A2. Line 3 was drawn from (A1) for $V_m = 0.22$ and $K_m = 0.1$. In this case $V_m/K_m = 2.2$, and line 1 is the tangent line to curve 3; the constant $k = 2.2$ of the linear plot is the maximal value if the process is nonlinear. In the limit $k \rightarrow 0$.

Not every cause of nonlinearity, of course, will permit the use of (A1). For example, an abrupt change in hemodynamics or firm binding of part of the substance to the biological substrate leads to kinetic modifications that do not lend themselves to such a simple description.

Industrial toxicology is most commonly concerned with small amounts of toxic substances that gain access to the body, and the laws of first-order kinetics described in Chapter 4 are usually obeyed. As already mentioned, nonlinear effects begin to be seen at relatively high concentrations of toxic substances. Other causes of nonlinearities occur rather irregularly and lead to deviations from linearity that are apt to be regarded as being due to chance. This may explain why pharmacokinetics developed for a long time on the basis of linear relationships. Many investigators were dissatisfied with the fact that the basic pharmacokinetic parameters, such as transfer constants and half-lives, are dose- or concentration-dependent. This fact, which is not amenable to description in terms of classical linear pharmacokinetics, can be readily described quantitatively in terms of the above concepts. This has led Wagner (1974) to suggest that in the future the parameters V_m and K_m may be widely applied in place of the presently used transfer rate constants and half-lives.

Let us use the nonlinearity concept to describe some particular cases. A very common case is the one in which foreign substances are disposed of by two parallel processes—through urinary excretion of unchanged substance and by metabolism. The first of these obeys first-order kinetics, while the second occurs in conformity with the Michaelis–Menten equation. As long as the concentration remains small, substance elimination can be described as shown in Chapter 4 (p. 142). When the concentration has risen to a certain level, however, the ratio between the two elimination processes is no longer constant and is concentration-dependent. To describe the overall process mathematically, consider a scheme similar to that shown on p. 142 except that one process (E) is nonlinear:

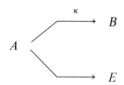

The system of equations describing the velocities of substance elimination by the two pathways (V_E and V_E) and taking cognizance of (A1) is as follows:

$$V_B = \kappa A$$

$$V_E = \frac{V_m A}{K_m + A}$$

(A2)

The ratio of the elimination velocities

$$\frac{V_B}{V_E} = \frac{\kappa}{V_m} (K_m + A)$$ (A3)

depends on the concentration (A).

If a known dose (D) has been introduced into the body, the amounts eliminated by the linear process (unchanged substance) and by the nonlinear process (by way of metabolism) can be found by integrating (A2). Without going into details, we will make use of the solutions presented by Piotrowski (1971):

$$B_t = \left(D + \frac{V_m}{\kappa} \right)(1 - e^{-\kappa t}) - V_m t$$

$$E_t = V_m t$$ (A4)

Dividing the first equation of (A4) by the second, we get

$$\frac{B_t}{E_t} = \left(D + \frac{V_m}{\kappa} \right) \cdot \frac{1 - e^{-\kappa t}}{V_m t} - 1$$ (A5)

Equation A5 indicates that the ratio of elimination pathways is dose-dependent. Other factors being equal, the elimination of unchanged substance increases with the dose. This increase is linear, as can be shown using a fixed value of time (i.e., by measuring the amount of unchanged substance excreted over a sufficiently long time t_E) and varying the dose. Then $(1 - e^{-\kappa t_C})/V_m t_E$ will be a constant quantity—suppose φ ($\varphi > 0$). The quantity $\varphi(V_m/\kappa) - 1$ is likewise constant—suppose ψ. Equation A5 now becomes

$$\frac{B}{E} = \varphi D + \psi$$ (A6)

This is an equation of a straight line, which was required to prove.

There are many instances where a substance is eliminated unchanged with increasing dose; some examples are shown in Table A1.

It may happen that a substance is eliminated by two independent metabolic pathways. A classical example is the parallel binding of benzoic acid or its derivatives to glucuronic acid and to glycine. The reaction with glycine is nonlinear; it will be rate limited by the store of free glycine when the amount of benzoic acid is sufficiently large. At the same time glucuronide formation usually obeys first-order kinetics. It is evident that the foregoing considerations fully apply to this case as well.

Table A1. Proportion of Partly Metabolizable Substances Excreted Unchanged, Depending on Dose

Substance and Animal	Mode of Elimination	Dose (mg/kg) and Amount (%) Excreted Unchanged			
		Low Dose	%	High Dose	%
Aniline, rabbits	Urine	0.1–1	<1	20–150	0.1–5.9
4,6-Dinitro-o-cresol, rats	Urine	5.8–7	1.9	35–45	7.7
Cyclohexane, rabbits	Expired air	0.3	0	360–390	25–38
Carbon disulfide, rats	Expired air	4	68	80	~100
Fluorobenzene, rats	Expired air	0.5	42	1.0	65

Source. Piotrowski (1971).

If both processes are nonlinear, the ratio of their velocities will be given by

$$\frac{V_B}{V_E} = \frac{V_{m,B}}{V_{m,E}} \cdot \frac{K_{m,E} + A}{K_{m,B} + A} \tag{A7}$$

A.2.2.   Uptake of Substances by Tissues

On p. 147 a two-compartment graphic model is shown in which the central compartment A simulates the blood, and B simulates the tissue into which the substance passes from A to accumulate to a certain limit and ultimately be eliminated into E. A mathematical description of substance transferences between the compartments by first-order processes is also presented. The variation in concentration in A and B and the elimination into E are described by system 50 of differential equations (p. 148) and depicted graphically in Figure A3.

Consider now nonlinear effects of substance accumulation in the above model. The linear uptake is described by curve B in Figure A3 and, in mathematical form, by (53) (p. 149). Substituting the values for c_1 and c_2 from (54) (p. 149) into this equation, we find the concentration in B at any time to be proportional to the dose introduced into A [in (54) A_0 is the dose]. By assigning numerical values to the parameters of (53), we can construct a series of plots of B against dose for different instants of time. One possible variant is shown in Figure A4.

The linear plots of Figure A4 conform to (53) and do not impose any

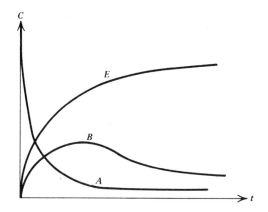

Figure A3. Variation in concentration of substance in a two-compartment open model when a given dose has been rapidly introduced into the central compartment A (blood); B is the peripheral compartment (tissue), freely communicating with A; elimination (E) is only from A.

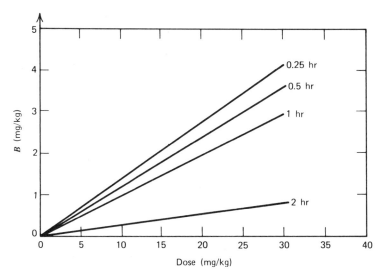

Figure A4. Plots of B (amount of substance in tissue) against dose for different times, using parameters chosen by Wagner (1974).

limitations on substance uptake by tissues as the dose is increased. In practice, however, such a situation is unrealistic, and the relationships illustrated in Figure A4 will hold only as long as the dose is relatively small. Actually, since there is only a certain amount of each kind of tissue in the body, there is also a limiting amount of substance (different for different substances) that can be taken up by any tissue. As can be seen from Figure A5, as the dose is raised to a sufficiently high level, further uptake slows down, becomes nonlinear, and tends to a limit.

Mathematical expressions for the case under consideration that take account of nonlinearity are rather complex, and the interested reader is referred to the original work of Di Santo and Wagner (1972) and Wagner (1974). Calculations can be done on a computer. The curves of Figure A5 were generated by computer.

Before 1972 there was virtually no literature concerning the measurement of foreign substances in various bodily tissues from a toxicokinetic point of view. The authors mentioned above have developed a theory of nonlinear uptake of foreign substances by tissues (here this theory has been briefly outlined in qualitative form), have carried out practical investigations, and have demonstrated the existence of nonlinear effects. The literature containing evidence of nonlinearities in foreign substance absorption, distribution, metabolism, and excretion and in the kinetics of substance action has been summarized by Wagner (1974).

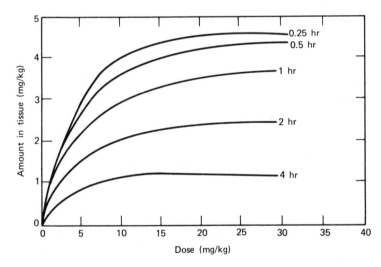

Figure A5. Uptake of substance by tissue as a function of dose for different times. (After Wagner, 1974.)

A.2.3. The Limit of Nonlinearity and Its Possible Use

It must be emphasized that in most situations nonlinear effects are of no consequence and can be disregarded in mathematical models. This is particularly true in industrial toxicology, where the amounts of foreign compounds entering the body tend to be small. Kinetic processes then occur within linear segments, and deviations from linearity are either nonexistent or negligibly small. Not infrequently the sensitivity of the analytical method used to obtain data on variations in foreign substance content in a test object is insufficient to permit detection of deviations from linearity. A pertinent example can be found in Di Santo and Wagner (1972): an assay sensitive to 0.05 μg/ml would not permit a decision as to whether a linear or a nonlinear mathematical model was more appropriate, although the drug elimination curves computed from the two models were different when the observation times were large enough.

In toxicokinetics, nonlinearity is more commonly manifested in the dependence of kinetic parameters on dose or concentration and also in their variation with time. By way of example here are results from three studies. The elimination constant of acetate given intravenously to dogs was found to decrease from 0.231 to 0.139 min^{-1} in the course of its clearance from the blood (Freundt, 1973). Eichelbaum et al. (1974) administered cyclohexylamine to healthy human subjects in a single oral dose of 2.5, 5.0, or 10.0 mg/kg. The plasma concentration reached its peak after 90 to 120 min, while the plasma half-life varied from 3.5 to 4.8 hr in proportion to the dose. The plasma elimination half-life of the herbicide 2,4,5-trichlorophenoxy acetic acid after intravenous injection to rats in doses of 5 and 100 mg/kg was 4.33 and 23.1 hr, respectively (Sauerhoff et al., 1976).

The reasons for such deviations are many and varied, as already mentioned. In the discussion that follows, examples will be given to show how toxicokinetics can be modified by various physiologic, pathologic, and other factors. Here we will only reiterate that not all causes of nonlinearity can be rationalized mathematically, as has been done, for instance, in the case of enzymatic metabolism.

Wagner (1974) has presented six criteria for the recognition of nonlinearities by proper conduct of the experiment and treatment of experimental data. Since these guidelines are adapted to the pharmacologic aspects of kinetics, they will not be reproduced here.

Worthy of consideration is the proposal of Sanotsky (1976) to use the transition to nonlinear effects as a characteristic of harmful action by poisons. He pointed out that at low exposure levels the elimination half-lives of poisons are independent of concentration or dose; at toxic and lethal concentration levels the half-life is appreciably longer, as can be seen from Table A2.

Table A2.   Dependence of Half-Life on Exposure Level

Substance and Elimination Route	Index Measured	Concentration		
		$C_{min} \times 10^{-1}$	C_{min}	C_{leth}
Methylene chloride, blood	Exposure level (mg/liter)	1	10	100
	Half-life (min)	45 ± 12	49 ± 8	120 ± 16
Carbon tetra-chloride, blood	Exposure level (mg/liter)	0.2	2	40
	Half-life (min)	190 ± 20	220 ± 25	460 ± 40
Benzene, expired air	Exposure level (mg/liter)	0.1	1.2	30
	Half-life (min)	80	160	575

Source.   Sanotsky (1976).

A prolongation of half-life in passing to higher exposure levels is regarded by Sanotsky as an indication of impaired detoxication. He therefore suggests that the bend in the plot of half-life as a function of exposure level be considered as marking the beginning of the area within which the substance exerts its harmful action on the organism. Similarly, the ratio of the metabolized portion of poison to that eliminated unchanged may significantly change with exposure level, so that up to 100 % of the poison may be metabolized at low exposure levels and very little or none at all at lethal levels. (Experiments with acetic esters confirming this are referred to on p. 133.) The concentration or dose range in which the metabolism of a given poison undergoes suppression is interpreted by the author as the area where the detoxication mechanisms are disrupted.

This approach is fully consistent with nonlinear toxicokinetics. One should not, however, lose sight of the fact that the causes of deviations from linear relationships of the type half-life $= f$ (dose) are multiple. Also, on the practical side, one should bear in mind the laboriousness of deriving such relationships and the uncertainty involved in establishing the point of transition to nonlinear effects.

A3.   FACTORS MODIFYING TOXICOKINETICS

This section discusses various factors affecting to differing degrees the magnitude of kinetic parameters. It is not our objective to attempt a review of the (now fairly numerous) studies concerned with the influences exerted on the toxicokinetics of xenobiotics by various characteristics of the organism, disease states, dosage form of compounds, and so on. Such a review would take too much space and would rapidly become outdated. Rather, our objective is to illustrate, with a limited number of examples, the various kinetics-modifying factors that constitute a certain system, and to describe individual quantitative aspects of their action. Where possible, the examples were taken from toxicological studies, but since these are rather few in number many examples had to be borrowed from pharmacological literature.

A.3.1. Factors That Depend on the Biological Object

Individual Features

Toxicokinetic differences due to individual characteristics are illustrated in Figures A6 and A7. It can be seen from Figure A6 that the extreme values of the degradation constant (κ) of butyl acetate in the blood of nine rabbits differ

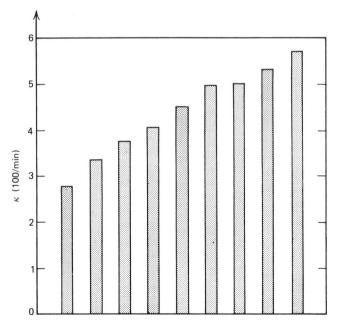

Figure A6. Rate constants for degradation of butyl acetate in the blood of nine different rabbits. (After Filov, 1963.)

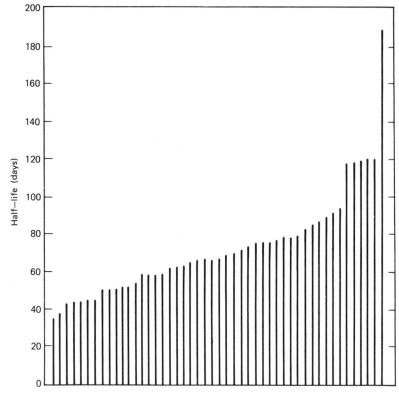

Figure A7. Half-lives of methylmercury in 48 persons. (Constructed from data of Al-Shahristani and Shihab, 1974.)

by a factor of 2. Hence the distribution of rabbits with respect to their abilities to metabolize butyl acetate may be presumed to be normal. Figure A7 shows, in similar form, the biological half-lives of methylmercury as determined by Al-Shahristani and Shihab (1974) by neutron activation analysis over a prolonged period in the hair of 48 persons who had ingested the poison with grain. The concentration of mercury in the hair varied in parallel with that in the blood, so that it was possible to judge mercury clearance from the body. As can be seen from the figure, the half-life varies widely from about 35 to 190 days, that is, fivefold, with an average of 72 days. The histogram constructed by the authors indicates that the distribution of mercury half-lives among the population studied is not a normal one. The half-life was not related to age or diet. A practical implication of such widespread half-life values is a comparable variation in the risk of being poisoned with methylmercury.

The causes of interindividual variations in kinetic parameters are varied.

Breckenridge and Orme (1973) have concluded from their kinetic study of warfarin absorption in man that the underlying causes are interindividual differences in amounts absorbed and in absorption rates.

Fagerström et al. (1975) have found the rate of mercury uptake from water by pikes per unit of body weight to be weight-dependent. A detailed study of warfarin elimination in rats has shown that the blood half-life of warfarin after intravenous injection varies from 6 to 18 hr but remains constant for each individual rat (Vacobi and Levy, 1974). Vesell et al. (1973) have found the plasma half-life of antipyrine to be also constant in individual dogs. To account for the observed interindividual differences in antipyrine half-lives, the authors studied these in relation to enzyme levels in hepatic microsomes and found the half-life to correlate inversely with the activities of aniline hydroxylase and ethylmorphine demethylase, but not with those of cytochrome P-450, cytochrome reductase, or NADPH oxidase. In other words, the activity of specific enzymes determines the life span of the substance in the body. This conclusion, though somewhat commonplace, is essential for our purposes here, for it indicates that toxicokinetic parameters may be genetically determined.

The role of genetic factors in the pharmacokinetics of foreign compounds has been explored by Vesell (e.g., 1974a, 1974b). The clearance of plasma from antipyrine and phenylbutazone in monozygotic (identical) and dizygotic (fraternal) twins is shown in Figure A8. Monozygotic twins possess identical genomes, while dizygotic ones share, on the average, one half of their genes. The twins were so selected as to minimize intertwin differences in environmental factors. Intertwin differences in plasma half-lives were found to be small or nonexistent among identical twins but appreciable among fraternal twins. It is appropriate to cite here an example of isoniazid disappearance from blood plasma (Mitchison, 1973). The main pathway of isoniazid disposition is its acetylation to inactive form. This process is genetically controlled. All human beings can be divided into two groups according to whether they inactivate isoniazid rapidly (about 40% of most populations examined) or slowly. The process of isoniazid absorption is very similar in slow and rapid inactivators, so that the peak concentrations of isoniazid were approximately the same and were reached at the same time in both groups. But thereafter the courses of the curves were very different, the half-life of isoniazid being 2.4 times greater in slow inactivators than in rapid ones.

In comparing the elimination of a substance in each pair of subjects the following considerations may be a useful guide (Nelson, 1965). If the elimination is first order, $C = C_0 e^{-\kappa t}$ for each subject. The difference between blood concentrations of the substance for each pair (subjects 1 and 2) at any time t is given by

$$\Delta C = C_1 - C_2 = C_{0,1} e^{-\kappa_1 t} - C_{0,2} e^{-\kappa_2 t}$$

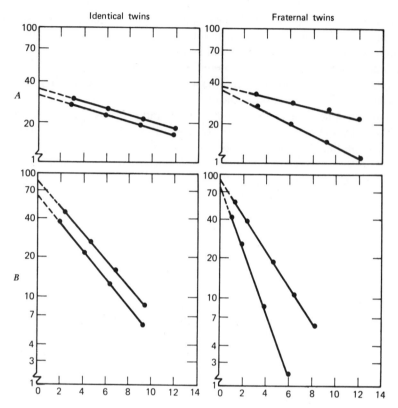

Figure A8. Clearance of plasma from antipyrine (*A*) and phenylbutazone (*B*) in identical and fraternal twins. *A*: a single oral dose of 18 mg/kg; *ordinate*, concentration (*μg*/ml plasma); *abscissa*, hours after administration. *B*: a single oral dose of 6 mg/kg; *ordinate*, concentration (*μg*/2 ml plasma); *abscissa*, days after administration. (After Vesell, 1974a.)

The quantity ΔC is a function of time and has a maximum. The time taken to attain this maximum (t_{max}) can be computed from the equation

$$t_{max} = \frac{\ln(\kappa_2 C_{0,2}/\kappa_1 C_{0,1})}{\kappa_2 - \kappa_1} \tag{A8}$$

Age

One avoids prescribing sulfonamides (and, incidentally, many other drugs) for newborn infants. On the other hand, the doses of sulfonamides prescribed for older children are higher, on a weight basis, than those used for adults. These empirically established rules of sulfonamide dosage are in accordance with pharmacokinetic data. The elimination of sulfonamides is much slower in newborns than in adults. During the first years of life the elimination rate increases sharply to exceed that in adults, and then decreases slowly with increasing age until it reaches the "normal" adult value by the age of about 20 years.

As pointed out by Gladtke (1973), pharmacokinetic parameters are highly variable in newborns and older infants—much more so than in adults. It has been shown, for example, that the plasma half-life of unchanged phenobarbital is independent of age in the age range between 20 and 60 years, being 75 hr on average. In persons aged over 75 it increases up to 100 hr (Traeger et al., 1974). Triggs et al. (1975) compared the pharmacokinetics of sulfamethizole, paracetamol, and phenylbutazone in groups of young (22 to 30 years) and elderly (73 to 91 years) individuals and found that, although the rate and degree of absorption of the drugs after oral administration were the same in both groups, their half-lives were different. Thus the half-life of sulfamethizole was 105 ± 5 min in the young group and 181 ± 13 min in the elderly group; the half-lives of paracetamol were 109 ± 7 and 130 ± 9 min, respectively. These differences were proportional to those in creatinine clearance and in certain body function indices. Triggs and Nation (1975) attribute such differences to age-related changes in degree of drug binding to proteins, in apparent volumes of distribution, and in renal and extrarenal clearances. In other words the distribution of foreign substances undergoes change with advancing age, and this affects their kinetic characteristics.

Sex

Typical results are those from experiments by Tomita (1971), who studied sex differences in the half-life of radioactive cadmium injected subcutaneously into mice as chloride in a dose of 1 μCi. The half-life was 21.5 days in males and 28.0 days in females. Similar differences are commonly seen in human beings. In women substances tend to be retained longer than in men, and their blood levels are higher accordingly. This is thought to be due to the higher proportion of "inert" fatty tissue in women, which acts as a depot. The role of fatty tissue in benzene toxicokinetics has been demonstrated in direct experiments by Sato et al. (1975): the more fat the animal contained, the more benzene was retained in the body and, incidentally, the more white blood cell abnormality was observed. This was true of both males and females. Retention was, however, greater in females, as were changes in leukocyte counts. Similar results were obtained in human subjects. The elimination of benzene from the blood obeyed the equation $C = 5.26e^{-0.00335t}$ in men and the equation $C = 4.14e^{-0.00198t}$ in women (C being the blood concentration of benzene in μg/ml, and t the time in min). The difference between these two equations is statistically significant. It can thus be seen that benzene disposition is more rapid in men than in women.

This does not, of course, apply to all xenobiotics. One example of a reverse relationship is given by Baker and Foulkes (1973): p-chlorophenyl-4-phenyl-3oxa-2,2-dimethylbutanoic acid, a hypolipidemic agent, was found to accumulate markedly less in female than in male marmosets. Also, nonpregnant females receiving standard doses of the compound on a weight basis showed blood levels three times those of their pregnant counterparts.

Species Differences

While, as shown above, the toxicokinetics of xenobiotics may be affected by interindividual and sex differences, one would expect still greater interspecies differences in their kinetic parameters. Here examples of such differences will be given first, followed by a brief discussion of their relevance to the extrapolation of experimental data from one species to another.

First let us take note of Table A3, which shows rate constants for butyl acetate metabolism by the blood in human beings and 11 animal species. It can be seen that the extreme values differ about twentyfold, that is, by a factor of 10 more than the largest intraspecies variation in κ in the same experiment (see Figure A6). We have failed to establish a straightforward relationship between the magnitude of κ and the biological characteristics of blood in the

Table A3. Constants for Butyl Acetate Degradation (κ) by Blood in Various Species (each figure is the average of two to four determinations in different individuals)

Species	κ (min^{-1})
Dogs	0.013
Sheep	0.014
Pigs	0.017
Frogs	0.023
Cows	0.026
Human beings	0.027
Cats	0.032
Rabbits	0.044
White rats	0.065
White mice	0.069
Pigeons	0.10
Guinea pigs	0.25

Source.   Filov (1963).

Table A4. **Constants for Absorption (k) and Elimination (κ) of Polychlorinated Biphenyls (Average Values) in Fatty Tissue of Young Pigs and Sheep**

Animal	k (day^{-1})	κ (day^{-1})
Pig	0.027	0.112
Sheep	0.010	0.064

Source. Borchard et al. (1976).

species studied, but an overall correlation is obvious: the blood of small animals is more active than that of larger ones. This may be attributed to higher metabolic activity in small animals. There are, however, deviations from this general pattern: bovine blood is more active than that of pig, sheep, and dog; the blood of pigeons and, especially, guinea pigs is more active than that of white mice; frog blood has relatively low activity.

A study on the toxicokinetics of polychlorinated biphenyls (PCB) in growing pigs and lambs (Borchard et al., 1976) has shown their elimination rate constants to be 0.691 and 0.302 day^{-1}, respectively. The time courses of PCB levels in fatty tissue were also followed (Table A4). The authors attribute the higher values of kinetic parameters in pigs to their more intensive growth.

Figure A9 shows kinetic blood level curves of fluorenone in dogs, rats, and rabbits, all given the same dose of the compound (Rentsch, 1974). It can be seen that fluorenone behavior in the blood may be very different in different species. Thus, whereas in rabbits it had disappeared from the blood after 4 hr, in dogs it remained in appreciable amounts after 24 hr. In this context mention may be made of the work of Kodama et al. (1975), who studied the various kinetic aspects of a single compound in experiments on rats, mice, rabbits, monkeys, and human subjects. Among the established interspecies similarities and dissimilarities in substance behavior was the following: after intragastric administration the blood level of unchanged compound was relatively high in rats and mice and low in rabbits and human subjects.

Such variations can be related to differences in enzymatic capacity to biotransform a particular xenobiotic. This is apparent, in particular, in Table A5, where the duration of biological effect and the biological half-life of hexobarbital are seen to be inversely correlated with the level of its inactivation by enzymes. It may be added that in man the half-life of hexobarbital was found to be 360 min.

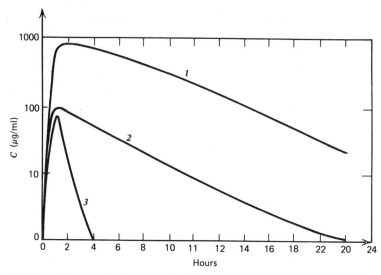

Figure A9. Kinetic curves for fluorenone in the blood of dogs (*1*), rats (*2*), and rabbits (*3*) after an oral dose of 200 mg/kg. (Adapted from Rentsch, 1974.)

The above examples of species differences seem to be sufficient for our purposes here. Sometimes such differences are small or even absent, but these cases are exceptions. Variations may exist even between very close groups, as is exemplified by data on half-lives of methylmercury in healthy individuals of different nationalities (Al-Shahristani and Shihab, 1974): 72 days in Iraqians, 65 days in Japanese, and 70 days in Swedes, on the average.

Table A5.   Duration of Action, Biological Half-life, and Level of Enzymatic Inactivation of Hexobarbital in Different Species

Species	Dose (mg/kg)	Duration of Action (min)	Half-life (min)	Activity of Inactivating Enzymes ($\mu g/(g\ hr)$)
Mouse	100	12 ± 8	19 ± 7	598 ± 184
Rabbit	100	49 ± 12	60 ± 11	196 ± 28
Rat	100	90 ± 15	140 ± 54	134 ± 51
Dog	50	315 ± 105	260 ± 20	36 ± 30

Source.   Part of the table published in Vesell (1974a).

The reasons for toxicokinetic variations among species are to be sought primarily in the biochemical status, which differs from one species to another. Many examples similar to those shown in Table A5 could be given. However, since this is not our objective, we will merely note that the rates of biotransformation and transfer of substances show an overall positive correlation with metabolic levels.

The subject considered here has a direct bearing on data transfer from one species to another, including human beings—a problem which has far-reaching practical implications. This problem is approached differently in each particular case, depending on the available data and on the task at hand. If one is contemplating the transfer of toxicity data for a substance, one first of all must make sure that the mechanisms by which its toxic action is brought about are identical or similar in the species concerned. The next essential step is to ascertain the relative efficiency of the detoxication mechanisms, and this brings one directly to a consideration of the relative speeds with which the blood and the body as a whole are cleared from the toxic substance, that is, to the question of its toxicokinetics. Let us consider this question with reference to the results of interesting research with methotrexate carried out by a group of American workers (Dedrick et al., 1970).

Methotrexate is a reasonably stable compound which is largely eliminated unchanged. Its mechanism of action in different species, at least in mammals, has been associated with the inhibition of dihydrofolate reductase. Figure A10 shows semilog plots of methotrexate plasma concentrations against time in mice, rats, dog, monkeys, and man constructed from data of different groups of investigators who used different doses and routes of administration (intravenous or intraperitoneal). Inspection of Figure A10 shows, first, that plasma concentrations vary over a wide range, from 0.0077 to 130 μg/ml. Next, for all species that were studied after receiving more than one dose (mice, rats, and man) the curves are roughly parallel and the plasma concentration at any time is approximately proportional to the dose for these species. Finally, the rate at which the plasma concentration declines is most rapid for mice and rats and least rapid for man.

A successful attempt was made to correlate these plasma concentration data by normalizing the variables plotted. This normalization was based on body weight relationships. The plasma concentration data were normalized by dividing by the dose per unit of body weight, while the time variable was normalized by dividing by an equivalent time as an empirical function of the fourth root of the body weight. The result obtained is shown in Figure A11. It can be seen that all the plots in Figure A10 that cover a plasma concentration range of 0.0077 to 130 μg/ml, a body weight range of 22 to 70,000 g, and a dose range of 0.1 to 450 mg/kg are superimposed to constitute a single plot in Figure A11. The resulting universal curve can be used for several purposes.

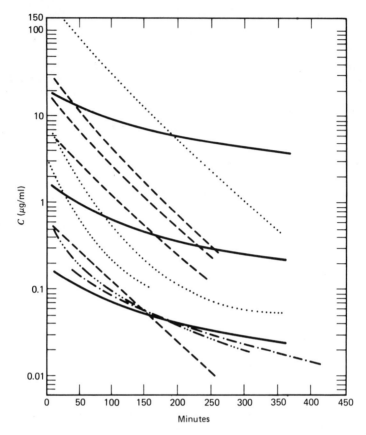

Figure A10. Variation in plasma concentrations of methotrexate in various mammalian species after different single doses were injected intravenously or intraperitoneally. Mouse, . . . ; rat, –––; monkey, ·–·; dog, –. . . ; man ––. (After Dedrick et al., 1970.)

For the purpose of comparing plasma clearances from methotrexate in the mouse and man, 1 min in the life of a mouse may be taken to be equivalent to about 8 min for man. This provides a rational basis for transferring pharmacokinetic data from mouse to man. The plot can be used also to calculate the half-life for methotrexate elimination from the blood. This quantity is related to body weight W by the relationship

$$T_{0.5} = \frac{0.693\sqrt[4]{W}}{k} \tag{A9}$$

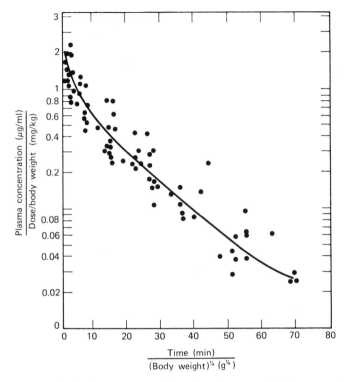

Figure A11.   Variation in plasma concentrations of methotrexate in different species in normalized coordinates. Dots are data points from which the plots of Figure 10 were constructed. (After Dedrick et al., 1970.)

where k is the slope. In Figure A12 blood half-lives of methotrexate are plotted in semilog coordinates as functions of body weight for different mammals. Dedrick et al. (1970) give an example of passing from mammals (mouse) to fish (stingray): 1 min of methotrexate concentration decline in the mouse is roughly equivalent to 16 min in the stingray.

A reliable interspecies transfer of data is possible only if the mechanisms of substance distribution are similar in the species considered. Similarly treated data for another substance may not fit into a single plot in normalized coordinates; this would suggest that the mechanisms by which the substance is distributed are different in different species (such differences may concern the degree of binding to plasma or tissue proteins, excretion pathways, etc.). The problem of animal data transfer to man is also discussed in the addendum of Chapter 1.

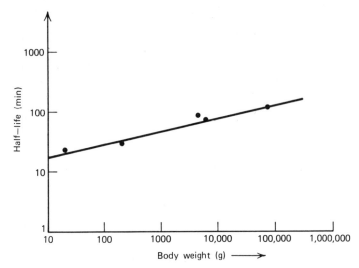

Figure A12. Plasma half-life of methotrexate plotted versus body weight for several mammals. (After Dedrick et al., 1970.)

A.3.2.   Effect of Physiologic Variables

The modifying effects of physiologic variables and disease states on the kinetics of substances in the body have been discussed by Dettli and Spring (1973), with separate consideration of influences on absorption, distribution, and elimination. Without repeating any of the materials contained in that publication, let us consider briefly the main physiologic and, in Section A3.3, pathologic factors that affect the kinetics of foreign substances.

Food Intake

The nature, composition, and amount of food can affect primarily the kinetics of substance absorption. This is obvious in the case of gastrointestinal absorption. Apart from the competitive relationships present during absorption, of importance here is the sorption of poisons by food particles and their possible chemical interactions. With other than oral routes of poison entry, the effect of food may be mediated through the change it causes, for example, in the blood flow. Shively and Vesell (1975) reported the human plasma half-lives of phenacetin and acetaminophen to be about 15% longer when the drugs were administered 6 hr before a meal than when they were given 2 hr after it.

   Komuro et al. (1975) studied the effect of fasting on distribution volumes of foreign substances in rats. Substance distribution and kinetic parameters were found to be affected by weight loss, increase in hematocrit, and decreases in volumes of plasma and interstitial fluid. Blood concentrations of the substances studied were higher in fasting than in control rats even though the intestinal absorption was depressed. This was due to decreased distribution volume (by 40% after 60 hr of fasting).

Exercise

Volume of circulating blood, blood flow rate, blood pressure, plasma protein concentration, renal blood flow, activities of various enzyme systems, and a number of other variables are all affected by changes in physical activity, whether it is increased or decreased. The kinetics of foreign compounds may vary accordingly. Alterations in the pharmacokinetics of drugs, depending on the patient's status, have been demonstrated in several clinical studies. One example is the study of Cadorniga et al. (1974) on the pharmacokinetics of ampicillin injected intramuscularly to outpatients and inpatients (Table A6). As can be judged from the table, limited exercise slows the absorption and somewhat accelerates the elimination of the compound.

Hemodynamic Factors

The role of hemodynamic factors in the kinetics of xenobiotics has been repeatedly emphasized above. The basic fact is that the rate of blood flow through an organ correlates directly with the rate of substance absorption into that organ. For details of the relationship of hemodynamic factors to the kinetics of foreign compounds in the body as a whole and in its individual parts, reference may be made to the excellent papers by Rowland (1975) and Wilkinson (1975).

Oxygen Tension

A rise in arterial oxygen tension was found by Cumming (1976) to result in a considerable shortening of the antipyrine half-life in human plasma (from

Table A6. Pharmacokinetic Parameters of Ampicillin in Outpatients and Inpatients Given 250 Mg of the Drug Intramuscularly

Parameter	Outpatients	Inpatients
Absorption constant	2.077 hr^{-1}	1.807 hr^{-1}
Latent period	0.109 hr	0.329 hr
Time taken to attain peak concentration	0.92 hr	1.29 hr
Peak concentration in blood	$2.57 \ \mu g/ml$	$2.70 \ \mu g/ml$
Elimination constant	0.478 hr^{-1}	0.542 hr^{-1}

Source.   Cadorniga et al. (1974).

18.4 ± 3.5 to 8.4 ± 1.0 hr). The physiologic effect of the drug increased in duration as oxygen tension was reduced.

Circadian Rhythms

In a study on six healthy human subjects with preliminarily synchronized diurnal activities, the urinary concentration of sodium salicylate was found to rise faster, to reach higher values, and to decline more rapidly in those who had received the drug at 19.00 or 23.00 hr than in those given it at 7.00 or 11.00 hr (Reinberg, 1975).

A.3.3. Effect of Disease States

Foremost among the various pathologic states that modifty toxicokinetics are those involving the liver or kidney, that is, the organs largely responsible for the metabolism and elimination of xenobiotics.

Liver Disease

The effects of liver disease on toxicokinetic parameters are well documented in numerous publications, so two or three examples will suffice here. In hepatectomized rats both distribution volumes and rate constants for intra-compartmental transfer were found to be strongly altered; for instance, the constant of pentobarbital elimination from the blood decreased from 0.0184 min^{-1} in health to 0.00098 min^{-1} after hepatectomy (Ossenberg et al., 1975). Table A7 shows the effects of some liver diseases in man on the half-life of anti-pyrine (Branch et al., 1973). The prolongation of antipyrine half-life in liver disease is apparently due to defective synthesis of microsomal enzyme pro-

Table A7. Effect of Liver Disease on the Half-Life of Antipyrine in Blood Serum

Disease	Half-life (hr)
Normal subjects	12.0 ± 1.7
Cirrhosis	33.8 ± 6.8
Chronic hepatitis	26.2 ± 11.2
Acute hepatitis	19.5 ± 6.0
Obstructive jaundice	17.8 ± 5.4

Source. Branch et al. (1973).

Table A8.   Kinetic Constants of Bromsulphalein in
Rats with Normal and Impaired Liver Function

Group	k (min^{-1})	κ (min^{-1})	f
Control	0.0435	0.0267	0.912
Rats given CCl_4	0.0523	0.0154	0.578

tein: phenobarbital induced enzyme synthesis with a resultant shortening of antipyrine half-life.

Of interest is the application of the one-compartment model to liver function studies in rats, using the Bromsulphalein test (Soloviyev et al., 1976). The absence of the gallbladder in this species permits evaluation of both excretory and absorptive functions of the liver from data on Bromsulphalein biliary excretion. For this purpose one can use an equation describing the absorption of a known dose D of substance in a one-compartment system (see Section 3.5):

$$\frac{dy}{dt} = \frac{k\kappa Df}{\kappa - k}(e^{-kt} - e^{-\kappa t})*$$ (A10)

where dy/dt is the excretion rate $(dy/dt \approx \Delta y/\Delta t)$, and f is the proportion of the dye excreted in bile. The excretory and absorptive functions of the liver are characterized by κ and k, respectively.

In these experiments liver function was impaired by carbon tetrachloride, and bile was sampled every 10 min in both the test and the control group ($\Delta t = 10$ min). The constants κ and k were calculated on a computer and are shown in Table A8; the changes in Bromsulphalein level in both groups are depicted in Figure A13. It can be seen from Table A8 and Figure A13 that liver disease alters Bromsulphalein kinetics in rats: the dye is eliminated more slowly, and the proportion excreted in bile decreases. The increase in absorption rate constant is attributed by the authors to diminished liver capacity for Bromsulphalein.

Kidney Disease

The urinary excretion of xenobiotics is reduced and their metabolism by certain pathways is slowed in renal abnormalities that are manifested in

---

* This equation differs somewhat from the derivative equation obtained from (32) (p. 137), but the difference is insignificant and so we reproduce the equation as given by Soloviyev et al.

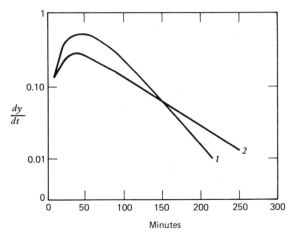

Figure A13. Variation in biliary excretion rate of Bromsulphàlein in intact rats (*1*) and in those with impaired liver function (*2*). (After Soloviyev et al., 1976.)

uremia, and these circumstances may strongly alter the pharmacokinetics of substances and influence their biological action. As far as the latter is concerned, the increased accumulation of compounds and their metabolites, involving a higher risk of toxicity, becomes of particular importance.

A sensitive indicator of renal function is the clearance of endogenous creatinine (C_{cr}). The elimination rate constant of a xenobiotic (κ) can be related to this clearance by a simple linear expression (Dettli, 1975):

$$\kappa = \kappa_{nr} + \alpha C_{cr} \tag{A11}$$

where κ_{nr} is the nonrenal elimination constant, and α is the constant of proportionality between renal excretion rate and C_{cr}.

In accordance with (A11) the elimination of xenobiotics may involve three main types of substances (Figure A14, lines 1, 2, and 3):

1. Substances that are eliminated in health entirely by the kidneys, so that $\kappa_{nr} = 0$ and $\alpha > 0$. In Figure A14 this is shown by the straight line passing through the origin of the plot of κ versus C_{cr}. The slope of this line is determined by α. It can be seen that a change in C_{cr} due to renal disease will immediately affect κ, and the more so, the greater the value of α.

2. At the other extreme, substances eliminated by nonrenal routes only ($\alpha = 0$ and $\kappa_{nr} > 0$). Here $\kappa = \kappa_{nr}$, and the elimination rate is independent of renal function.

3. Substances eliminated by both renal and nonrenal routes ($\alpha > 0$ and $\kappa_{nr} > 0$), as happens most commonly.

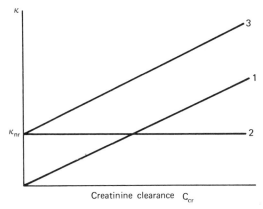

Figure A14. Plots of elimination constants for xenobiotics against endogenous creatinine clearance with three types of elimination. See text for explanation.

Alternatively, the elimination half-life may be considered instead of the elimination constant. The former is related to creatinine clearance by the expression

$$T_{0.5} = \frac{0.693}{\kappa} = \frac{0.693}{\kappa_{nr} + \alpha C_{cr}} \tag{A12}$$

This relationship is nonlinear and so less preferable for practical use.

The above equations are based on the one-compartment body model. Using the same model, consider now the plasma level of creatinine. In a steady state this level (C_0) is related to creatinine clearance (C_{cr}) and the rate of endogenous creatinine formation ($C_{0,form}$) by the simple relationship

$$C_0 = \frac{C_{0,form}}{C_{cr}} \tag{A13}$$

in which $C_{cr} = V\kappa_{cr}$, where V is the apparent volume of distribution in the body and κ_{cr} is the constant for creatinine urinary excretion in health. Hence $C_0 = C_{0,form}/V\kappa_{cr}$. The elimination half-life of creatinine is related to the above parameters by the relationship

$$T_{0.5} = \frac{0.693}{\kappa_{cr}} = \frac{0.693 \times V}{C_{cr}} = \frac{0.693 \times VC_0}{C_{0,form}} \tag{A14}$$

For the average healthy human being aged between 20 and 50 years with a body weight of 70 kg and a body surface area of 1.73 m^3, C_{cr} is 150 ml/min and V is 50 liters. Hence the normal half-life of creatinine is 3.85 hr.

Table A9.   Effect of Reduced Renal Function on the Blood Half-Life ($T_{0.5}$) and Steady-State Level of Creatinine

		f			
Parameter	1 (normal)	0.5	0.25	0.1	0.05
$T_{0.5}$ (hr)	3.85	7.7	15.4	38.5	77
C_0 (mg %)	1.06	2.11	4.2	10.6	21.1

Source.   Chiou and Hsu (1975).

In renal insufficiency the half-life becomes longer, with a decrease in κ_{cr} by the factor f, which is a fraction of the normal renal function. The blood level of creatinine also rises. Chiou and Hsu (1975) have reported numerical relationships between half-life and C_0 as a function of f (Table A9).

It is noteworthy that the smaller f is, the more time is required to reach C_0. Thus the time taken to reach $0.95C_0$ increases from 1 to 14 days as f decreases from 0.5 to 0.05.

Blood levels of creatinine make it possible to judge renal function only if creatinine is in a steady state and its formation in the body is normal. In the absence of steady state (patients with acute or unstable renal insufficiency) or in cases where creatinine formation is impaired an equation such as (A13) is unacceptable.

Thyroid Dysfunction

Vesell et al. (1975) reported changes in the plasma half-lives of various compounds in persons with impaired thyroid function (Table A10). The decrease in half-life occurring in hyperthyroidism was attributed by the authors to accelerated metabolism of substances in hepatic microsomes, and its pro-

Table A10.   Relationship of Half-Life ($T_{0.5}$) to Hyper- and Hypothyroidism

Compound	$T_{0.5}$ in Human Plasma (hr)		
	In Health	In Hyperthyroidism	In Hypothyroidism
Antipyrine	11.9 ± 1.4	7.7 ± 1.2	26.4 ± 4.0
Propylthiouracil	6.7 ± 1.0	4.3 ± 0.7	24.7 ± 3.4
Methimazole	9.3 ± 1.4	6.9 ± 0.6	13.6 ± 4.8

Source.   Vesell et al. (1975).

longation in hypothyroidism was ascribed to delayed biotransformation. When thyroid function was normalized, the half-life likewise returned to normal.

Experimental Polyarthritis

Kaiser and Forist (1974) induced polyarthritis in rats by intracutaneous injection of *Mycobacterium butyricum*. Intact rats were given a single oral dose of 4,5-bis(*p*-methoxyphenyl)-2-phenylpyrrole-3-acetonitrile at the rate of 52.1 mg/kg, while polyarthritic rats were given a total of 29 doses of the compound for a total dosage of 2.4, 6.8, or 11.4 mg/kg (in different groups). The half-life of the substance was found to be 11.3 hr in intact rats and 5.4 hr in those with polyarthritis. It is worthy of note that the half-life was independent of dose in the diseased animals (suggesting that the elimination was first order).

Thermal Trauma

In normal rats the elimination from blood of intravenously administered calcium is describable by a four-exponential equation (Movshev, 1968):

$$Ca(t) = 0.587e^{-0.83t} + 0.235e^{-0.12t} + 0.148e^{-0.022t} + 0.03e^{-0.0024t}$$

On the third day after a burn involving 20% of the body surface area, a five-exponential equation was required to describe calcium elimination:

$$Ca(t) = 0.648e^{-1.04t} + 0.112e^{-0.12t} + 0.128e^{-0.06t}$$
$$+ 0.098e^{-0.017t} + 0.014e^{-0.001t}$$

On day 15 postburn a fifth term was still required, but the elimination process proceeded more slowly than on the third day. A similar pattern of postburn changes was observed for calcium absorption into bone.

A.3.4. Factors Associated with Dosage Form

In pharmacology the pharmacokinetics of drugs is known to be affected by dosage form. This subject is especially dealt with in biopharmaceutics, where pertinent information can be found. The dose-dependent kinetics of xenobiotics was discussed in sufficient detail in Section A2 on nonlinear toxicokinetics, so only two aspects will be considered here: the dependence of toxicokinetics on the dosing regimen and its dependence on the route of substance entry into the body.

Table A11 shows variations in the blood concentration of dimethylformamide during 9 days of exposure by inhalation. The concentration is seen to

Table A11.   Blood Levels of Dimethylformamide in Rats during Repeated Exposures to Two Different Concentrations

Inhaled Concentration (mg/m^3)	Blood Level (mg %) on Day		
	1	3	8
400	7.85 ± 0.18	0.36 ± 0.20	0.17 ± 0.05
40	0.04 ± 0.01	0.05 ± 0.01	0.02 ± 0.01

Source.   Muraviyeva et al. (1975).

fall off, the decline being much steeper with the higher inspired concentration. An acceptable explanation for this finding is that dimethylformamide induces metabolizing enzymes, the degree of induction being more or less proportional to the amount of the poison. This may also account for the significant decrease observed in the plasma half-life of carbamazepine in man: after a single dose the half-life was 35.6 ± 15.3 hr, but after multiple doses it shortened to 20.9 ± 5.0 hr (Eichelbaum et al., 1975). Understandably, such an effect is far from being of general occurrence. The very existence of linear toxicokinetics and linear pharmacokinetics as fields of knowledge with certain rules and laws depends on a degree of stability of the parameters used.

The effects of route of administration on several kinetic characteristics of substances, primarily on their distribution, excretion, and metabolism, have been reviewed by Gibaldi and Perrier (1974). Here is an example of such an effect, taken from Notari et al. (1974): the half-life of oxytetracycline elimination from horse blood was 6.36 hr with rapid intravenous injection, 13.0 hr with intramuscular injection but only 3.5 hr when the drug was administered by continuous infusion.

Toxicokinetics may also depend on the solvent in which the substance is applied to a biological object. In rats, for example, as much as 80 % of oral hexachlorobenzene was absorbed when the poison was administered in oil but only 6 % when it was given in aqueous solution (Koss and Koransky, 1975). Similar examples were also adduced in Chapter 3 (Section 6.1), where they were interpreted in terms of thermodynamic activity and of the thermodynamic capacities of the phases between which the substance is transferred.

A.3.5.   Effect of Temperature

The results of studies relating to the role of temperature in pharmacokinetics have been summarized by Ballard (1974) in a theoretically oriented review. Most of the studies cited there were conducted on animals under conditions of hypo- or hyperthermia, that is, were concerned with the effects of altered body temperature; others considered the role of environmental temperature variations. Environmental temperature may, first of all, affect the physicochemical properties of substances before these enter the body. It can also affect body temperature to a certain degree. Lastly, temperature changes both in the environment and in the body may have direct effects on physiologic and biochemical processes within the organism, and these in turn may influence pharmacokinetics. A lowering of body temperature prolongs the period of absorption and the entire cycle of substance passage through the body. This explains the greater tolerance (an increase in the absolute value of the LD_{50}) to some xenobiotics shown by animals chronically exposed to cold. As regards the distribution of substances, a process in which protein binding has an important role to play, an increase in temperature results in weakened binding and in a shift in equilibrium, so that a greater fraction of the substance remains in free form, a circumstance that has a bearing on its ultimate fate in the body.

The relatively small number of studies on the impact of temperature on the kinetics of xenobiotics in the body performed so far does not permit detailed predictions for individual compounds. Yet the overall trend is beyond doubt: inhibition of life processes leads to retardation of pharmacokinetic processes, and vice versa.

A.3.6. Toxicokinetic Aspects of Interaction between Xenobiotics

Examples

In pharmacology it has long been known that one drug may strongly alter the efficiency of another in the body. In most cases such modifying effects depend on changes in the kinetic parameters of the drugs involved. Since the introduction into common practice of measurement of blood concentrations of drugs and their metabolites, many examples have accumulated to show how a chemical compound may influence the kinetics of other compounds. Here are some examples. In a study on workers occupationally exposed to the insecticides lindane and DDT, the blood half-lives of antipyrine and phenylbutazone were found to be decreased (Kolmodin-Hedman, 1974). Thus the mean half-life of antipyrine was 7.7 hr (range: 2.7 to 11.7 hr), compared with 13.1 hr (range: 5.2 to 35 hr) in the control. Table A12 gives half-life values for antipyrine* in individual subjects before and after phenobarbital administration, and it can be seen that phenobarbital reduced the time of antipyrine circulation in practically all of them.

---

* Antipyrine is a convenient compound to use in studying modifying effects in pharmacokinetics because its half-lives in the blood of healthy human beings are highly reproducible.

Table A12. Effect of Phenobarbital on Antipyrine Half-Life

| Subject | Half-life (hr) | | Percentage Decrease in Half-life |
	Before Phenobarbital	After Phenobarbital	
D. E.	13.6	9.6	29.4
A. M.	8.0	6.3	21.2
B. J.	18.2	8.4	53.8
B. F.	10.8	7.3	32.4
F. D.	12.0	10.5	14.2
P. D.	9.3	9.3	0
C. K.	17.5	5.5	68.6
N. R.	14.5	5.8	60.0
H. H.	12.3	9.2	25.2
P. M.	6.5	5.5	15.4
E. W.	15.0	6.9	54.0
E. E.	9.0	6.9	23.3

Source.   Vesell (1974a).

Figure A15 illustrates the kinetics of urinary excretion of yttrium in rats and the effect on this process of the calcium salt of ethylenediaminetetraacetic acid (Ca EDTA). Yttrium chloride was injected into a caudal vein concomitantly with Ca EDTA given intraperitoneally. It follows that Ca EDTA greatly increases yttrium excretion—and the more so, the higher its dose.

Rauws (1974) has studied the pharmacokinetics of thallium in rats after intravenous injection. Preliminary intragastric administration of Prussian blue resulted in a 1.5- to 2-fold increase in thallium elimination rate. Prussian blue also shortened the half-life of thallium from about 4 days to 2.

Numerous examples of the modifying effects of various compounds on the pharmacokinetics of antibiotics can be found in Yakovlev et al. (1976).

Causes of Modifying Effects; Some Models

There is no single cause for changes in pharmacokinetics brought about by chemical compounds. The causes are varied; some of them are fairly specific. In the above example with thallium the explanation is that in rats this metal is repeatedly released and reabsorbed through the intestinal wall (entero-enteral cycle). Prussian blue sharply reduces the efficiency of this cycle with the resultant acceleration of thallium elimination in the feces.

The more common causes of changes in kinetic parameters include, among others, interference with biotransformation processes, induction of

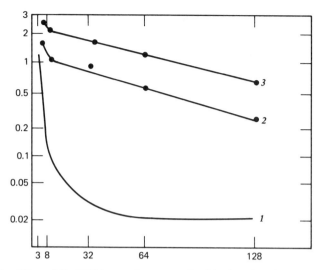

Figure A15. Effect of Ca EDTA on urinary excretion kinetics of yttrium in rats. *Ordinate,* yttrium content in urine (% of injected amount); *abscissa,* days. *1,* Excretion in the absence of complexone; *2,* excretion after a complexone dose of 10μM; *3,* excretion after a complexone dose of 200 μM. (After Bazhenov and Menshikova, 1974.)

enzymes that cross-metabolize the xenobiotics, competition among xeno-biotics for binding sites (e.g., for binding by serum albumin), interference by one xenobiotic with renal excretion of another, and complex formation. As yet there is no general theory of pharmacokinetic modification by xenobiotics, and only particular aspects of such a theory have been developed; some of these are discussed below.

Following Dettli (1974), let us express the elimination constant κ through the clearance Cl and the distribution volume V:

$$\kappa = \frac{Cl}{V} \qquad (A15)$$

Clearance in turn can be related to such parameters of glomerular filtration in the kidneys as the plasma flow rate in the glomeruli F and the filtration fraction p:

$$Cl = F \cdot p \qquad (A16)$$

Incorporating (A15) and (A16) into the simplest equation of elimination kinetics, we have

$$-\frac{dC}{dt} = \kappa C = \frac{Cl}{V} C = \frac{F \cdot p}{V} C \qquad (A17)$$

On the basis of the well-known physicochemical rule that the filtration or diffusion of one molecular species is not influenced by the presence of another noninteracting molecular species, we can state that direct interactions between substances are unlikely to occur in the process of glomerular filtration. But, as follows from (A17), this process depends on F and p, which are in turn proportional to the intraglomerular pressure and the time of contact. Therefore any substance influencing intraglomerular blood flow or pressure may be expected to influence its own elimination and that of other substances. Examples are hypotensive agents and thiazide diuretics.

In the process of tubular reabsorption, a foreign substance will gradually concentrate through removal of water and will therefore tend to diffuse back into the tubular capillaries. Such simplification is sufficient for our purposes, and no consideration will be given, for example, to active transport. It is essential, however, that direct interactions between foreign substances are as unlikely as in the case of glomerular filtration. The most important factor from the viewpoint of possibility of reabsorption is that the cellular membranes are more permeable to nonpolar than to polar molecules. Acidic or basic compounds undergo dissociation to varying degrees; the ionized moiety is usually more polar then the neutral molecule and will therefore permeate less through the tubular wall. The extent of tubular reabsorption thus depends on the degree of ionization of the xenobiotic in the tubular lumen.

According to the law of mass action the fraction of neutral molecules φ depends on the pH of the solvent. The introduction of acidifying or alkalinizing agents into the solvent will therefore affect the elimination of xenobiotics capable of electrolytic dissociation. To consider the quantitative aspect of this process, let us take a hypothetical acidic compound AH, which dissociates according to the scheme $AH \rightleftharpoons A^- + H^+$. Using the mass action law, we can write $[A^-][H^+] = K_a[AH]$, where K_a is the dissociation constant. The fraction of neutral molecules can now be expressed as

$$\varphi = \frac{[AH]}{[A^-] + [AH]} + \frac{[H^+]}{[H^+] + K_a}$$
$$= \frac{1}{1 + K_a/[H^+]} = \frac{1}{1 + 10^{pH - pK_a}}$$

$$(A18)$$

Here K_a characterizes the strength of the acid, and its value decreases with increasing strength. When $K_a = [H^+]$, $\varphi = 0.5$ (K_a is the hydrogen ion concentration at which half of the molecules of the substance are ionized; pH and pK_a are the negative logarithms of $[H^+]$ and K_a). The value of φ decreases with rising urine pH; hence the urinary excretion of acidic substances will be faster in alkaline than in acidic urine. When the urine pH is raised, say from 5 to 8 by the administration of an alkalinizing agent, we have

$$\frac{\varphi_{pH^5}}{\varphi_{pH^8}} = \frac{1 + 10^{8 - pK_a}}{1 + 10^{5 - pK_a}}$$

It follows from this equation that the effect of alkali administration on the φ ratio diminishes with increasing pK_a of the substance to become negligibly small for very weak acids ($pK_a > 8$).

The same considerations apply also to the influence of urine pH variation on the renal excretion of basic compounds ($BOH \rightleftharpoons B^+ + OH^-$).

Consider now the elimination of a xenobiotic by two independent routes, say in the urine (κ_1) and by metabolism (κ_2). In this case the overall elimination rate constant κ will be the sum of κ_1 and κ_2. If an interacting substance jointly present with the xenobiotic influences only one elimination pathway, say κ_1, its effect on the overall elimination will be of no practical consequence when $\kappa_1 \ll \kappa_2$. Thus, if $\kappa_1 = 10\%$ and $\kappa_2 = 90\%$ (i.e., $\kappa_1 = 0.1\kappa$ and $\kappa_2 = 0.9\kappa$), and κ_1 increases under the influence of the interacting substance by 100%, κ will increase by only 10%. If the reverse is true (i.e., $\kappa_1 = 0.9\kappa$ and $\kappa_2 = 0.1\kappa$), the increase in κ_1 by 100% will raise the overall rate constant κ by 90%.

Many xenobiotics are believed to be excreted into urine by a process of active transport. The role of carrier is played by macromolecules present in the tubular wall and reversibly binding xenobiotic molecules. The same is true of biliary excretion of xenobiotics. Clearly, if the transport system is nonspecific, the substances that bind to the carrier molecules will lessen the possibility of the binding of other substances. A mathematical analysis for this case is presented in Dettli (1974), as well as for the case of metabolism. Here we will merely note that the enzyme system responsible for the biotransformation of xenobiotics is unspecific. Therefore interactions among xenobiotics may affect their metabolism and, consequently, their kinetics in the body. The degree of mutual influence of two xenobiotics can be described by the equation

$$-\frac{dC_1}{dt} = \frac{v_{1,max}}{V_1} \cdot \frac{C_1}{C_1 + K_1(1 + C_2/K_2)} \tag{A19}$$

where $-(dC_1/dt)$ is the decrease in xenobiotic concentration in the body through metabolism; V_1 is the distribution volume of the xenobiotic; $v_{1,max}$ is its maximum metabolic rate (the enzyme system is saturated with the xenobiotic); K_1 is the dissociation constant of the xenobiotic-enzyme complex; C_2 is the concentration of the second foreign substance whose effect on the metabolism of the first xenobiotic is being studied; K_2 is the dissociation constant of the second substance-enzyme complex.

A well-known example of the effect of one substance on the metabolism of another is provided by the administration of ethyl alcohol in cases of acute poisoning with ethylene glycol. The toxicity of ethylene glycol is due mainly to its enzymatic conversion to oxalic acid, leading to severe crystalluria. This metabolic process is competitively inhibited by ethanol with the result that ethylene glycol is slowly eliminated unchanged.

It should be pointed out that a xenobiotic may induce enzymes which then become involved in the metabolism of that xenobiotic and of others. In describing the influence of substance 2 on the toxicokinetics of substance 1 by (A19), enzyme induction corresponds to $v_{1,max}$.

Let us turn now to the case where a substance is absorbed in a constant dose D at regular intervals τ. If the dose D is not eliminated completely during these intervals, the substance will gradually accumulate in the body. After a sufficiently large period it will reach a steady state which can be described by the equation

$$C_\infty = \frac{D/\tau}{\kappa V} \tag{A20}$$

where κ is the elimination constant, and V is the distribution volume of the substance. When a substance is eliminated by enzymatic transformation, enzyme induction may increase the value of κ and thereby lower the steady-state level of the substance in the body (C_∞). On the other hand, when the metabolism (or the tubular secretion) of substance 1 is inhibited by substance 2, κ will decrease by a factor $(1 + C_2/K_2)$, where C_2 and K_2 are as in (A19). The steady-state level will then increase in conformity with the equation

$$C_{1,\infty} = \frac{D_1/\tau}{\kappa V/(1 + C_2/K_2)} \tag{A21}$$

It should be noted, however, that the foregoing considerations are valid only when the process of enzymatic degradation is far from being saturated. As saturation phenomena appear, the elimination process no longer obeys first-order kinetics and the value of C_∞ progressively increases.

Various considerations relating to the effect of one xenobiotic on the absorption and distribution of another, to the interactions of chronically administered substances, to the kinetics of displacement of a substance from its protein binding sites by its own metabolites, and to some other facets of substance-substance interactions are contained in the papers by Dettli (1974) and Rowland (1974).

A Model for Complexone Action

An effective method of accelarating the elimination of toxic metals from the body is complexone therapy. The complexone binds the metal, preventing it from exerting its toxic action and promoting its accelerated excretion in the urine. Complexone therapy therefore depends on the interference of one xenobiotic—a nontoxic (within limits) organic compound forming reasonably stable complexes with heavy metals—with the toxicokinetics of another xenobiotic.

Following Popov and Bezel (1974), let us make logical assumptions that will allow us to construct a deterministic model of complexone action and that will reflect the behavior in the body of complexone and poison as known from previous experience. A toxic metal incorporated into the organism is assumed to be present there in two forms, labile and deposited. The first of these (C_1) can be eliminated by natural mechanisms of excretion. Physically, this is the fraction of the metal present in the blood and possibly in the interstitial and cellular fluids. The other form (C_2) is eliminated from the body only through conversion to the labile form and is the fraction of the metal residing in organs and tissues and bound to biomolecules. The complexone binds to the labile form of the metal.

The naturally occurring turnover of metal can be represented by the two-compartment model shown in graphic form on p. 147. Transferences of the metal between the compartments are described by system 50 of equations, shown on p. 148.

In the presence of a complexone the model has to be made more complex. Since the complexone is also present in two forms—free and metal-bound—we introduce two more compartments, in which the complexone is present in concentrations C_5 and C_4, respectively. Complexone action will be simulated by the four-compartment model shown in Figure A16 and allowing for the movement of both the metal and the complexone. In this model the constant k has a special role to play. It is derived on the assumption that the rate of formation of the metal-complexone complex is proportional to the product of concentrations of labile metal and free complexone, that is,

$$\frac{dC_4}{dt} = kC_1C_5 \qquad (A22)$$

The formation of such a complex in the organism is a rather complicated process depending on many factors, the main ones being the rate constant for the chemical reaction between complexone and metal (K), the constant of stability of the complex formed (K_{stab}), the complexone dose (D), and the competition for the complexone among endogenous metals (Comp); there are also

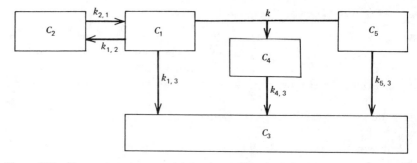

Figure A16. Four-compartment model for the modification of metal by complexone. C_1, concentration of labile metal; C_2, concentration of deposited metal; C_3, concentration of metal in excreta; C_4, concentration of metal-bound complexone; C_5, concentration of free complexone; k_{ij}, rate constants for transferences of metal or complexone among compartments and to excreta k, rate constant for formation of metal-complexone complex.

several factors of subsidiary importance. All these factors are implicit in the constant k:

$$k = f(K, K_{stab}, D, \text{Comp}, \ldots) \qquad (A23)$$

The system of equations describing changes in concentrations of the toxic metal and complexone in all compartments of the model is as follows:

$$\left. \begin{aligned} \frac{dC_1}{dt} &= -(k_{1,2} + k_{1,3})C_1 + k_{2,1}C_2 - kC_1C_5 \\[1.5em] \frac{dC_2}{dt} &= k_{1,2}C_1 - k_{2,1}C_2 \\[1.5em] \frac{dC_3}{dt} &= k_{1,3}C_1 - k_{4,3}C_4 \\[1.5em] \frac{dC_4}{dt} &= -k_{4,3}C_4 + kC_1C_5 \\[1.5em] \frac{dC_5}{dt} &= -k_{5,3}C_5 - kC_1C_5 \end{aligned} \right\} \qquad (A24)$$

Popov and Bezel (1974) used this model to describe the elimination from the body of the radioactive isotope yttrium-91 in the presence of the complexone EDTA or DTPA. Parameters for the model were determined from published data on yttrium-91 toxicokinetics in the absence of complexone and on complexone pharmacokinetics; the rate constant for elimination of the metal-complexone complex was taken to be equal to that of the complexone itself.

Under such conditions $k_{1,3} = 1.127$ days^{-1}, $k_{2,1} = 0.030$ day^{-1}, $k_{1,2} = 0.248$ day^{-1}, and $k_{4,3} = k_{5,3} = 16.6$ days^{-1}. For a particular metal, complexone, species, and so on, the factor k is, as follows from (A23), a function of complexone dose: $k = f(D)$. Using different values of k, Popov and Bezel obtained a set of solutions for system A24 with various complexone doses. The calculations were done on a computer.

The efficiency of complexone action E was determined from the relative amount of the toxic metal eliminated during 24 hr after complexone administration. The model makes it possible to estimate the efficiency of the complexone, depending on its dose and the time of its application after intake of the metal, as well as to assess the role of changes in the elimination half-life of complexone. As an example Figure A17 presents plots of this efficiency against complexone dose for different times of complexone administration.

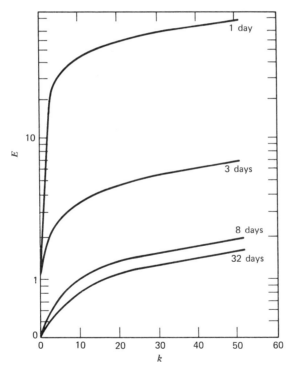

Figure A17. Dose dependence of complexone efficiency (E) at different times after complexone administration, the dose being expressed in terms of k. *Ordinate*, E (% of administered amount); figures at curves denote time of complexone administration after injection of metal. (From Popov and Bezel, 1974.)

These plots are nonlinear and show a tendency to saturation: as D increases, that is, as $k \to \infty$, $E \to E_{max}$. At E_{max} the complexone will remove all labile metal, that is to say, the metal from compartment 1, and also all of the metal that has passed from deposited to labile form over 24 hr (i.e., from compartment 2 to compartment 1):

$$E_{max} = C_1(t) + \int_t^{t+1} k_{2,1} \cdot C_2(t)dt \qquad (A25)$$

The curve E_{max} is the limiting estimate of the efficiency of any complexone.

It has been shown also that slowing the elimination of complexone from the body has the same impact on its efficiency as increasing the dose.

Mention should be made of a multicompartment model of complexone therapy for chronic mercury poisoning using meso-dimercaptosuccinic acid. The compartments of this model simulate bodily organs or systems essential for the pathogenesis of mercury intoxication, such as the blood plasma and interstitial fluids, liver, kidneys, and nervous tissues. The model is described by a system of linear differential equations:

$$\left. \begin{aligned} \frac{dC_1}{dt} &= \sum_{i=1}^{n-1} k_{i,1}C_i - \sum_{j=1}^{n-1} k_{1,j}C_1 \\ &\vdots \\ \frac{dC_n}{dt} &= \sum_{i=1}^{n-1} k_{i,n}C_i - \sum_{j=1}^{n-1} k_{n,j}C_n \end{aligned} \right\} \qquad (A26)$$

where $(n - 1)$ is the number of compartments, C_i is the mercury concentration in the ith compartment, and $k_{i,j}$ are the constants of mercury transference from the ith to jth compartment.

The complexone-mercury interaction was simulated on the basis of a commonly used equation of chemical kinetics. The dynamics of complexone in the body with different modes of administration was described by simple first-order kinetic equations.

The above model was employed to consider various regimens of complexone administration, thus making it possible to assess the efficacy of the treatment courses used.

A.3.7. Chemical Structure, Physicochemical Properties, and Toxicokinetics

Changing the structure of a molecule may of course affect not only its biological activity but also its fate in the body. If the structural modification does not involve the active site of the molecule, on which the effect of its interaction with the biological substrate depends, the main cause of biological activity modification will be a change in the transport-distribution relationships, that is, in the toxicokinetic parameters. In designing a new compound with the desired biological efficiency, consideration needs to be given to such factors as its capacity to reach the site of action; the duration of effect, which often depends on the time the substance remains in the site of action; and the rate and pathways of its removal from the body. One way to meet these requirements is to develop formulations (transport forms) of compounds or their precursors which, in the process of biotransformation, will be converted to active compounds where and when appropriate. A complete theory regarding the influence of the structure and properties of chemicals on their kinetics in the body is yet to be developed, but the relationships that are known have been treated in a systematic way in several surveys and theoretical reviews, notably in those by Ariëns (1971), Notari (1973), and Lien (1974), with special reference to the needs of pharmacology. In this section we confine ourselves to a few examples and considerations, without repeating the information contained in these publications.

A striking example of the impact that a structural change in a molecule may have on its toxicokinetics occurs when a mercury atom is inserted in the aromatic ring; sharp changes ensue in all kinetic parameters and in the distribution of the substance in the body. In particular the substance begins to show an affinity for hepatic tissue (Deckart et al., 1975). This example is among those entailing radical changes in the molecular structure, but kinetic parameters may be influenced by even relatively minor modifications involving isomerism. For example, the warfarin enantiomers have different half-lives in rats. The half-life of one of them varies in different animals from 4.9 to 9.6 hr, and that of the other, from 7.7 to 21.6 hr (Vacobi and Levy, 1974). It is interesting that the ratio of these half-lives remains strictly constant (1.87) in each individual animal.

In regard to series of congeneric compounds, regular changes in the physicochemical properties in such series (e.g., increasing the radical by adding methylene or methyl groups) entail regular changes in kinetic parameters. The relationships between properties and activity discussed in Chapter 7 serve as guidelines when looking for similar relationships between properties and toxicokinetic parameters. The as yet small number of studies along this line are cited in the publications mentioned above. In particular, a relationship has been discovered between the alkyl chain length of p-aminobenzoate esters and their ability to pass across membranes. This is a parabolic relationship similar to the one embodied in Hansch's equation for correlating biological efficiency and lipophilic character in congeneric series. Breimer and Rekker (1974) have presented parabolic equations relating the percentage absorption of xenobiotics in the body and their lipophilicity. Some of these authors' equations include other physicochemical properties along with lipophilicity.

Let us consider in some detail the relations between the absorption of xenobiotics in various animal species and man and their partition coefficients (Liublina, 1973). This question bears directly on the establishment of hygienic standards for airborne toxic substances based on data from experiments with laboratory animals.

In such an experiment it is common practice to take into account only the observed biological response, on which basis the appropriate standard is set up. Yet the process whereby the organism of a small laboratory animal is saturated with a toxic compound differs from that occurring in man. Moreover this process depends on the physicochemical properties of the inhaled substance. We will discuss here the relation between animals and man in this respect by considering the roles played by the partition coefficient λ and the elimination (degradation) rate constant κ in the saturation of the body with a volatile xenobiotic. We recall that this process depends on pulmonary ventilation, distribution volume of the substance in the body, its blood/air partition coefficient, its biotransformation rate, exposure conditions (concentration in the air and its fluctuations, duration of contact with contaminated air), and some other factors.

In Filov's review (1967) an equation is shown relating the absorption rate constant k to pulmonary ventilation V_{pulm}, partition coefficient λ, and volume of distribution V:

$$k = \frac{V_{pulm}}{\lambda V} \tag{A27}$$

If we suppose that the distribution occurs into the aqueous phase of the organism and that the substance penetrates inside the cells, an adult person weighing 70 kg may be considered to have a V of 42 liters (see p. 118). As a first approximation the distribution volume is proportional to the body

Table A13. Values of Some Parameters Characterizing Mammals of Different Weights and Affecting Toxicokinetics

Species	P (kg)	V_{pulm} (liters/min)	V (liters)	k (min^{-1})
Human adult	70	8.4	42	$0.2/\lambda$
Human infant	4	1	2.4	$0.41/\lambda$
White rat	0.2	0.113	0.12	$0.92/\lambda$
White mouse	0.025	0.0235	0.015	$1.6/\lambda$

weight of an animal in the same ratio as that for an adult human being; this means that $V = (42/70)P = 0.6P$.

Table A13 gives values of some observed or calculated parameters that characterize a human adult, a 4-kg human infant, and small laboratory animals (rat and mouse) and that are relevant to toxicokinetics. The volume of pulmonary ventilation corresponds to moderate physical exercise. It can be seen that the absorption rate constant for the human adult is 4.7 times smaller than that for the rat and eight times smaller than that for the mouse. The respective figures for the infant are 2.3 and 4. These relationships, based on approximate calculations, indicate that the saturation process in laboratory animals is substantially different from that in man.

The processes of substance accumulation in the above mammals were then calculated (Liublina, 1973) using (26) (see p. 131) for different values of λ (1, 10, 100, 1000, 10,000) and of κ ($\kappa = 0$, $\kappa = 0.01k$, $\kappa = 0.1k$, $\kappa = k$, $\kappa = 10k$, $\kappa = 100k$). The results are illustrated in Figure A18, where the accumulation of substance in man with 7-hr exposure is compared to that in the rat and mouse with 4-hr exposure, that is, the period of exposure commonly used in chronic toxicity tests designed to establish a maximum allowable concentration in the air of work areas.*

It follows from Figure A18, which consists of four sets of curves, that the 4-hr exposure of laboratory animals is quite sufficient for this purpose. At λ values of 100 or more, the concentration of a substance with $\kappa \leq k$ that has accumulated in the human body after 7 hr will be considerably lower than that in the rat after 4 hr and much lower than that in the mouse after the same period. As the degradation rate constant κ increases, the value of λ has to be progressively greater to assure the absence of difference in accumulation between mouse and man. Thus, whereas for slowly metabolized substances ($\kappa \leq k$) a λ value of 100 is associated with a large difference in accumulation between man and laboratory animals, for substances having $\kappa = 10k$ and the same λ (100) this difference is insignificant, and for those with $\kappa = 100k$ there is no difference even at $\lambda = 1000$. Hence it may be concluded that for substances with $\kappa \leq k$ a value of $\lambda \geq 100$ should determine a substantially different degree of accumulation in man than in experimental animals. In such cases the experimenter has an additional safety margin, for he considers that the test substance may be toxic for animals because more of it will have accumulated over 4 hr than in man over 7 hr of exposure. The higher the λ value, the greater is this safety margin.

---

* These calculations are of course very approximate, since different media of the body have different partition coefficients in respect to air. If the substance is sufficiently fat-soluble, it continues to saturate the fat depots long after the arterial blood has been rapidly saturated. Nevertheless such calculations give an idea of the relative times taken to saturate man and experimental animals.

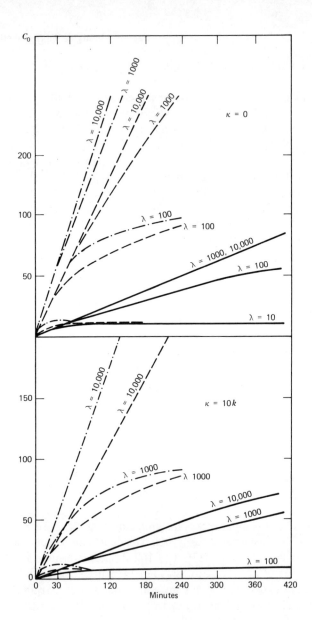

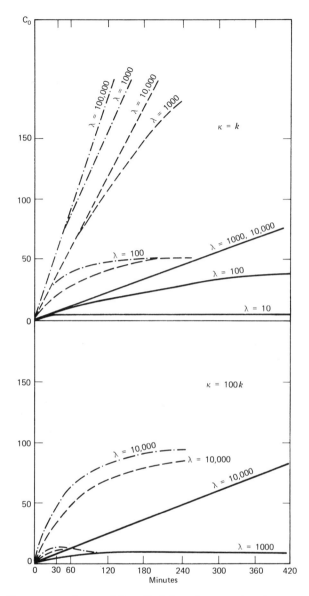

Figure A18. Time courses of accumulation of substance in man, rat, and mouse, with different values of the partition coefficient (λ) in the case of inhalation of inert gas or vapor ($\kappa = 0$) and the inhalation of vapors of substances having $\kappa = k$, $\kappa = 10k$, and $\kappa = 100k$. *Abscissa*, exposure time; *ordinate*, concentrations in the body as multiples of concentration in air (C_0). Solid lines refer to adult man; dashed lines, to rat; and dot-and-dash lines to mouse. The lower line in each group of plots is formed by superimposing the curves for man, rat, and mouse.

217

A4. SOME MORE PARTICULAR ASPECTS OF TOXICOKINETICS

This section contains examples of toxicokinetic studies and of the application of kinetics to problems of industrial toxicology. The examples selected are not representative of the main tasks or of any particular system in this area of research and are intended only as illustrations of toxicokinetics.

A.4.1. Examples of Studies on the Toxicokinetics of Heavy Radioactive Elements

Studies on the kinetics of passage through the body of heavy radioactive isotopes (including the transuranic ones) with various routes of absorption constitute an important area of work in the establishment of hygienic standards.

An example of a detailed study is that of Pavlovskaya et al. (1974) on the kinetics of isotopes of the thorium series (thorium-228, radium-224, and lead-212). Rats were given, by intragastric intubation, 10^{-6} Ci/kg of thorium-228 chloride in equilibrium with the daughter radionuclides, and bone, liver, kidneys, spleen, and blood were assayed for these three radionuclides 3, 6, 12, 48, and 72 hr and 30 days thereafter, using a gamma spectrometer for the determinations.

No equilibrium between the radionuclides was found to occur in the organs and tissues during the first 3 days after dosing. Thorium-228 absorption occurred into bone tissue almost exclusively. Radium-224 was likewise taken up mainly by bone, where its level was about 3-, 20-, 50-, and 50-fold as high as in the kidneys, spleen, blood, and liver, respectively. The highest level of lead-212 occurred in the kidneys. Taking the content of lead-212 in the kidneys 6 hr postadministration as 100, its contents in the liver, bone, blood, and spleen were, respectively, 32, 23, 14, and 1. Blood absorption of the radionuclides continued for 3 to 6 hr postadministration.

The observed disequilibration was due primarily to differences in the absorption of the radionuclides from the gastrointestinal tract, as well as to their different affinities for the tissues studied.

As an illustration, Figure A19 shows the time courses of the radionuclides in bone tissue. Curves for the absorption and elimination of isotopes from the skeleton and various organs, coupled with data on their levels in the blood, make it possible, on the one hand, to represent these processes in the form of kinetic equations (as was done by the authors) and, on the other, to gain a clear idea of their transit through the organism. Thus, in the study under consideration, the elimination of lead-212 from the blood was described by a three-exponential curve, with $^{1}T_{0.5} = 11$ hr, $^{2}T_{0.5} = 38$ hr, and $^{3}T_{0.5} = 10$

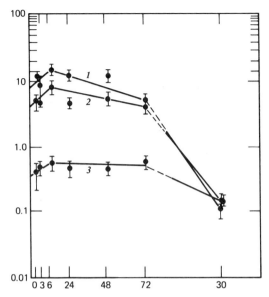

Figure A19. Time courses for absorption in and elimination from rat skeleton of ^{228}Th. (*3*), ^{224}Ra. (*1*), and ^{212}Pb. (*2*) after intragastric introduction of thorium chloride equilibrated with daughter radionuclides. *Abscissa*, 0 to 72 hr; 30 days. *Ordinate*, content of isotopes (% of administered amount).

days. The slowing of clearance is associated with lead redistribution in the body. Lead clearance from the liver in the interval between 3 hr and 30 days was described by a similar curve with $^1T_{0.5} = 15$ hr, $^2T_{0.5} = 36$ hr, and $^3T_{0.5} = 6$ to 7 days. Renal excretion of radium-224 6 hr postadministration was a biexponential function: $Q = 2.46e^{-1.2t} + 0.53e^{-0.2t}$, and so on.

Chronic exposure to an isotope makes it possible to determine the onset of equilibrium and the extent of the isotope accumulation in organs and tissues. One example is a study on the dynamics of curium-244 accumulation in tissues with chronic administration for 256 days into the stomach (Semenov, 1975) and subcutaneously (Moskalev et al., 1974). Figure A20 shows curves of curium accumulation in the liver and skeleton, drawn by us from Semenov's data. It can be seen that the curium-244 attained a steady-state concentration in the liver by day 64. The same was true of its uptake into the kidneys, lungs, spleen, and muscles, via both routes of administration. Accumulation in the skeleton, however, by far exceeded that in the other tissues and is very unlikely to have attained a steady state by day 256. At the same time the theoretically calculated accumulation of curium-244 as a multiple of its dose was in accord with experimental data only for the liver and kidneys,

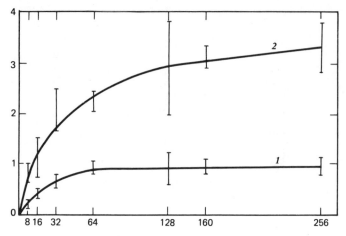

Figure A20.   Accumulation kinetics of ^{244}Cu. in rat liver (*1*) and skeleton (*2*) with chronic administration. *Abscissa*, days of administration; *ordinate*, tissue content (% of daily dose).

not for the skeleton. This may be explained by changes that occur in the sorptive properties of bone under the impact of radiation and of the isotope already taken up.

Since radioactive isotopes can penetrate the blood through intact skin and may be retained for a long time in the surface skin layer, the study of skin clearance from isotopes is of considerable importance. Simakov et al. (1976) studied the elimination from skin of alpha emitters in experiments with young pigs, whose skin is most similar to human skin both morphologically and physiologically. A curve of neptunium-237 clearance from skin is shown in Figure A21. This curve was used to calculate two elimination half-lives of neptunium. The rapidly eliminated fraction of the isotope (40%) is removed from the skin to the environment with a half-life of less than 24 hr. The slowly eliminated fraction (60%) is removed to the organism and has a half-life of 20 days. Table A14 compares relevant toxicokinetic parameters of four alpha emitters.

A.4.2.   The Toxicokinetics of Mercury

Although mercury is one of the most ancient poisons, whose toxicology could be expected to have been thoroughly studied by the present time, it continues to receive the attention of research toxicologists. Among a number of complex problems of mercury biology is the relationship between the

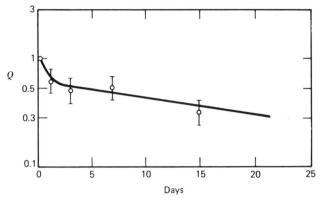

Figure A21. Decline of ^{237}Np. in pig skin with time. Q, relative proportion of ^{237}Np. in skin.

amount of mercury excreted in the urine and its content in the air of work areas. Attempts to develop an exposure test for mercury from urinary excretion data have met with failure. Yet mercury is known to concentrate in the kidneys to a greater extent and to be retained there longer than elsewhere in the body.

The possible reasons for such failure are discussed in detail by Piotrowski (1971), who points out, in particular, the possibility of mercury binding in the organism (including the blood) in the form of various compounds having different kinetic parameters and showing wide interindividual differences, both quantitative and qualitative; a further factor is said to be the dose dependence of mercury toxicokinetics related to possible renal function impairment.

Table A14. Half-Lives for Elimination of Alpha Emitters from the Skin and the Proportion of Their Rapidly (*1*) and Slowly (*2*) Eliminated Fractions

Emitter	Half-life of (*1*) (hr)	Half-life of (*2*) (days)	Proportion of (*1*)	Proportion of (*2*)
^{210}Po	24	15	0.7	0.3
^{237}Np	24	20	0.4	0.6
^{239}Pu	13	5	0.8	0.2
^{241}Am	13	5	0.8	0.2

Source. Simakov et al. (1976).

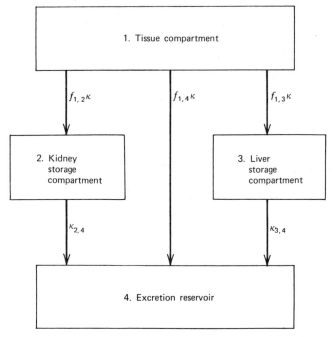

Figure A22. Four-compartment model for the elimination of mercury from the body. See text for explanation. (After Cember, 1969.)

Confining ourselves to the kinetic aspect of the problem, let us consider a model of mercury elimination from the body (Cember, 1969) which is pertinent to the preceding discussion. The postulated model is shown schematically in Figure A22. It has four compartments: a central compartment, 1 (tissues), that includes all body organs and tissues except the kidneys and liver; a long-term storage compartment, 2 (the kidneys), from which the stored mercury is cleared slowly; a short-term storage compartment, 3 (the liver); and an excretion reservoir compartment, 4, in which both urinary and fecal mercury accumulates. The mercury leaves the central compartment by three parallel pathways: to the long-term storage compartment to the excretion reservoir; to the short-term storage compartment to the excretion reservoir; and directly to the excretion reservoir. The direct path includes filtration in the kidneys, biliary secretion, and secretion by the intestinal mucosa. Denote the total initial amount of mercury in compartment 1 by D (which is equal to the dose injected, e.g., intraperitoneally); the amounts of it in the four compartments by Q_1, Q_2, Q_3, and Q_4; and the fractions of it cleared from the central compartment by the three pathways by $f_{1,2}, f_{1,3}$, and $f_{1,4}$, with $f_{1,2} + f_{1,3} +$

$f_{1,4} = 1$. Finally, $\kappa_{2,4}$ and $\kappa_{3,4}$ are the constants of mercury clearance from the kidneys and liver, respectively, and κ is the constant of mercury elimination from the central compartment.

If the transfer of mercury to the compartments is assumed to be governed by first-order kinetics, the toxicokinetics of mercury in the model is described by the following system of differential equations:

$$
\left.
\begin{aligned}
\frac{dQ_1}{dt} &= -\kappa Q_1 \\[2mm]
\frac{dQ_2}{dt} &= f_{1,2}\kappa Q_1 - \kappa_{2,4}Q_2 \\[2mm]
\frac{dQ_3}{dt} &= f_{1,3}\kappa Q_1 - \kappa_{3,4}Q_3 \\[2mm]
\frac{dQ_4}{dt} &= f_{1,4}\kappa Q_1 + \kappa_{2,4}Q_2 + \kappa_{3,4}Q_3
\end{aligned}
\right\}
\tag{A28}
$$

This system can be solved by setting the initial conditions: at $t = 0$, $Q_1 = D$, and $Q_2 = Q_3 = Q_4 = 0$. In general form the solutions to the differential equations are as follows:

$$
\left.
\begin{aligned}
Q_1 &= De^{-\kappa t} \\[2mm]
Q_2 &= \frac{Df_{1,2}\kappa}{\kappa_{2,4} - \kappa}(e^{-\kappa t} - e^{-\kappa_{2,4}t}) \\[2mm]
Q_3 &= \frac{Df_{1,3}\kappa}{\kappa_{3,4} - \kappa}(e^{-\kappa t} - e^{-\kappa_{3,4}t}) \\[2mm]
Q_4 &= D\Bigg[\left(f_{1,4} + \frac{f_{1,2}\kappa_{2,4}}{\kappa_{2,4} - \kappa} + \frac{f_{1,3}\kappa_{3,4}}{\kappa_{3,4} - \kappa}\right)(1 - e^{-\kappa t}) \\[2mm]
&\quad + \frac{f_{1,2}\kappa}{\kappa - \kappa_{2,4}}(1 - e^{-\kappa_{2,4}t}) + \frac{f_{1,3}\kappa}{\kappa - \kappa_{3,4}}(1 - e^{-\kappa_{3,4}t})\Bigg]
\end{aligned}
\right\}
\tag{A29}
$$

The numerical values of the toxicokinetic parameters were estimated by Cember from his previously published experimental data on the mercury contents in rat organs and excreta measured over a period of 70 days after a single injection of mercury in the form of nitrate. The parameters determined from these data had the following values: $f_{1,2} = 0.45$; $f_{1,3} = 0.16$; $f_{1,4} = 0.39$;

$\kappa = 0.46$ day^{-1}; $\kappa_{2,4} = 0.035$ day^{-1}; and $\kappa_{3,4} = 0.31$ day^{-1}. Inserting the parameter values in (A29) yields the concrete numerical expressions of the equations for the rat. In particular, the overall urinary and fecal excretion of mercury is given by

$$Q_4 = D[0.02(1 - e^{-0.46t}) + 0.48(1 - e^{-0.035t}) + 0.49(1 - e^{-0.31t})] \quad (A30)$$

The total amount of mercury in the rat at any time is equal to the sum of the contents in the individual compartments: $Q = Q_1 + Q_2 + Q_3$. Substituting the values for Q_1, Q_2, and Q_3 into this equation from (A29) and inserting the numerical values for the parameters, we have

$$Q = D[e^{-0.46t} + 0.48(e^{-0.035t} - e^{-0.46t}) + 0.49(e^{-0.31t} - e^{-0.46t})] \quad (A31)$$

Equations A30 and A31 make it possible to test the model experimentally. For this purpose Cember (1969) injected rats with a single intrapetitoneal dose of ^{203}Hg-tagged mercuric chloride at dose levels of 25, 50, and 100 μg mercury kg body weight. The total elimination of mercury in the urine and feces, followed for 23 days after these different doses, was found to occur in conformity with (A30). Similarly, the decline of mercury in the rat body occurred in accordance with (A31).

The model just discussed differs from one that could be used to simulate the process of mercury passage through the human body upon inhalation of mercury/vapors. Such a model has yet to be developed. The above model, however, may be found useful for this purpose; moreover, it is valuable per se in that it draws attention, for example, to the intestinal excretion of mercury.

In Cember's model the central compartment includes all organs and tissues save the liver and kidneys which are directly involved in excretion. The kinetics of mercury clearance from individual tissues is also of interest. According to Iverson et al. (1973), who studied mercury clearance from 17 different tissues in the guinea pig, this process is well described by a biexponential curve whose kinetic characteristics were found to be fairly similar for all the tissues sampled. The rapid phase of excretion occurred with a $T_{0.5}$ of 2 to 3 days, and the slow phase, with a $T_{0.5}$ of 15 to 16 days, $T_{0.5}$ being independent of dose in the dose range 1 to 10 mg/kg of mercury administered orally. The distribution of mercury in the body was nonuniform. Its level was highest in the kidneys and lowest in the blood, the difference being about 200-fold.

Somewhat in contrast to this, Matsubara-Khan (1974) has found that the elimination of subcutaneously administered mercury from most organs in the mouse* can be satisfactorily described by a monoexponential expression.

---

* The behavior of mercury in the mouse is similar to that in the guinea pig.

It cannot be ruled out, however, that a biexponential model may be applicable in that case too (Matsubara-Khan presents only the conclusions reached, without adducing numerical experimental data).

A.4.3.   Trichloroethylene and Its Metabolites

In view of the wide application of trichloroethylene in various industries, its metabolic fate has been the object of much research. In particular, many authors tried to develop exposure tests that could be used to judge the level of exposure to trichloroethylene from urinary excretion data on its metabolites (these studies were reviewed by Gadaskina and Filov, 1971). The attempts met with little success, however, for reasons that have been partly disclosed by studying the toxicokinetics of trichloroethylene and its metabolites.

The main pathway of trichloroethylene biotransformation is the formation of unstable chloral hydrate; this rapidly yields trichloroethanol, which is partly eliminated in the urine as glucuronide and partly converted to trichloroacetic acid, which is likewise excreted in the urine:

$$Cl_2C=CHCl \longrightarrow Cl_3C-CH=O \cdot H_2O \longrightarrow Cl_3C-CH_2OH$$

trichloroethylene $\qquad$ chloral hydrate $\qquad$ trichloroethanol

$$\longrightarrow Cl_3C-COOH$$

trichloroacetic acid

$$Cl_3C-CH_2-O-C_6H_9O_6$$

trichloroethanol glucuronide

A clear understanding of the dynamic relationships between trichloroethylene and its metabolites in the body can be gained from the paper of Müller et al. (1974), who investigated the kinetics of these compounds in man. After administration of trichloroethylene, chloral hydrate, or trichloroethanol, the decline of blood concentration of trichloroethanol followed a similar pattern in all three cases and was described by an exponential equation; the average half-life in the blood was 13 hr (range: 12.4 to 14.3 hr). In contrast, the equation for the blood concentration decline of trichloroacetic acid, as well as its half-life, depended on the precursor used. The results are shown in Table A15. The urinary excretion of trichloroacetic acid was likewise precursor-dependent and followed a similar pattern.

One should agree with Müller et al. in that the observed dependence of trichloroacetic acid elimination on the precursor and dosing regimen is determined by the fate of the precursor, its capacity for retention in tissues, the duration of its circulation in body fluids, and so on. It follows, then, that

Table A15. Elimination of Trichloroacetic Acid from Human Blood after Inhalation of Trichloroethylene or Parenteral Administration of Chloral Hydrate, Trichloroethanol, or Sodium Trichloroacetate

What and How Administered	Regression Equation	Half-life (hr)	Equation Number	Significance of Difference between Equation in Preceding Column and Equation			
				2	3	4	5
Trichloroethylene, 50 ppm, 6 hr daily for 5 days	$y = -0.0070x + 4.027$	99.0	1	$p > .1$	$p < .005$	$p < .005$	$p < .001$
Trichloroethylene, 100 ppm, 6 hr daily for 10 days	$y = -0.0081x + 4.615$	85.6	2		$p < .005$	$p > .1$	$p < .005$
Chloral hydrate, 15 mg/kg	$y = -0.0111x + 3.874$	62.5	3			$p > .1$	$p > .1$
Trichloroethanol, 10 mg/kg	$y = -0.0106x + 3.333$	65.4	4				$p > .1$
Sodium trichloroacetate, 3 mg/kg	$y = -0.0137x + 3.195$	50.6	5				

Source. Müller et al. (1974).

neither the urinary excretion of trichloroacetic acid nor the overall elimination of both metabolites can provide a quantitative basis for judging what the previous exposure to trichloroethylene has been in a situation where its concentration in the work environment fluctuates during a working day and from day to day, as it does in practice. In experiments on rats Garrett and Lambert (1973) found the toxicokinetic parameters of trichloroacetic acid and its precursors to depend appreciably also on hematocrit value, amount and composition of blood proteins, and other variables.

A5. ENVIRONMENTAL TOXICOKINETICS (ECOLOGICAL TOXICOKINETICS)

Before coming into contact with and acting on living organisms, chemical agents spread in the environment from natural or anthropogenic sources. Today the latter sources predominate; moreover, an overwhelming majority of chemical compounds now circulating in the biosphere are man-made and do not occur naturally on our planet. One example is the various pesticides. Research into the time-related migration of compounds in the environment has become a major challenge, for it underlies the practical task of reducing as much as possible the impact of compounds on man at present and in future. An important part of this research is the quantitative mathematical description of migrational processes. For this purpose use can be made of the mathematical tools of kinetics as applied to toxic compounds foreign to the organism, that is to say, of toxicokinetics.

With these considerations in mind we can take a wider view of toxicokinetics than we have done hitherto by regarding it as consisting of two parts: individual toxicokinetics, whose objects of study are man and animals (only this part has been considered here so far), and environmental toxicokinetics. Environmental toxicokinetics—a concept introduced by Ariëns (1969)—may also be called ecological toxicokinetics. Alternatively, one could avoid the term "toxicokinetics" by using, say, "migrational kinetics" instead to mean the same thing.

Environmental toxicokinetics is the kinetics of distribution and conversion of toxic chemicals in the biosphere. It deals not with individuals but with populations and complexes of populations in their environment, which includes the air, soil, surface waters and groundwaters, as well as other types of biomass.

Among the main problems of concern to environmental toxicokinetics are the long-term exposure to low concentrations (sometimes extending throughout the lifetime of individuals) and the associated long-continued accumulation of substances in the tissues of biological objects, as well as the multiplicity and complexity of various exposures.

The basic method of mathematical modeling of environmental toxicokinetics is compartmental analysis, which permits the creation of a model for the environment whereby processes of transfer of chemical agents can be described mathematically. By way of example consider briefly a model for mercury toxicokinetics in the soil and atmosphere (Abramovsky et al., 1976).

The premise underlying the system of interrelated compartments in this model is that the sources of mercury in the biosphere are, first, the naturally occurring soil and rock weathering processes (q_{nat}) and, second, the anthropogenic processes resulting from human economic activities (q_{anthr}). The model then appears as shown in Figure A23, where Q denotes the amounts of mercury in the different media, τ with subscripts denotes the times of mercury elimination from soil (s) and atmosphere (a) to water (w) and of mercury transfer between soil and atmosphere, k is the fraction of anthropogenic mercury entering the atmosphere, and f is the fraction of mercury transferred from atmosphere to soil. Mercury accumulates in the aqueous medium. In this model the mercury balance is described by three differential equations that are mathematical models of mercury environmental toxicokinetics:

$$
\left.
\begin{aligned}
\frac{dQ_a}{dt} &= kq_{anthr} + \frac{Q_s + Q_s^{anthr}}{\tau_{sa}} - \frac{Q_a}{\tau_a} \\[2mm]
\frac{dQ_s}{dt} &= q_{nat} + f\frac{Q_a}{\tau_a} - \frac{Q_s}{\tau_{sa}} - \frac{Q_s}{\tau_{sw}} \\[2mm]
\frac{dQ_s^{anthr}}{dt} &= (1 - k)q_{anthr} - \frac{Q_s^{anthr}}{\tau_{sa}} - \frac{Q_s^{anthr}}{\tau_{sw}}
\end{aligned}
\right\}
\qquad \text{(A32)}
$$

To be able to use these equations for calculating mercury accumulation and thus for forecasting global and local mercury contamination, the parameters of the model must first be evaluated. Such evaluation is a highly important step and requires, on the one hand, field measurements of mercury in the different media, as well as information on its global amounts, and, on the other, the application of boundary and initial conditions. Here only the main premises used in determining the parameters will be indicated.

A logical initial condition is the absence of anthropogenic sources. If $q_{anthr} = 0$, the system is in equilibrium:

$$
\frac{Q_a^0}{\tau_a} = \frac{Q_s^0}{\tau_{sa}}
\qquad \text{(A33)}
$$

Consideration of the balance gives

$$
f\frac{Q_a^0}{\tau_a} + q_{nat} = \frac{Q_s^0}{\tau_{sa}} + \frac{Q_s^0}{\tau_{sw}}
\qquad \text{(A34)}
$$

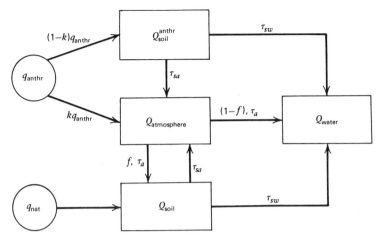

Figure A23. A compartmental model for the movement of mercury in the environment. See text for explanation.

and, from (A33) and (A34),

$$q_{\text{nat}} = \frac{Q_s^0}{\tau_{sw}} + (1 - f)\frac{Q_a^0}{\tau_a} \tag{A35}$$

To estimate q_{nat}, the two terms on the right side of (A35) must of course be determined. The first of these was estimated for the Lake of Baikal and gave a value of $\approx 4.8 \times 10^3$ tons/year. From measurements of mercury contents in the air above continents and oceans and from data on the distribution of this element by height and in areas of industrial emissions, it was found that $Q_a \approx 3.5 \times 10^2$ tons, $Q_a^0 \approx 3 \times 10^2$ tons; the estimate for soil was $Q_s^0 \approx 4 \times 10^6$ tons. When these estimates are used, $q_{\text{nat}} \approx 7 \times 10^3$ tons/year. From the same equations, $\tau_{sw} \approx 9 \times 10^2$ years and $\tau_{sa} \approx 4 \times 10^2$ years; from field measurements, $\tau_a \approx 3 \times 10^{-2}$ years; f was taken to be 0.8 and $0 \leq k \leq 1$.

Once the parameter values are known, practical calculations of global mercury toxicokinetics can be undertaken. Without delving into these calculations, we will give only their main result. Considering that the maximum allowable concentration of mercury in the ambient air is 3×10^{-7} g/m^3 (in the USSR), it has been shown from the above model that, in order for this concentration to be exceeded, the anthropogenic mercury emissions will have to be increased by two orders of magnitude, that is, to exceed the present level by a hundred times. A much less optimistic conclusion is reached, however, if one takes into account other media in addition to the atmosphere.

Indeed, the mercury contents in local bodies of water may well exceed the permissible levels even at the present rate of q_{anthr} emission to the atmosphere. Without polluting the atmosphere itself to impermissible levels, the atmospheric emissions of mercury may create health hazards by contaminating soils and, especially, water bodies.

Mathematical methods as applied to environmental toxicokinetics have already received well-deserved recognition in the pesticide area in connection with the wide use of pesticides and because of the availability of data on their migration from zones of application to the environment and on their fates, as determined by meteorological and other environmental factors (Spynu and Ivanova, 1976). Some rewarding results have been reported, and the mathematical models employed for this purpose suggest that environmental toxicokinetics is successfully developing.

Worthy of consideration in this context is the paper, now more than 10 years old, by Robinson (1967), devoted to the toxicokinetics of organochlorine pesticides in ecological systems and discussing principles of modeling with reference to the content of foreign substance in animal tissues and in ecosystems. The proposed model is based on postulates consistent with experimental evidence and very similar to those used in the individual toxicokinetics discussed above. The first postulate is that the concentration of organochlorine pesticides in any tissue is a function of the daily intake. For a particular compound, it can be written as $C_{\alpha i} = f_{\alpha i}(a)$, where $C_{\alpha i}$ is the concentration of the compound in the ith tissue of an animal of species α, and a is the daily intake. The next postulate concerns the distribution relationships in the body and states that the concentrations in different tissues are functionally related: $C_{\alpha i} = f'_{\alpha i k}(C_{\alpha k})$, where i and k refer to different tissues.

Furthermore, the pesticide concentrations in the tissues of course depend on the time of exposure: $C_{\alpha i} = f''_{\alpha i}(t)$. This, as we know, is a curvilinear relationship that tends to an upper limit with increasing t. Also, the concentration $C_{\alpha i}$ can have a maximum. Its decline with t may depend on many factors (these are discussed in Section A3), for example, on the induction of xenobiotic-degrading enzymes.

When exposure ceases, the rates of decrease in concentration in the tissues at a given time are proportional to the concentrations at that time:

$$\frac{d(C_{\alpha i})}{dt} = -f'''_{\alpha i}(C_{\alpha i})$$

An ecosystem may be defined as the sum total of living organisms and abiotic components in an area which interact to produce an exchange of materials and energy between the living and nonliving components. The living organisms can be divided into three main groups: the producers (autotrophic organisms), the consumers (heterotrophic organisms), and the decomposers (saprophytes), which are heterotrophs that break down complex compounds of dead protoplasm and release simpler compounds that may be used by the autotrophs. The interaction among these groups thus conditions a cyclic exchange of matter and energy within the ecosystem. The latter may be regarded as a certain supersystem, with the trophic levels corresponding to the producers, consumers, and decomposers. Individual species form subsystems of the trophic levels, and individual organisms are members of these subsystems.

The total biomass in a given trophic level is $\sum_{jk} m_{ijk}$, and the content of a particular pesticide in this level is $\sum_{jk} m_{ijk} x_{ijk}$, where m_{ijk} is the body weight of the kth member of the jth species in the ith trophic level, and x_{ijk} is the average concentration of the pesticide in the body of this individual. At a given instant of time the total amount of the pesticide in the ecosystem is $(\sum_{ijk} m_{ijk} x_{ijk} + W)$, where W is the mass of the pesticide within the abiotic components (soil, water, air). The total mass of the pesticide in the ith trophic level may increase through transfer from the $(i - 1)$th trophic level and may decrease either by degradation or by transfer to the $(i + 1)$th level.

The total biomass in the ith level may increase as a result of migration into the ecosystem, reproduction, and growth of the organisms in that level. The main factors responsible for decreases in the biomass are migration from the ecosystem, death of individuals, and loss of weight through starvation. Precise information on these processes is usually lacking. Nevertheless a model can be constructed if the ecosystem is regarded as a black box with transfer functions defined as the ratio between the input and output of mass or energy or pesticide residues; the trophic levels may be regarded as compartments of the black box.

Changes in the biomass will have concomitant effects on the total mass of the pesticides. For example, migration of individuals from the ecosystem will decrease both the biomass and the pesticide mass in their trophic level. Growth of organisms will increase the biomass, and the food required for growth may result in a transfer of pesticides to the level where such growth occurs. The death of individuals will decrease the biomass in the ith level with a concurrent reduction in the mass of the pesticide. The pesticide will eventually be incorporated into the saprophytes (with or without some degradation) or returned to the abiotic components.

Suppose that the transfer of biomass from the $(i - 1)$th level in time Δt to the ith level, as a result of activities of the consumers in the latter level, is given by $\sum_{jk} \Delta m_{(i-1)jk}$, and let the increase in biomass in the ith level consequent to this consumption be given by $\sum_{ik} \Delta m_{ijk}$. Then $\sum_{jk} \Delta m_{(i-1)jk} > \sum_{jk} \Delta m_{ijk}$, which involves losses. The higher the ecologic productivity, the smaller is this inequality. The amount of the pesticide in the ith trophic level is $(\sum_{jk} \Delta m_{(i-1)jk} - \sum_{jk} \Delta m_{ijk}) x_{(i-1)jk}$. The concentration in the ith level will rise unless the rate of loss of the pesticide from that level is equal to or greater than the rate of gain. The rate of loss from the ith level is a function of the concentration in that level (losses depend on biochemical degradation or the death of organisms): $dx_{ijk}/dt = -m(x_{ijk})$. This relationship is of course much more complex than one describing the elimination of substance from tissues.

The foregoing consideration is general enough to be taken as a basis for modeling. In Robinson's view this could be helpful in interpreting the ecological implications of the use of organochlorine pesticides and their consequent occurrence in the environment. It is evident, however, that great care should be exercised in arriving at conclusions about the behavior of pesticides in ecosystems, for such conclusions may well be based on small numbers of observations or on data regarding differences between samples from different trophic levels collected at different times.

The environment is highly varied and complex. The application of the principles of compartmental analysis permits the creation of mathematical models to describe environmental toxicokinetics. But even the simplest compartmental models, which disregard many factors of subsidiary importance, lead to fairly complex equations which as a rule cannot be solved analytically. To solve such equations recourse must be had to numerical methods using a computer. There are at least two aspects of computer application. First, it is possible to solve equations based on the sum total of the available factual (experimental, hygienic) data. Second, an analogue computer can represent a compartment model with all its intrinsic relationships. Toxicokinetics can then be computer simulated, and the result obtained can be either put to immediate use as appropriate or, preferably, compared to the available data about the process concerned. If the comparison yields divergent results, the simulated compartmental system is inadequate for the purpose at hand. This may happen because the postulates underlying the model are unduly simple or faulty. The model will then have to be revised, and the revised version again represented by computer, and so on (iterative procedure). The repeated running of the model enables one to attain the required degree of representation of the real toxicokinetic system. In the process of such machine experimentation many aspects of the problem can be formulated more precisely or clarified to the point where even the problem itself may have to be restated. Only very simple problems, whether pertaining to environmental or individual toxicokinetics, can be solved without recourse to a computer.

A6. THE DYNAMICS OF UPTAKE OF XENOBIOTICS INTO TISSUES: ELEMENTS OF A THEORY

A theory of the dynamics of uptake of xenobiotics into tissues should formulate the most general relationships governing this process and applicable to all cases. This theory should provide a methodological basis for solving various problems, including practical ones, relating to the accumulation of exogenous compounds in tissues.

A theory that would satisfy the above requirements is rather difficult to construct because the biological objects themselves—the various bodily tissues—are highly complex structures whose functional characteristics (e.g., sorptive properties) depends on many variables, including the often elusive effects of regulatory mechanisms. Complexity of the object should not, however, preclude efforts aimed at developing such a theory. Clearly, an analytical approach is appropriate here, that is, a mental simplification of the object and its characteristics, followed by a description of the simplified variant. The simplified model must nevertheless reflect all the essential features of the object. Subsequently the model may be made more complex to any desired degree, imparting to it additional, previously discarded attributes and approximating it to the real object. One reservation needs to be made: the model should be made more sophisticated by including in it only qualities of significance for the construction of the theory, omitting those known to be of minor importance.

Mention should be made of a highly interesting book by Lightfoot (1974) on mass transport phenomena in living systems, where a theory of these phenomena is evolved from the perspective of physiology. Although the transfer of xenobiotics is not specifically considered, in many cases the concepts expounded are applicable to xenobiotics as well. We refer to the concept of mass transfer across membranes, including biomembranes, and that of convective mass transfer. One of our earlier publications (Filov, 1970) was devoted to a consideration of the elements of a theory of xenobiotic uptake in tissues based on concepts of sorption in a volume. These elements are presented below in a somewhat modified form.

When one considers the movement of a substance to the site of action in a target tissue, it is possible to distinguish at least two phases of this process. One is the movement of the substance to the tissue in the bloodstream. The other is its penetration into and its retention in the tissue, that is, its sorption. The causes or mechanisms of sorption are varied. It may be a physical absorption or a chemisorption determined by particular chemical interactions. Insofar as we are interested in the dynamics of substance uptake in the tissue, we may, to a first approximation, disregard the mechanism of sorption and treat sorption as a single process resulting in loss of the substance from the blood and its gain in the tissue. (The gain of substance implies a more or less firm binding of it to the tissue structures.)

The analysis which follows is in no way concerned with the first of the two phases mentioned above, which is a subject to be dealt with by the kinetics of substance distribution in the body. We made an attempt to describe the basic dynamics of substance uptake in the living tissue, supposing that the substance spreads within a given tissue from the capillaries which permeate the tissue or bathe areas thereof. For such a description we drew on the ideas and methods underlying the theory of sorption dynamics as described by Rachinsky (1964) and Timofeyev (1962). This considers tissue as a macroscopically homogeneous medium with isotropic properties. A substance is introduced into the tissue in the capillary blood flow, the blood being regarded as the mobile phase, to use a term from physicochemical kinetics. Similarly, structures of the tissue proper that sorb the substance by virtue of certain physical or chemical forces are regarded as the immobile phase. The proposed model has broad analogies in medicine and biology: take any organ (liver, thyroid, etc.) or any tissue (muscle, brain, tumor, etc.).

The main premises rendering the model amenable to a relatively simple mathematical description are the following. Consideration is confined to substances that are degraded very slowly (if at all). Degradation can then be neglected, for it will not occur for a reasonably long time postsorption. This, however, applies only to the bulk of substance molecules and not to a very small portion of substance, that portion being the smaller the slower the degradation rate. It is further assumed that only one substance having a low concentration is transferred from blood to tissue and that the blood-tissue system has a constant temperature.

We are now in a position to draw up an equation of substance balance in the model. It is more convenient to use the rectangular coordinates x, y, and z, introducing first the following designations. As usual, t is the time; n is the volume concentration of substance in the blood per unit volume of tissue; m is the volume concentration of substance within the tissue proper (i.e., in the immobile phase), also per unit volume of tissue; $\mathbf{u}$ is the vector of linear velocity of substance flow in the tissue. The quantities n, m, and $\mathbf{u}$ are functions of coordinates and time.

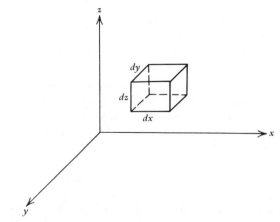

Figure A24.   The elementary volume $dx\,dy\,dz$ in x, y, z coordinates.

Consider an infinitesimal tissue volume in the form of a box with the sides dx, dy, and dz corresponding to the parallel coordinate axes (Figure A24). This volume will be equal to the product $dx\,dy\,dz$. Being a vector quantity, the flow of substance in the volume can be resolved into three components directed along the axes u_x, u_y, and u_z. Consider now the amount of substance entering the volume for an infinitesimal time dt through the wall $dy\,dz$; it is equal to $u_x n\,dy\,dz\,dt$. Over the same time the amount of substance exiting from the volume through the opposite wall will be $u_x n\,dy\,dz\,dt +$ $(\delta/\delta x)(u_x n\,dy\,dz\,dt)dx$.

The change in amount of substance in the above volume over time dt, as a result of the flow in the direction of the x axis, will be equal to the amount that has entered through the wall $dy\,dz$ minus the amount that has exited through the opposite wall, that is, to

$$- \frac{\delta}{\delta x}(u_x n\,dy\,dz\,dt)dx \quad \text{or} \quad -\frac{\delta}{\delta x}(u_x n)\,dx\,dy\,dz\,dt.$$

The same reasoning can be applied to the change in amount in an infinitesimal small volume due to substance flow in the directions of the y and the z axis. In the former case the change will be $-(\delta/\delta y)(u_y n)dx\,dy\,dz\,dt$, and in the latter, $-(\delta/\delta z)(u_z n)dx\,dy\,dz\,dt$.

The total change in amount of substance due to the flow $\mathbf{u}$ in the volume $dx\,dy\,dz$ will be given by the sum of changes due to the flows along the coordinate axes:

$$-\left[\frac{\delta}{\delta x}(u_x n) + \frac{\delta}{\delta y}(u_y n) + \frac{\delta}{\delta z}(u_z n)\right]dx\,dy\,dz\,dt$$

which can be written in more compact form as

$$- [\operatorname{div}(\mathbf{u}n)]dx\,dy\,dz\,dt$$

The change in amount of substance due to the flow $\mathbf{u}$ involves corresponding changes in amount of substance within the mobile and immobile phases (i.e., in the blood and tissue). In other words, the total gain or loss of substance in the volume $dx\,dy\,dz$ will be equal exactly to the sum of gains or losses of substance in the mobile and immobile phases of the system. In the elementary volume of blood the change in amount of substance will be $(\delta n/\delta t)dt\,dx\,dy\,dz$, and in that of tissue, $(\delta m/\delta t)dt\,dx\,dy\,dz$.

The overall balance of substance in the volume $dx\,dy\,dz$ will therefore be

$$- [\operatorname{div}(\mathbf{u}n)]dx\,dy\,dz\,dt = \frac{\delta n}{\delta t}dx\,dy\,dz\,dt + \frac{\delta m}{\delta t}dx\,dy\,dz\,dt$$

or, after eliminating the superfluous terms,

$$\frac{\delta n}{\delta t} + \frac{\delta m}{\delta t} + \text{div}(\mathbf{u}n) = 0 \qquad (A36)$$

This balance equation is based on a consideration of only a purely mechanical flow $\mathbf{u}$ of the sorbed substance. However, to make the picture more complete, account may be taken of the change in amount of substance in the volume $dx\, dy\, dz$ due to diffusion and convection of the substance molecules. Since the system is isothermic, this change will be given by the equation

$$\left(\frac{\delta n}{\delta t}\right)_{\text{diff}} dx\, dy\, dz\, dt = \Delta n D_{\text{mol}}\, dx\, dy\, dz\, dt \qquad (A37)$$

where D_{mol} is the molecular diffusion coefficient, and Δ is the Laplacian operator. (This equation follows from the diffusion theory as developed, e.g., in the monograph of Landau and Livshits, 1954.)

The complete balance equation taking into account the diffusive-convective transfer of substance is

$$\frac{\delta n}{\delta t} + \frac{\delta m}{\delta t} + \text{div}(\mathbf{u}n) = \Delta n D_{\text{mol}} \qquad (A38)$$

However, as already mentioned, there is no need to take account of all possible factors in describing this process to a first approximation. Therefore, if the phenomena of substance transfer by diffusion and convection are neglected, as they may be, the balance equation will simplify to (A36).

If a given tissue takes up several substances that satisfy the conditions specified above, the sorption process will be described, in the general case, by a system of k equations, where k is the number of substances:

$$\frac{\delta n_i}{\delta t} + \frac{\delta m_i}{\delta t} + \text{div}(\mathbf{u}n_i) = \Delta n_i D_{\text{mol}\,i}, \qquad \text{at } 1 \leq i \leq k \qquad (A39)$$

This balance equation can in theory be used to calculate m at any time and at any point in the tissue. To do this it should be written in integral form relative to m, which will require appropriate integration under specified initial and boundary conditions. In practice, however, this is hardly possible because of the many unknowns in this equation and because of the analytical difficulties due to the fact that the solution of partial differential equations remains an insufficiently developed area of mathematics. As a rule one has to solve such equations by way of their simplification and with frequent recourse to approximate methods of solution.

One example of simplification is provided by a one-dimensional problem assuming undirectional flow of substance in the tissue. (This case corresponds to a degree to the spread of drug in a tissue from the depot preliminarily created in that tissue.) The balance equation for this problem involving the spread of substance along an imaginary x axis is as follows:

$$\frac{\delta n}{\delta t} + \frac{\delta m}{\delta t} + \frac{\delta}{\delta x}(un) = \frac{\delta^2 n}{\delta x^2} D_{mol} \tag{A40}$$

If the substance flow along the x axis occurs at a constant rate ($u = $ constant), the equation simplifies to

$$\frac{\delta n}{\delta t} + \frac{\delta m}{\delta t} + u\frac{\delta n}{\delta x} = \frac{\delta^2 n}{\delta x^2} D_{mol} \tag{A41}$$

The initial and boundary conditions for this equation can be formulated, and it can then be solved when additional relationships between the unknowns are found. The problem of solving such equations arises, for example, in areas of study directly bordering on the theory of chromatography. But for the purely biological problem under discussion these equations are too simplistic, although one possible aspect of their application in the case of drug distribution from depots has been indicated above.

As already stated, in addition to purely mathematical difficulties, equations of substance balance in tissue are difficult to solve because of the many unknowns. These difficulties can be overcome only by finding additional functional relationships between the unknowns. For this purpose one should first of all consider kinetic dependencies that relate concentrations of substance in blood and tissue to time. Kinetic equations not only can help in solving balance equations but also have a role to play by themselves, characterizing the time dependence of drug uptake by tissues.

The rate of substance sorption by tissue is defined by the increment in amount of sorbed substance per unit of time. Obviously, other factors being equal and constant, the sorption rate will decrease with time because of the progressive tissue saturation by the sorbed substance. In general form the time dependence of sorption rate can be expressed by the differential equation $dm/dt = f(t)$ or by its integral form, $m = f'(t)$. These equations reflect the time course of sorption and, when represented graphically, give a clear picture of the process (Figure A25).

A useful quantity is the relative sorption γ, which is the ratio of the concentration of sorbed substance at a given time m to the maximal concentration of sorbed substance m_∞, determined by the sorptive capacity of the tissue: $\gamma = m/m_\infty = \varphi(t)$. The region of relative sorption values of relevance to the

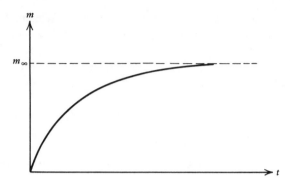

Figure A25.   A kinetic curve for sorption: m, concentration of sorbed substance; t, time.

tissue uptake of xenobiotics appears to lie, in many cases, somewhere at the beginning of the kinetics curve (i.e., $\gamma \ll 1$).

The foregoing discussion has concerned the essentials of sorption kinetics. Now we proceed to a more detailed consideration of our model of blood-bathed tissue, taking cognizance of the constraints imposed on it. The kinetics of substance sorption will now depend on the concentration of already sorbed substance m, on the concentration of substance in the mobile phase n, and on the rate of substance flow $\mathbf{u}$, as well as on the remaining parameters that determine the diffusive-chemical stage of sorption and that are designated here by the symbol K. Taking into account the dependencies just listed, we can write an equation of sorption kinetics in general form as

$$\frac{\delta m}{\delta t} = F(n, m, \mathbf{u}, K) \tag{A42}$$

Here the partial derivative $\delta m/\delta t$ means that, in our model, m is dependent not only on time but also on the coordinates.

If $\mathbf{u}$ and the factors included in K remain constant, which for our model of living tissue is very probable, as is the previously introduced condition of temperature constancy, the equation of sorption kinetics becomes much simpler, for the sorption rate now depends solely on the concentrations of the substances sorbed in the mobile and immobile phases:

$$\frac{\delta m}{\delta t} = F(n, m) \tag{A43}$$

It should be borne in mind that the dynamic sorption process we are concerned with, taking into account the previously introduced constraints, is reversible, that is, there is desorption as well as sorption. Therefore the rate of sorption is in fact the difference between the rate of sorption proper and the rate of desorption:

$$\frac{\delta m}{\delta t} = \left(\frac{\delta m}{\delta t}\right)_{sorp} - \left(\frac{\delta m}{\delta t}\right)_{desorp} \tag{A44}$$

With the course of time, if the flow of sorbed substance in the tissue is constant, the quantitative difference between sorption proper and desorption will progressively decrease so that ultimately these processes will become equilibrated; in theory this will happen at $t = \infty$, and in practice, after a time interval peculiar to each particular substance. Once such equilibration has been reached, the tissue and blood concentrations of substance become constant, and their ratio, which characterizes the model and substance selected, is called the distribution ratio or distribution (partition) coefficient. The equilibration results in the sorption rate, as measured by the amount of substance sorbed per unit of time, becoming equal to zero: $\delta m/\delta t = 0$. Substituting zero for the derivative $\delta m/\delta t$ in a sorption kinetics equation will give an equation of sorption statics: $F(m, n) = 0$ or, in integral form, $m = \psi(n)$.

In some cases equations of sorption statics, instead of those of sorption kinetics, can be included in a system of differential equations describing the dynamics of substance uptake in tissue. This will also be a simplification whose degree is difficult to assess a priori for a biological system such as tissue, although it is probably quite justifiable in certain situations.

If we consider the tissue uptake of more than one substance simultaneously, the system of equations of sorption kinetics (or statics) will consist, as in the case of balance equations, of k equations equal to the number of substances:

$$\frac{\delta m_i}{\delta t} = F_i(n_1, n_2, \ldots, n_i, \ldots, n_k, m_1, m_2, \ldots, m_i, \ldots, m_k)$$

or

$$m_i = \psi_i(n_1, n_2, \ldots, n_i, \ldots, n_k), \quad \text{at } 1 \le i \le k$$

The formulation of specific forms of equations for sorption kinetics or statics is fairly complex. In the theory of sorption kinetics this is done by the use of special procedures that make it possible to find approximate forms of the equations (Timofeyev, 1962). These procedures will not be discussed here; they can be found in the original literature or, for the sorption of substance by living tissues, have to be specially developed.

It can be seen that the substance flow rate **u** is a quantity essential for describing the dynamics of substance uptake in tissue. This quantity appears in equations of substance balance in tissue and in the general equation of substance sorption kinetics. The dependence of substance balance in tissue and of substance sorption kinetics on **u** shows the importance of the distribution of the flow rate in tissue both in space and in time, since $\mathbf{u} = \mathbf{u}(x, y, z, t)$. Hence, to supplement the equations describing the dynamics of substance uptake in tissues, it is expedient to turn to the theory of physicochemical hydrodynamics, where relationships can be found for the spatiotemporal distribution of the substance flow rate. First of all, the well-known continuity equation may prove useful: $\delta\rho/\delta t + \mathrm{div}(\rho\mathbf{u}) = 0$, where ρ is the density of the mobile phase. In the case we are concerned with, this equation appreciably simplifies to div $\mathbf{u} = 0$, since the blood concentration of substance has been postulated above to be low and so its change cannot affect the density; moreover, blood can be dependably regarded as an incompressible liquid. Both these conditions lead to $\rho = \rho(x, y, z, t) = $ constant.

The latter equation can at once be used to simplify the balance equation (Rachinsky, 1964):

$$\frac{\delta n}{\delta t} + \frac{\delta m}{\delta t} + \mathrm{div}(\mathbf{u}n) = \Delta n D_{\mathrm{mol}} \qquad (A45)$$

The third term on the left-hand side of (A45) is resolvable into components: $\mathrm{div}(\mathbf{u}n) = \mathbf{u}\,\nabla n + \mathrm{div}\,\mathbf{u}$, where ∇ is the nabla operator. But since div $\mathbf{u} = 0$, $\mathrm{div}(\mathbf{u}n) = \mathbf{u}\,\nabla n$, which can be written into the balance equation to give

$$\frac{\delta n}{\delta t} = \frac{\delta m}{\delta t} + \mathbf{u}\,\nabla\,n = \Delta n\,D_{\mathrm{mol}} \qquad (A46)$$

Another useful equation from the field of hydrodynamics is the one describing the movement of a viscous liquid. This equation for liquids of constant density is comparatively simple and is called the Navier–Stokes equation; it will not be discussed here.

The above equations of substance balance and sorption (and possibly statics) and of mobile-phase hydrodynamics appear to be quite sufficient for describing the dynamics of xenobiotic uptake in tissues. The specific forms these equations take may be very complex, as may be their solutions, which will undoubtedly require a computer. The equations may be greatly simplified to a form amenable to solution by standard procedures. In many cases, however, the simplification will have to be done at the cost of substantial simplification of the model as a whole. This cost may prove to be prohibitively high if the model no longer represents the essence of the biological process it was designed to describe.

As an example, a one-dimensional problem involving substance movement in one direction only may be cited. The balance equation for such a problem has been written above, and it is not difficult to give the remaining equations of substance uptake dynamics for this case. The resulting equations can be solved, but the value of such a model for the biological phenomenon under consideration is uncertain; anyway, the model will be a far cry from reality.

It is true, though, that consideration of a far-from-reality model need not be such a useless exercise as might seem at first glance. It may well provide a foundation on which the elements of an edifice adequately representing the real object can be gradually erected at a later time.

Apart from equations, which define the course of substance uptake in general form, of great importance for a more detailed characterization of this process or, to be more exact, for the correct description of its development, is the formulation of the initial and boundary conditions. The initial conditions should be understood to mean the values of all pertinent parameters at $t = 0$, that is, at the time when consideration of the process is started. The boundary conditions are the values of the same parameters at the boundaries of the model, both external (the border between the tissue in question and the surrounding tissues) and internal (between the phases if the model is a multiphasic one; the capillary blood and the tissue proper may be regarded as different phases).

Although the initial and boundary conditions may vary widely, depending on the model simulating the physical essence of a particular tissue, the course of substance uptake in the tissue will be defined quite unequivocally by these conditions. Despite the need for an individual approach to the formulation of initial and boundary conditions, it is possible to point out some of the basic conditions. If one is concerned with a one-dimensional problem, the conditions are relatively easy to define. Since, however, unidimensional models should be looked upon with suspicion, we will not do this here; moreover, these conditions are very similar to those formulated in the theory of unidimensional chromatography (Rachinsky, 1964).

Understandably, the conditions will depend on how the substance gets into the organism. The simplest case seems to be one where the blood level of a xenobiotic is kept constant. Such constancy, within limits of course, is seen fairly commonly (e.g., when a substance is absorbed periodically from the environment, when a drug enters the blood from a depot set up in some tissue, or when a slow-release drug is absorbed over a time). Then, as a first approximation, it may be taken that, at $t = 0$, $n = n_0$, and $m = 0$,

$$x, y, z = 0, \qquad t \geq 0, \qquad n = n_0, \qquad m = f(t)$$

$$x, y, z \leq \infty, \qquad t \to \infty, \qquad n = n_0, \qquad m = kn$$

where k is the distribution coefficient.

If the blood level of a substance varies, the law governing this variation must be known in order to formulate the conditions. Thus after a rapid intravenous injection the decline in concentration has been shown in many studies to obey an exponential law (or, to be more precise, to be defined by the sum of several exponentials). The initial and boundary conditions will include this law, so at $t = 0$, $n = n_0$, and $m = 0$

$$x, y, z = 0, \qquad t \geq 0, \qquad n = n_0 e^{-\alpha t}, \qquad m = f'(t)$$

$$x, y, z \leq \infty, \qquad t \to \infty, \qquad n = \to 0$$

If the blood level of an administered substance rises as a result of continued absorption, the rise will also occur exponentially, and the initial conditions will include the expression $n = n_0(1 - e^{-\alpha t})$.

Thus, in the foregoing consideration of the essentials of the dynamics of tissue uptake of foreign substances, a physicomathematical approach was chosen and applied to a biphasic sorption model. This model of necessity represents a considerable simplification of the real system; moreover, the possibility of its further simplification has been indicated (this concerns the case of unidimensional sorption). As a result, it has been possible to formulate a strict balance equation for the uptake of sorbed substance into tissue; to give general forms of kinetic equations for sorption; to point out the desirability of using, in certain cases, equations of sorption statics; and to utilize some of the basic equations of hydrodynamics in the description of the sorption process. Furthermore, the main types of boundary and initial conditions have been indicated that characterize the dynamics of substance uptake in such typical cases as after a single intravenous administration, in the initial period after a single oral administration, and when the blood concentration is maintained at a constant level.

The elements mentioned above appear to be basic to a theory of the dynamics of substance sorption by tissues at the phenomenological level. No attempt has been made to approach this topic from a molecular-statistical point of view, which would necessarily entail consideration of the specific forces of molecular interaction between substance and tissue and, in addition, would require the use of other concepts relating to the mechanism of substance-tissue interaction. Such an approach is beyond the scope of this addendum.

The foregoing consideration is probably not the only one possible, and it has been undertaken in the most general terms. It may be said that we have formulated the problem of constructing a theory of the dynamics of uptake of stable xenobiotics in tissue and have outlined ways of tackling that problem. No specific applications have been discussed because such a theory has not yet been developed to a sufficient degree and because relevant experimental data are lacking. In our view a necessary stage of work along this line must be the development of suitable forms of kinetic equations. Prerequisites for these are at hand. In particular, in the field of toxico- and pharmacokinetics, very interesting equations have been proposed, some of which may be applied without substantial modification to describe the dynamics of substance uptake into tissue.

A7. TASKS AND PROSPECTS

Toxicokinetic investigations entail a quantitative approach to the problems of toxicology. Study of the kinetic relationships governing the passage of toxic compounds through the body places the problem of the action of poisons on organs and tissues and on the organism as a whole on a strictly quantitative basis. Thus a knowledge of the fate of a substance in the body and of the time courses of the levels of that substance and of its metabolites in the various tissues and in the blood, coupled with a comparison of the observed effects, enables one to express the action of the substance in quantitative terms.

This general task of toxicokinetics predetermines its more particular, including practical, applications. Here are some of them.

1. *Study of mechanisms of toxic action.* In the last analysis this task is to be solved at the molecular-biochemical level. The initial stage, however, usually begins with a study of the kinetic parameters that characterize the passage of a given poison through the organism and its particular systems, and it is often the kinetics of poisons that leads to an understanding of the biological effects they produce. A kinetic analysis can yield useful information about the fate of the poison in the body.
2. *Prophylaxis and treatment of intoxications.* One way to prevent or minimize toxicity is to assure timely removal of the offending substance or its toxic metabolites from the body. A knowledge of the kinetics of metabolism and elimination of substances can provide a basis for control of the removal of the toxic principle.
3. *Cumulative action studies.* In the case of cumulative actions resulting from material cumulation which involves the accumulation of xenobiotics only, the problem is a purely kinetic one. The kinetic approach may be also of value in the event of functional cumulation; for example, the half-life of a cumulative effect may serve as a measure of its magnitude.
4. *Transfer of data from animals to man and explanation of individual differences in responses to poisons.* Until very recently the problem of interspecies transfer of experimental toxicity data was tackled without regard to toxicokinetic characteristics. Today such transfers often cannot be considered valid unless the kinetics both of the xenobiotic and of the toxic effect are taken into account.

5. *Prediction of a toxic process with repetitive exposures from data of toxicity studies involving a single exposure or a limited number of exposures.* This process has two intimately iterrelated aspects: kinetic and physiological.
6. *Rational assessment of toxicity parameters.* The parameters currently used to assess the toxicities of xenobiotics have inherent limitations. One of the current attempts to introduce dynamic characteristics into toxicological parameters concerns the development of cumulation coefficients based on kinetic concepts. Toxicokinetic methods when combined with those presently used will undoubtedly permit a more objective establishment of maximum permissible levels of harmful substances in the air, water, and other media.
7. *Pollution control.* The need to assay biological materials for toxic compounds or their metabolites has raised questions as to what samples, how many samples, and how often samples should be collected for such assays. If a rational system of sampling is to be developed, the toxicokinetics of pollutants must be known, including their half-lives in the body. Toxicokinetic information will be found valuable also in the planning of air sampling programs for work environments.

In regard to the outlook for toxicokinetics in the near future, the kinetics of toxic effect should be mentioned first. This area of research, where much remains to be done, has several important aspects. Foremost among these is the assessment of bodily responses as they relate to the concentrations of poison in the biological media and, more particularly, in the sites of action (receptor sites). As a result the receptors themselves may become more of a reality. Information for this can be provided by experiments in which the biological effect and blood levels of a xenobiotic are measured as functions of varying dose. A logical premise on which to base subsequent conclusions is that the biological effect of a xenobiotic is proportional to the degree to which it occupies the receptor sites. Then, if the maximum value of the biological effect is not proportional to the dosage, it may be concluded that the affinity of the substance for the receptor sites is high and that the receptor sites are relatively saturated with the substance for a wide range of its concentrations in the organism. If the effect is proportional to the dose, the implication is that the affinity is low and the receptors are present in excess numbers. If the decay of the biological effect parallels the decline of the blood level of the xenobiotic, it may be inferred that the receptor sites reside in the blood (or, to be more precise, in the central compartment of the body model). A long delay in onset of the maximum effect suggests that the receptors are located in a deep compartment.

In most practical situations the action of a xenobiotic can be adequately judged from measurements of its concentration in the blood. If, however, the biological activity of a substance is determined by the amount of its metabolites, which cannot be measured, determination of the blood concentration of the substance will not give any meaningful quantitative information. By reasoning along similar lines Barth et al. (1976) have developed a quantitative scheme for a theory of interaction between biologically active compounds and receptors. The scheme covers the transport of substances to the receptor sites, substance-receptor interactions, conformational changes in the receptors, and the production of a "stimulus" that precurses the biological effect. If worked out in more detail, this scheme may well contribute to the advancement of toxicokinetics.

Toxicokinetics depends for much of its progress on the development of mathematical models used to simulate the passage of xenobiotics through the organism. Current models often include nonlinear effects as well. The elaboration of any more or less sophisticated model is a fairly involved scientific endeavor, since, as a rule, there are no ready solutions from which to proceed. To develop such a model, the toxicologist has to enlist the cooperation of a mathematician. Here the predicament with which the toxicologist is confronted is that he has to deal with mathematical abstractions, among which he can easily lose sight of the objective he has set himself in the first place.

ADDENDUM REFERENCES

Abramovsky, B. P., Yu. A. Anokhin, V. A. Ionov, I. M. Nazarov, and A. Kh. Ostromogilsky, The global balance and maximum permissible atmospheric emissions of mercury, in *Vsestoronniy Analiz Okruzhaiushchei Prirodnoi Sredy. Trudy II Sovetsko-Amerikanskogo Simpoziuma, Gonolulu, Gavayi, 20–26 Oktiabria 1975 g. [Comprehensive Analysis of the Environment. Proceedings, Second Soviet-American Symposium, Honolulu, Hawaii, 20–26 October, 1975]*, Gidrometeoizdat, Leningrad, 1976.

Al-Shahristani, H., and K. M. Shihab, Variation of biological half-life of methylmercury in man, *Arch. Environ. Health*, **28**, 342–344 (1974).

Ariëns, E. J., A molecular approach to the modulation of pharmacokinetics: modification of metabolic conversion by molecular manipulation, *Pure Appl. Chem.*, **19**, 187–217 (1969).

Ariëns, E. J., Modulation of pharmacokinetics by molecular manipulation, in E. J. Ariëns, Ed., *Drug Design*, Vol. 2, pp. 1–127, Academic Press, New York, 1971.

Baker, S. B. de C., and D. M. Foulkes, Blood concentrations of compounds in animal toxicity tests, in D. S. Davies and B. N. C. Prichard, Eds., *Biological Effects of Drugs in Relation to Their Plasma Concentrations*, pp. 41–50, Macmillan, London, 1973.

Ballard, B. E., Pharmacokinetics and temperature, *J. Pharm. Sci.*, **63**, 1345–1358 (1974).

Barth, A., R. Franke, and D. Börnert, Theoretische Aspekte der Ermittlung von Parametern der Wirkung von biologischaktiven Verbindungen, *Pharmazie*, **31**, 396–401 (1976).

Bazhenov, A. V., and G. A. Menshikova, Dependence of [91]yttrium elimination from the body on the dose and time of application of calcium EDTA, in *Metabolizm Radioizotopov v Zhivotnom Organizme. Trudy Instituta Ekologii Rastenii i Zhivotnykh Uralskogo Nauchnogo Tsentra Akad. Nauk SSSR*, Vol. 89, pp. 37–42, Sverdlovsk, 1974.

Bezel, V. S., B. V. Popov, and I. E. Okoneshnikova, A model for the chemotherapy of chronic mercury intoxication, in *Matematicheskaya Teoriya Biologicheskikh Protsessov* (*Tezisy Dokladov 1 Konferentsii*), pp. 303–305, Akad. Nauk SSSR, Kaliningrad, 1976.

Borchard, R. E., M. E. Welborn, L. E. Hansen, R. P. Link, and R. H. Teske, Apparent pharmacokinetics of PCB components in growing pigs and lambs when fed a ration containing Apoclor 1254, *Arch. Environ. Contam. Toxicol.*, **4**, 226–245 (1976).

Branch, R. A., C. M. Herbert, and A. E. Read, Determinants of serum antipyrine half-lives in patents with liver disease, *Gut*, **14**, 569–573 (1973).

Breckenridge, A., and M. Orme, Kinetics of warfarin absorption in man, *Clin. Pharmacol. Ther.*, **14**, 955–961 (1973).

Breimer, D. D., and R. F. Rekker, Chemische Structur en Farmacokinetik, *Chem. Weekbl.*, **70** (44), F10–F12 (1974).

Cadorniga, R., I. Arias, and I. Migoya, Variation de la farmacocinetica de la amplicilina sodica en funcion del ejercicio fidico, *Il Farmaco, Ed. Prat.*, **29**, 386–394 (1974).

Cember, H., A model for the kinetics of mercury elimination, *Am. Ind. Hyg. Assoc. J.*, **30**, 367–371 (1969).

Chiou, W. L., and F. H. Hsu, Pharmacokinetics of creatinine in man and its implications in the monitoring of renal function and in dosage regimen modification in patients with renal insufficiency. *J. Clin. Pharmacol.*, **15**, 427–434 (1975).

Cohen, Y., Les radioéléments en pharmacocinétique, *Bull. Inf. Sci. Techn. CEA*, No. 147, 55–62 (1970).

Cohen, Y., Les radioéléments en pharmacocinétique, *Prod. Probl. Pharm.*, **26**, 28–36 (1971).

Cumming, J. F., The effect of arterial oxygen tension on antipyrine half-time in plasma, *Clin. Pharmacol. Ther.*, **19**, 468–471 (1976).

Deckart, H., H. Herzmann, H. Flentje, A. Blottner, and K. D. Schwartz, Pharmakokinetik radiojodmarkierter organischer Merkuriverbindungen, *Strahlentherapie*, **74**, 134–141 (1975).

Dedrick, R. L., Animal scale-up, in T. Teorell, R. L. Dedrick, and P. G. Condliffe, Eds., *Pharmacology and Pharmacokinetics*, pp. 117–145, Plenum Press, New York, 1974.

Dedrick, R. L., K. B. Bischoff, and D. S. Zaharko, Interspecies correlation of plasma concentration history of methotrexate, *Cancer Chemother. Rep.*, Part 1, **54**, 95–101 (1970).

Dettli, L., Pharmacokinetic aspects of drug interactions, in L. E. Cluff and J. C. Petrie,

Eds., *Clinical Effects of Interaction between Drugs*, pp. 39–68, American Elsevier, New York, 1974.

Dettli, L., Elimination kinetics and drug dosage in renal insufficiency patients, *Triangle*, **14** (3/4), 117–123 (1975).

Dettli, L., and P. Spring, The modifying effects of physiological variables and disease upon pharmacokinetics and/or drug response, in *Pharmacology and the Future of Man. Proceedings, 5th International Congress on Pharmacology, San Francisco, 1972*, Vol. 3, pp. 165–173, Krager, Basel, 1973.

Devissaguet, J.-Ph., and R. Le Verge, Principles généraux des calculateurs analogiques. Applications pharmacocinétiques et biopharmaceutiques, *Thérapie*, **30**, 7–20 (1975).

Di Santo, A. R., and J. G. Wagner, Potential erroneous assignment of nonlinear data to the classical linear two-compartment open model, *J. Pharm. Sci.*, **61**, 552–555 (1972).

Eichelbaum, M., J. H. Hengstmann, H. D. Rost, T. Brecht, and H. J. Dengler, Pharmacokinetics, cardiovascular and metabolic actions of cyclohexamine in man, *Arch. Toxikol.*, **31**, 243–263 (1974).

Eichelbaum, M., K. Ekbom, L. Bertilsson, V. A. Ringberger, and A. Rane, Plasma kinetics of carbamazepine and its epoxide metabolite in man after single and multiple doses, *Eur. J. Clin. Pharmacol.*, **8**, 337–341 (1975).

Fagerström, T., R. Kurten, and B. Asell, Statistical parameters as criteria in model evaluation: kinetics of mercury accumulation in pike *Esox lucius*, *Oikos*, **26**, 109–116 (1975).

Filov, V. A., Esterase activity in the blood of animals of various species, *Biull. Eksp. Biol. Med.*, **4**, 45–46 (1963).

Filov, V. A., Dynamics of uptake of foreign chemicals into tissues: Elements of a theory, in N. V. Lazarev, A. A. Golubev, and E. T. Lykhina, Eds., *Aktualniye Voprosy Promyshlennoi Toksikologii*, pp. 7–20, Institut Gigiyeny Truda i Profzabolevaniy, Leningrad, 1970.

Filov, V. A., Mathematical aspects of pharmakokinetics and toxicokinetics, in *Farmakologiya. Khimioterapevticheskiye Sredstva. Toksikologiya. Problemy Farmakologii*, Vol. 5, pp. 9–80, VINITI: *Itogi Nauki i Tekhniki* Series, Moscow, 1973.

Filov, V. A., Pharmacokinetics and toxicokinetics, *Farmakol. Toksikol.*, **37**(4), 490–493 (1974).

Filov, V. A., The place of mathematical methods in pharmacokinetics, in *Materialy po Matematicheskomy Obespecheniuy i Ispolzovaniyu EVM v Mediko-Biologicheskikh Issledovaniyakh*, pp. 190–191, Institut Medistinskoi Radiologii, Obninsk, 1976.

Freundt, K. J., On the pharmacokinetics of the ethanol metabolite acetate: elimination from the blood and cerebrospinal fluid, *Arzneimittelforsch.*, **23**, 949–951 (1973).

Gadaskina, I. D., and V. A. Filov, *Prevrashcheniya i Opredeleniye Promyshlennykh Organicheskikh Yadov v Organizme* [*Conversions and Determination of Industrial Organic Poisons in the Body*], Meditsina, Leningrad, 1971.

Gadaskina, I. D., N. D. Gadaskina, and V. A. Filov, *Opredeleniye Promyshlennykh*

Neorganicheskikh Yadov v Organizme [*Determination of Industrial Inorganic Poisons in the Body*], Meditsina, Leningrad, 1975.

Garrett, E. R., and H. J. Lambert, Pharmacokinetics of trichloroethanol and metabolites and interconversions among variously referenced pharmacokinetic parameters, *J. Pharm. Sci.*, **62**, 550–572 (1973).

Gibaldi, M., and D. Perrier, Route of administration and drug disposition, *Drug Metab. Rev.*, **3**, 185–199 (1974).

Gladtke, E., Pharmacokinetics in relation to age, *Boll. Chim. Farm.*, **112**, 333–341 (1973).

Hattingberg, H. M., Darstellungsweise pharmakokinetischer Modelle durch Analogrechner, *Arzneimittelforsch.*, **23**, 1162–1167 (1973).

Horning, M. G., J. Nowlin, M. Stafford, K. Lertratanangkoon, K. R. Sommer, R. M. Hill, and R. N. Stillwell, The use of gas chromatographic-mass spectrometric computer systems in pharmacokinetic studies, *J. Chromatogr.*, **112**, 605–615 (1975).

Iverson, F., R. H. Downie, C. Paul, and H. L. Trenholm, Methyl marcury: acute toxicity, tissue distribution and decay profiles in the guinea pig, *Toxicol. Appl. Pharmacol.*, **24**, 545–554 (1973).

Kaiser, D. G., and A. A. Forist, Pharmacokinetics of 4,5-bis(*p*-methophenyl)-2-phenylpyrrole-acetonitrile in normal and polyarthritic rats, *J. Pharm. Pharmacol.*, **26**, 563–565 (1974).

Kodama, R., T. Sonoda, H. Vano, K. Noda, and H. Yde, Metabolism of 1-(3-trifluoromethylphenyl)3-(2-hydroxyethyl)quinazoline-2,4(1H,3H)-dione (H-88). II. Absorption, distribution and excretion in rat, mouse, rabbit, monkey and man, *Xenobiotica*, **5**, 601–609 (1975).

Kolmodin-Hedman, B., Decreased plasma half-lives of antipyrine and phenylbutazone in workers occupationally exposed to lindane and DDT, in P. L. Morselli, S. Garattini, and S. N. Cohen, Eds., *Drug Interactions*, pp. 249–257, Raven Press, New York, 1974.

Komuro, T., S. Kitazawa, and H. Sezaki, Fasting and the volume of drug distribution in the rat, *Chem. Pharm. Bull.*, **23**, 909–916 (1975).

Koss, G., and W. Koransky, Studies on the toxicology of hexachlorobenzene. I. Pharmacokinetics, *Arch. Toxikol.*, **34**, 203–212 (1975).

Kozlov, S. T., and E. A. Rudzit, Use of chromatography-mass spectrometry in pharmacokinetic studies (a review), *Farmakol. Toksikol.*, **39**(6), 750–755 (1976).

Landau, L. D., and E. M. Livshits, *Mekhanika Sploshnykh Sred* [*The Mechanics of Continua*], Izdatelstovo Tekhniko-Teoreticheskoi Literatury, Moscow, 1954.

Lehninger, A. L., *Biochemistry*, Worth, New York, 1972.

Lien, E. J., The relationship between chemical structure and drug absorption, distribution and excretion, *Med. Chem.*, **4**, 319–342 (1974).

Lightfoot, E. N., *Transport Phenomena and Living Systems*, John Wiley, New York, 1974.

Liublina, E. I., Comparative accumulation of foreign substances in man and laboratory animals in relation to some properties of their inspired vapors and gases, *Gig. Sanit.*, **9**, 29–33 (1973).

Matsubara-Khan, J., Compartmental analysis for the evaluation of biological half-lives of cadmium and mercury in mouse organs, *Environ. Res.*, **7**, 54–67 (1974).

Mitchison, D. A., Plasma concentrations of isoniazid in the treatments of tuberculosis, in D. S. Davies and B. N. C. Prichard, Eds., *Biological Effects of Drugs in Relation to Their Plasma Concentrations*, pp. 169–182, Macmillan, New York, 1973.

Moskalev, Yu. I., G. A. Zalikin, and A. I. Semenov, Kinetics of ^{244}Cm accumulation in organs and tissues with chronic exposure to this isotope, *Gig. Sanit.*, **6**, 41–43 (1974).

Movshev, B. E., Metabolism of ^{45}Ca in intact rats and in rats with burns, *Voprosy Meditsinskoi Khimii*, **14**(1), 12–16 (1968).

Müller, G., M. Spassovski, and D. Henschler, Metabolism of trichloroethylene in man. II. Pharmacokinetics of metabolites, *Arch. Toxikol.*, **32**, 283–295 (1974).

Muraviyeva, S. I., G. N. Zayeva, K. P. Stasenkova, and N. N. Ordynskaya, Urinary excretion of dimethyl formamide in relation to the level and duration of exposure, *Gig. Tr. Prof. Zabol.*, **12**, 36–39 (1975).

Nelson, E., Kinetic considerations in pharmacokinetic studies of drug metabolism, *Life Sci.*, **4**, 949–953 (1965).

Notari, R. E., Pharmacokinetics and molecular modification: implications in drug design and evaluation, *J. Pharm. Sci.*, **62**, 865–881 (1973).

Notari, R. E., *Biopharmaceutics and Pharmacokinetics. An Introduction*, Marcel Dekker, New York, 1975.

Notari, R. E., D. R. Kavaliunas, and H. W. Bockborader, Apparent biological half-life values determined by administration of drug by methods other than rapid intravenous injection, *J. Pharm. Pharmacol.*, **26**(12), Supp., 62–63 (1974).

Ossenberg, F.-W., M. Peignoux, D. Bourdiau, and J.-P. Benhamou, Pentobarbital pharmacokinetics in the normal and in the hepatectomized rat, *J. Pharmacol. Exp. Ther.*, **194**, 111–116 (1975).

Pavlovskaya, N. A., A. V. Provotorov, and L. G. Makeyeva, Behavior of ^{228}thorium and its daughter isotopes in the rat with peroral administration, *Gig. Tr. Prof. Zabol.*, **5**, 36–39 (1974).

Piotrowski, J., *The Application of Metabolic Excretion Kinetics to Problems of Industrial Toxicology*, U.S. Department of Health, Education and Welfare, Government Printing Office, Washington, D.C., 1971.

Popov, B. V., and V. S. Bezel, A mathematical model of complexone action, in *Metabolizm Radioizotopov v Zhivotnom Organizme. Trudy Instituta Ekologii Rastenii i Zhivotnykh Uralskogo Nauchnogo Tsentra Akad. Nauk SSSR*, Vol. 89, pp. 48–52, Sverdlovsk, 1974.

Rachinsky, V. V., *Vvedeniye v Obshchuyu Teoriyu Dinamiki Sorbtsii i Khromatografii* [*Introduction to a General Theory of Sorption Dynamics and of Chromatography*], Nauka, Moscow, 1964.

Rauws, A. G., Thallium pharmacokinetics and its modification by Prussian blue, *Naunyn-Schmiedeberg's Arch. Pharmakol.*, **284**, 295–306 (1974).

Rauws, A. G., Bromide pharmacokinetics: a model for residue accumulation in animals, *Toxicology*, **4**, 195–202 (1975).

Reinberg, A., Rythmes circadiens des paramètres de l'excrétion urinaire du salicylate chez l'homme adulte sain, *C. R. Acad. Sci.*, **D280**(14), 1697–1699 (1975).

Rentsch, G., The use of pharmacokinetic systems for the interpretation of long-term experiments: A new approach to toxicology, in *Proceedings, European Society for the Study of Drug Toxicity*, Vol. 15, 1974, pp. 323–329, Excerpta Medica, Amsterdam, 1974.

Rescigno, A., and J. S. Beck, Compartments, in R. Rosen, Ed., *Foundations of Mathematical Biology*, Vol. 2, pp. 255–322, Academic Press, New York, 1972.

Robinson, J., Dynamics of organochlorine insecticides in vertebrates and ecosystems, *Nature*, **215**, 33–35 (1967).

Roncucci, R., M.-J. Simon, G. Jacques, and G. Lambelin, Stable isotopes in drug metabolism and pharmacokinetics, *Eur. J. Drug Metab. Pharmacokinet.*, **1**, 9–20 (1976).

Rowland, M., Kinetics of drug-drug interactions, in T. Teorell, R. L. Dedrick, and P. G. Condliffe, Eds., *Pharmacology and Pharmacokinetics*, pp. 321–337, Plenum Press, New York, 1974.

Rowland, M., Hemodynamic factors in pharmacokinetics, *Triangle*, **14**(3/4), 109–116 (1975).

Sanotsky, I. V., Use of equations for elimination kinetics of poisons and their metabolites in establishing thresholds of harmful action, in *Primeneniye Matematicheskikh Metodov dlya Otsenki i Prognozirovaniya Realnoi Opasnosti Nakopleniya Pestitsidov vo Vneshnei Srede i Organizme. Materialy Vtorogo Simpoziuma*, pp. 48–50, Institut Gigieny i Toksikologii Pestitsidov, Polimernykh i Plasticheskikh Mass, Kiev, 1976.

Sato, A., T. Nakajima, Y. Fujiwara, and N. Murayama, Kinetic studies on sex difference in susceptibility to chronic benzene intoxication—with special reference to body fat content, *Brit. J. Ind. Med.*, **32**, 321–328 (1975).

Sauerhoff, M. W., W. H. Braun, G. E. Blau, and P. J. Gehring, The dose-dependent pharmacokinetic profile of 2,4,5-trichlorophenoxy acetic acid following intravenous administration to rats, *Toxicol. Appl. Pharmacol.*, **36**, 491–501 (1976).

Semenov, A. I., Kinetics of ^{244}Cm exchange during chronic peroral administration, *Gig. Sanit.*, **8**, 111–113 (1975).

Shively, C. A., and E. S. Vesell, Temporal variations in acetaminophen and phenacetin half-life in man, *Clin. Pharmacol. Ther.*, **18**, 413–424 (1975).

Simakov, A. V., R. Ya. Sitko, and M. A. Khodyreva, Effective elimination half-lives of alpha emitters from the skin, *Gig. Sanit.*, **1**, 36–38 (1976).

Soloviyev, V. N., T. T. Yegorenko, and A. A. Firsov, Application of a mathematical pharmacokinetic model to liver function studies in white rats using the Bromsulphalein test, *Lab. Delo*, **9**, 538–542 (1976).

Spynu, E. I., and L. N. Ivanova, Some approaches to mathematical modeling and monitoring of environmental pollution with pesticides, in *Primeneniye Matematicheskikh Metodov dlya Otsenki i Prognozirovaniya Realnoi Opasnosti Nakopleniya Pestitsidov vo Vneshnei Srede i Organizme. Materialy Vtorogo Simpoziuma*, pp. 5–8, Institut Gigiyeny i Toksikologii Pestitsidov, Polimernykh i Plasticheskikh Mass, Kiev, 1976.

Teorell, T., R. L. Dedrick, and P. G. Condliffe, Eds., *Pharmacology and Pharmacokinetics*, Plenum Press, New York, 1974.

Timofeyev, D. P., *Kinetika Adsorbtsii [Adsorption Kinetics]*, Izdatelstvo Akad. Nauk SSSR, Moscow, 1962.

Tomita, K., Sex difference of the time of biological half-life of cadmium injected subcutaneously to mice, *Jap. J. Int. Health*, **13**, 46–47 (1971).

Traeger, A., R. Kiesewetter, and M. Kunze, Zur Pharmakokinetik von Phenobarbital bei Erwachsenen und Greisen, *Dtsch. Gesundheitswes.*, **29**, 1040–1042 (1974).

Triggs, E. J., and R. L. Nation, Pharmacokinetics in the aged: a review, *J. Pharmacokinet. Biopharmac.*, **3**, 387–418 (1975).

Triggs, E. J., R. L. Nation, and J. S. Ashley, Pharmacokinetics in the elderly, *Eur. J. Clin. Pharmacol.*, **8**, 55–62 (1975).

Vacobi, A., and G. Levy, Pharmacokinetics of the warfarin enantiomers in rats, *J. Phamacokinet. Biopharmac.*, **2**, 239–255 (1974).

Vesell, E. S., Factors causing interindividual variations of drug concentrations in blood, *Clin. Pharmacol. Ther.*, **16**, 135–148 (1974a).

Vesell, E. S., Application of pharmacokinetic principles to the elucidation of polygenically controlled differences in drug response," in T. Teorell, R. L. Dedrick, and P. G. Condliffe, Eds., *Pharmacology and Pharmacokinetics*, pp. 261–280, Plenum Press, New York, 1974b.

Vesell, E. S., C. J. Kee, G. T. Passananti, and C. A. Shively, Relationship between plasma antipyrine half-lives and hepatic microsomal drug metabolism in dogs, *Pharmacology*, **10**, 317–328 (1973).

Vesell, E. S., J. R. Shapiro, T. Passananti, H. Jorgensen, and C. A. Shively, Altered plasma half-lives of antipyrine, propylthiouracil, and methimazole in thyroid dysfunction, *Clin. Pharmacol. Ther.*, **17**, 48–56 (1975).

Wagner, J. G., A modern view of pharmacokinetics, in T. Teorell, R. L. Dedrick, and P. G. Condliffe, Eds., *Pharmacology and Pharmacokinetics*, pp. 27–68, Plenum Press, New York, 1974.

Wilkinson, G. R., Pharmacokinetics of drug disposition: hemodynamic considerations, *Ann. Rev. Pharmacol.*, **15**, 11–27 (1975).

Yakovlev, V. P., D. A. Kulikova, and E. A. Rudzit, Pharmacokinetic interference between chemotherapeutic and pharmacologic preparations, *Antibiotiki*, **21**(10), 945–954 (1976).

5

CUMULATION OF POISONS: QUANTITATIVE EVALUATION

The term "cumulation" came to toxicology from pharmacology, where since the late eighteenth century it has been used with reference to sudden enhancement of the action of a drug repeatedly administered for a prolonged period. A distinction should be drawn between material cumulation (accumulation of the poison itself) and functional cumulation (summation of the changes caused by the poison). A cumulative effect may result from material and/or functional cumulation. In toxicology cumulative effects are studied at two levels: the lethal level, where a specified dose or concentration kills test animals after being administered a number of times; and the threshold level, where a visible or measurable effect is noted after administration for a number of times of a specified dose or concentration that previously produced no such effect. A chronic industrial poisoning is the result of functional or, sometimes, both material and functional cumulation.

Evaluation of the cumulative properties of harmful substances is a matter of particular importance for industrial toxicology. Thus the degree of cumulation is a major consideration when data obtained in a long-term (chronic) animal experiment with a given substance are used to arrive at an estimate of the maximum allowable concentration of that substance in the air of workplaces.

1. EVALUATION AT THE LETHAL LEVEL

Until recently, the quantitative evaluation of cumulation in industrial toxicology was confined almost exclusively to the lethal level, and a number of methods for such evaluation of experimental data are available. Most of these methods measure the effects from repeated administration of a poison by the oral route to small laboratory animals in a dose which is a definite fraction of the median lethal dose (LD_{50}). Functional cumulation is characterized by a coefficient of cumulation (K_{cum}) which reflects, in one way or another, the time of death of test animals repeatedly exposed to equal or regularly increasing doses.

Here we will discuss only the more commonly used methods of cumulation measurement based on the LD_{50}.* The latter is a more reliable quantity than the LD_{100} or LD_0, on which some other methods depend for the calculation of K_{cum}.

In the USSR the most widely used method is that of Kagan and Stankevich (1964), which defines K_{cum} as the ratio of the summated median lethal dose ($\sum LD_{50}$) given in the course of an experiment with repeated exposure to the single-exposure LD_{50} :

$$K_{cum} = \frac{\sum LD_{50}}{LD_{50}}$$

The cumulative effect may of course vary with the frequency of exposure and the size of the repeated dose. It is common practice to use daily exposures to a dose which is a certain fraction of the single-exposure LD_{50}. The daily dose may range from 0.2 to 0.01 of this LD_{50}, the fractions 0.1, 0.05, 0.02 being used most frequently.

As a rule, Kagan employs not one but two, three, or more different fractions of the LD_{50} in the course of an experiment. This enables him to follow changes in K_{cum} when the daily dose is later reduced and thus to predict, to a certain extent, the cumulative properties of the poison in question at low levels of doses or concentrations.

An important advantage of Kagan and Stankevich's method is the possibility of determining the confidence limits of the cumulation coefficient, thus giving it a certain probability. Moreover, this coefficient can be calculated at any dosage level, that is, not only for lethal doses but also for those producing some other selected response. When several cumulation coefficients have been obtained for different repeated doses, their values are plotted as a function of the fractional doses used. As will be shown later, such a plot makes it possible to draw important conclusions.

Kagan recommends that, in addition to K_{cum}, the degree of cumulation be also characterized by the critical dose, that is, the highest daily dose which can be used without producing a cumulative effect. Also, he has proposed calculating, as a further index of cumulative properties, the slope (tangent α) of the straight line giving the relation between the lethal effect and the dose used in the chronic experiment and determining the integral coefficient $(1/LD_{50}) \cdot$ tangent α (Kagan, 1965).

According to the classification proposed by Medved et al. (1968), based on the cumulation coefficients as calculated by Kagan and Stankevich's method, cumulation is described as extremely high ($K_{cum} < 1$), strongly marked

---

* Various methods for the determination of cumulation coefficients have been reviewed by Sidorov (1967); see also Ulanova et al. (1970).

($K_{cum} = 1$ to 3), moderate ($K_{cum} = 3$ to 5), or slight ($K_{cum} > 5$). To assure comparability of the cumulation coefficients Ulanova et al. (1970) advised using a daily dose equal to 0.1 of the LD_{50}.

In establishing hygienic standards for harmful substances present in bodies of water, cumulation is often assessed by the method of Cherkinsky et al. (1964), who recommended standardization of experimental conditions. In their method 0.2 of the LD_{50} is administered to 10 animals daily for a total of 20 days, and K_{cum} is calculated from the equation

$$K_{cum} = \frac{D_{cum}}{LD_{50}\,n} \cdot \frac{50}{a}$$

where D_{cum} is the total dose given to all animals (both those that died and those that have survived), n is the number of animals and is equal to 10, and a is the percentage of animals that have succumbed during the 20 days. A co-efficient of less than 5 points to strongly marked cumulation, and one of 20 or more indicates that no animals should die.

In this, as well as in other methods for the determination of K_{cum}, the times of death of test animals are recorded. After 20 days the surviving animals are given a single LD_{50} and the number of animals that have died is counted. If more than half of the animals have died, cumulation is considered to have taken place; if less than half, it is concluded that habituation to the poison has developed. A similar procedure was used by Pravdin (1960).

The advantage of Cherkinsky's method is that it is not very time-consuming and that a numerical value of K_{cum} can be obtained even if only one of the animals has died. The disadvantages are that it is necessary to standardize the experimental conditions to make the cumulation coefficients comparable, and (more serious) that the cumulation coefficient obtained is less informative than the one given by Kagan's method, since its probable accuracy is not stated.

Lim et al. (1961) proposed a "subchronic toxicity" test in which adminis-tration of a substance is started by giving a dose of about 0.1 of the LD_{50} for the first 4 days, and then the dosage is increased after every 4-day period by a factor of 1.5, the highest dose (1.12 of the LD_{50}) being used on days 25 through 28. The test requires 24 ± 4 days, a period which the authors consider to be adequate to bring out both cumulation and tolerance. An advantage of Lim's method is the nearly constant and relatively short duration of the experiment. The cumulation coefficient can be calculated as in Kagan and Stankevich's method, although its meaning will of course be different because of the differ-ent dosing regimen.

As a matter of fact the dosing regimen used in Lim's method helps to reveal the capacity of the organism to adapt itself to the poison. Studies carried out by the Laboratory of Toxicology at the Leningrad Institute of Industrial

Hygiene and Occupational Diseases have demonstrated the importance of the exposure regimen for the evaluation of habituation (or tolerance) to harmful substances. From the viewpoint of habituation, that is, the absence of responses to higher and higher concentrations or doses, the most effective exposure regimen has been found to be the one in which a daily dose is increased after being repeated two to four times (Liublina and Minkina, 1969). A cumulation coefficient estimated from Lim's test therefore corresponds to the maximum strain on the adaptive capabilities of the organism.

Thus each of the three methods described above has its advantages and disadvantages, and the method of choice will depend on the purpose at hand. It should be remembered, however, that a cumulation coefficient obtained by any one of these methods is not comparable to that calculated by any other.

Working with pesticides, Kagan has shown that the relationship between the degree of functional cumulation and the daily fractional dose may be different for different groups of chemicals. Thus increasing the daily dose of organochlorine pesticides (e.g., from 0.05 to 0.1 of the LD_{50}) also increased the $\sum LD_{50}/LD_{50}$ ratio, so that less of the poison was required to kill half of the test animals when a smaller daily dose was used.

The reverse was true for organophosphorus pesticides: the summated LD_{50} and, consequently, the K_{cum} decreased when the daily dose was raised and increased when it was lowered (Kagan, 1970). Other kinds of relationships between K_{cum} and daily dose were also noted. Thus the K_{cum} of tetramethylthiuram disulfide was independent of the magnitude of the daily dose, while the K_{cum} of aldrin and dieldrin initially decreased when the dose was reduced and then increased as it was reduced further (Medved et al., 1968).

The cumulation coefficients calculated by any of the above three methods are not very convenient in that a smaller coefficient corresponds to a greater degree of cumulation. The inverse ratio would seem to be desirable, but since Kagan and Stankevich's method has been worked out in detail and is widely used, it is better, instead, to supplement the concept of K_{cum} with that of the degree of cumulation expressed as the percentage ratio of LD_{50} to $\sum LD_{50}$ (Table 21).

It will be seen from this table that Medved's classification is not uniform in that the moderate cumulation category covers a smaller range of degree of cumulation estimates than do the other categories. A uniform classification built on the principle of arithmetic or geometric progression would be preferable. Medved's classification, which has come into wide use in the USSR and so should not be replaced by another, can be made more uniform if the boundary between categories 2 and 3 is shifted by substituting $K_{cum} = 2.2$ for $K_{cum} = 3$ in category 2 and $K_{cum} > 2.2$ for $K_{cum} > 3$ in category 3, as shown on the right side of Table 21, where the percentage degree of cumulation between the categories differs by a factor of 2.2.

Table 21. The Classification of Cumulative Action According to Medved et al. (1968) and Its Proposed Modification

Category of Cumulation	According to Medved et al.		Modified Version	
	Cumulation Coefficient	Degree of Cumulation (%)	Cumulation Coefficient	Degree of Cumulation (%)
1. Extremely high	<1	>100	<1	>100
2. Strongly marked	1–3	100–34	1 –2.2	100–46
3. Moderate	>3–5	33–20	>2.2–5	45–20
4. Slight	>5	<20	>5	<20

The cumulation coefficient gives an indication of the order of magnitude of the factor of safety F_s, a quantity by which the threshold concentration as found in a chronic experiment (C_{chr}) is divided to obtain the maximum allowable concentration (MAC). Kagan found the correlation coefficient between K_{cum} (as calculated by Kagan and Stankevich's method) and F_s to be 0.6 (1970); later, when a computer was used for the calculation, a more precise figure of 0.65 was obtained (Kagan et al., 1972). The K_{cum} is related to F_s by the equation

$$F_s = 2.26K_{cum}^2 - 39.2K_{cum} + 177.32$$

This equation was derived from data used in establishing hygienic standards for pesticides. The safety factors thus calculated have values of more than 20, even though the cumulation may be slight.*

Sidorov (1971) has suggested that the cumulative effect of a poison can be estimated from its biological action zone, defined as LC_{50}/C_{chr} (Sanotsky, 1964). Obviously, the wider this zone the more marked is the cumulation. Sidorov has proposed taking into account not only the cumulative properties of poisons (K_1), but also the species differences in sensitivity to poisons (K_2), and, if applicable, such long-term effects as blastomogenic, mutagenic, and sensitizing (K_3); he has derived the equation

$$MAC = \frac{C_{chr}}{K_1 \cdot K_2 \cdot K_3}$$

giving values of these three coefficients (Sidorov, 1971).

* $F_s = 20$ when $K_{cum} = 6$. In the above equation K_{cum} should not exceed 10; otherwise F_s will increase rather than decrease with increasing K_{cum}.

Shtabsky (1971) has proposed assessing cumulative properties on the basis of the times of death of animals with single and repeated administration of the poison and estimating the maximum permissible dose from the ratio of the numbers of deaths at different times.

2. EVALUATION AT THE THRESHOLD LEVEL

Since even a cumulation coefficient calculated at the lethal level can furnish information of value for arriving at an estimate of the maximum permissible dose or concentration, the determination of such coefficients at the threshold level would be expected to provide much more valuable information. Unfortunately, only a few studies have been undertaken at the threshold level so far. Usually a K_{cum} determined at the lethal level does not give any indication of the K_{cum} at the threshold level because the sites and nature of action of many industrial poisons on acute exposure are different from those on chronic exposure. Thus, as pointed out by Kagan et al. (1968), although the K_{cum} of carbathion at the lethal level is 15 (i.e., there is practically no cumulation; see Table 21), long-term exposure to this pesticide at the level of 5 mg/kg (0.01 LD_{50}) causes chronic poisoning of test animals.

Of special interest in this context are the results of Weil et al. (1969), which indicate a very high correlation ($r = 0.95$) between the minimal effective doses of pesticides and surfactants fed in diets to rats daily for a period of 7 days ($D_{7\text{-day}}$) and the same daily doses fed for 90 days ($D_{90\text{-day}}$). Calculations showed that the $D_{90\text{-day}}$ was equal to 1/3 of the $D_{7\text{-day}}$ when the doses were expressed in terms of ED_{50} and to 1/6.2 of the $D_{7\text{-day}}$ when they were expressed in terms of ED_{95}.

In this study the minimal effective doses fed to rats over a period of 2 years were found to correlate closely with the same doses given for 90 and 7 days: $D_{2\text{-year}} = D_{90\text{-day}}/1.8$ and $D_{2\text{-year}} = D_{7\text{-day}}/5.4$ at the ED_{50} level, and $D_{2\text{-year}} = D_{90\text{-day}}/5.7$ and $D_{2\text{-year}} = D_{7\text{-day}}/35.3$ at the ED_{95} level. The correlations of these doses with the LD_{50} were unsatisfactory. The possibility of translating the results of a 7-day test into a prediction of the 90-day or even 2-year results at the minimal effective dose level and the impossibility of going to long-term results from the lethal dose level serve to reemphasize the importance of estimating cumulation at low levels and demonstrate the feasibility of forecasting the results of a long-term experiment from those of a short-term test. At present, the need for estimating cumulation at low levels is no longer questioned.

Whenever one is dealing with cumulation, it is necessary to take account of adaptation processes which tend to develop in response to continued administration of any agent capable of altering an important bodily function—not necessarily to the extent of taking that function outside the physiological limits but even in cases where these limits are approached. Adaptation and cumulation represent a dialectical unity of opposites, cumulation signifying an augmentation of functional alterations, and adaptation, their diminution. The capacity for adaptation is inherent in any living organism, just like the capacity for self-preservation and reproduction. The term "adaptation" is used collectively to mean the processes of adjustment in response to most diverse influences; these processes may vary widely in duration from extremely short, measured by fractions of a second, to very prolonged, lasting weeks or even years.

In industrial toxicology the term "habituation" is often used to denote a decrease or disappearance of responses to a poison occurring after repeated exposures to it. In 1938 Lazarev wrote that "generally speaking, there can be no habituation to those poisons which have a cumulative action, irrespective of whether the cumulation is material or functional" (p. 380). Nowadays, however, habituation is seen as a phase in chronic intoxication and, as such, has been shown to occur in response to a variety of industrial poisons, whatever their cumulative properties.

Liublina et al. (1965, 1971) have shown that the blood of animals in the phase of habituation to a harmful substance administered by inhalation contains less of that substance than the blood of control animals exposed to it for the first time under identical conditions. On the other hand, animals which have already passed the habituation phase as a result of continued exposure and so have become more sensitive to the poison tend to accumulate more poison in the blood than the control animals.

Thus habituation involves some mechanisms enabling smaller concentrations of the harmful substance to be contained in the blood, while the subsequent increase in sensitivity to the substance is associated with its increased concentration in the blood. Experiments by Dobrynina (1968) have indicated that the postexposure decline in the blood concentration of acetone proceeds at a faster rate in mice habituated to the poison than in nonhabituated mice. It therefore appears that a poison is destroyed and eliminated more rapidly in animals in the habituation phase than in nonhabituated animals.

Habituation may be associated with metabolic alterations such as occur when a long-acting harmful substance (e.g., a narcotic) becomes a constant participant in tissue metabolism. Or there may be synthesized specially induced enzymes capable of degrading xenobiotics; a case in point is the elaboration of "tabunase" in response to long-continued administration of low doses of a tabun-type organosphorus compound. Also, habituation may be associated with inhibition of enzymic activity; one example is inactivation of enzyme systems during habituation to morphine. Furthermore, the organism may begin producing specific antibodies, for instance, in the sustained administration of arsenic or copper acetate. Sequestration of metals may likewise be involved in habituation to them. When a stimulus of low intensity acts on nerve tissue, habituation may be a manifestation of the pro-dromal phase of parabiosis; this occurs on exposure to a variety of stimuli, including industrial poisons. Low-level exposure to a threshold stimulus may lead to that stimulus becoming a subthreshold one as the result of an increase in lability* and some decrease in excitability—a feature typical of habitua-tion. The latter may also occur by other mechanisms.

In experiments conducted for the purpose of determining cumulation co-efficients, we are usually concerned with the result of cumulation and habitua-tion, both at the lethal and at the threshold level. Depending on the intensity and frequency of exposure, we may get, with one and the same substance, a picture of predominant habituation or a one where cumulation prevails. This is the reason why experiments using different and small doses are necessary if the cumulative properties of a poison are to be assessed correctly.

Habituation has been shown to be particularly marked in the case of in-halation exposure to organic solvents at the level of lethal concentrations. Thus Loit (1964), in his attempt to devise a simple, short experiment to eluci-date the cumulative properties of volatile organic solvents, encountered such strong habituation that repeated exposures to concentrations approaching the LC_{50} failed to kill even 50% of the mice. To obtain comparative data on cumulative properties of the solvents, he had to employ much harsher ex-posure conditions than those normally used to calculate the LC_{50} from single-exposure data.

At present, the cumulative properties of volatile substances are evaluated, for the most part, in oral or intraperitoneal rather than inhalation studies, al-though inhalation exposures are of course much more common in industrial settings.

As yet there does not exist any generally accepted and not time-consuming method for studying the cumulative properties of industrial poisons on a relatively small number of animals, even at the lethal level of exposure. Attempts to estimate cumulation coefficients at the threshold level in-volve additional difficulties. For one thing, there arises the question of the criterion of harmful action to be used. For another, there is the problem of habituation, which tends to occur at the threshold level in contrast to the lethal level, where experiments are often too short for habituation to develop. Moreover, it is only on rare occasions that the probable accuracy of threshold doses is determined, a circumstance which of course complicates the study.

---

* The lability of nerve tissue is characterized by the number of nerve impulses conducted per unit of time.

Furthermore, working at the threshold level requires a control group of animals and a preliminary determination of the $D_{min\ 50}$. Also, a certain initial period is needed to obtain baseline data on the indices to be measured, so that the animals can be properly allocated to the test and control groups.

Some experience with the estimation of K_{cum} at the threshold level has already been gained, however. Thus Rabotnikova (1966) from the Leningrad Institute of Industrial Hygiene and Occupational Diseases studied the cumulative properties of eight oxides of metals from the second group of the periodic table. In this study on mice, baseline data were obtained by determining body weight, summated threshold index* (according to Speransky, 1965), muscle strength (by Speransky's method, 1962), duration of hexenal (hexobarbital) narcosis, acidic resistance of erythrocytes, erhythrocyte counts, hemoglobin content, color index, and blood levels of SH groups. Metal oxides were then injected intraperitoneally twice a week in the form of emulsion (in sunflower seed oil) in the amount of 0.2 ml, each dose being equal to 0.5 of the threshold value. The range of tests used (most of them were nonspecific, although some, such as the determination of SH groups, may be regarded as specific for metal ions) made it possible to determine, over a 4-week period, phasic changes in many of the indices studied, for all of the eight oxides. For instance, the initial decrease in SH groups was followed by restoration of their contents to baseline level after four injections of beryllium oxide; muscle strength returned to baseline level after four injections of magnesium oxide; and so on. There were signs of nonspecifically increased resistance in mice, including increased hemoglobin content, color index, and erythrocyte resistance. For some of the oxides, however, signs of unfavorable responses to continued exposure were apparent toward the end of the third and during the fourth week. Examples are reduced erythrocyte resistance in the case of beryllium oxide and increased duration of narcosis in mice given cadmium or barium oxide.

Rabotnikova calculated the cumulation coefficient each time from data on the index for which a threshold effect had been attained first rather than from data on the same indices for every oxide. In our view this principle is justified, as is the use of not one but several indices in calculating cumulation coefficients. The cumulation coefficients at the threshold level calculated by Kagan and Stankevich's method ($K_{cum\ min}$) proved to be small—not more than 3.0 for all the oxides studied, being between 1.5 and 1.0 for BeO, BaO, and CdO; this means that the degree of cumulation was 34% at its lowest level and attained 100% (see Table 21).

Rabotnikova's experiments demonstrated the possibility and utility of

---

* An indicator of the CNS function.

estimating cumulation coefficients at the threshold level from data of short-term experiments, even for practical evaluations of industrial poisons. They also showed the great importance of habituation, which was later confirmed in a number of studies into the cumulative properties of various harmful substances administered at different dose levels (e.g., Krasovsky and Korolev, 1969; Krasovsky et al., 1970a,b); Krasovsky and Shigan, 1970, 1971; Shtabsky, 1969; Liublina, 1973a).

Gizatullina (1970, 1971) studied the cumulative properties of three organophosphorus and two organochlorine compounds to see whether the relationship between the K_{cum} and a daily fractional dose at the threshold level is similar to or different from that at the lethal level. The compounds were administered to rats intraperitoneally five times a week, using the following dosing schedules: (1) $0.25 D_{min\ 50}$; (2) $0.5 D_{min\ 50}$; and (3) increasing the dose by 50% on every odd injection, the starting dose being equal to $0.2 D_{min\ 50}$. The third treatment was designed to show how $K_{cum\ min}$ was affected by escalating doses.

The experiments included the determination of some specific indices: cholinesterase activity in the case of organophosphorus compounds, and summated threshold index and Bromsulphalein test for liver function in the case of organochlorine compounds. Preliminarily, fluctuations in cholinesterase activity were measured in intact animals, making it possible to regard the subsequent reduction in this activity by 12.5% as having been caused by the exogenous inhibitor.

A comparison of mean cholinesterase activities showed that the K_{cum} was higher (i.e., the degree of cumulation was lower) with the increasing dose schedule than with the $0.5 D_{min\ 50}$ schedule, for all three organophosphorus compounds considered (triphenyl phosphite, trioctyl phosphite, and metaphos). As for the $0.25 D_{min\ 50}$ regimen, it was not possible to calculate the K_{cum} because the mean cholinesterase activity began returning to normal even before the lower limit of threshold inhibition had been reached. Of particular interest are the results obtained for triphenyl phosphite (Figure 33). Although this experiment lasted for 4 weeks, it was found possible to calculate the $K_{cum\ min}$ as early as in the second week (except for the treatment with $0.25 D_{min\ 50}$). During the third and fourth weeks the mean cholinesterase activity returned to the baseline level in the treatments with 0.5 and $0.25 D_{min\ 50}$. The summated threshold index was, however, significantly lower than in the control. The weight of animals receiving constant doses of organophosphorus compounds did not differ from that of the control.

It is worth noting that in another study (Brzezicka-Bak and Bojanowska, 1969), where other organophosphorus compounds were administered orally for 9 weeks in a daily dose of $0.1 LD_{50}$, the cholinesterase activity in the whole

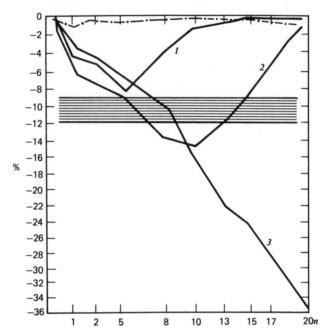

Figure 33. Percentage inhibition of cholinesterase activity in the blood of rats plotted against the number of exposures (n) to triphenyl phosphite in three different dosage regimens. *Curve 3*, treatment with increasing doses (the first and last doses, expressed as multiples of the threshold value, are equal to 0.2 and 31); *curve 2*, constant doses equal to 0.5 ED_{50}; *curve 1*, constant doses equal to 0.25 ED_{50}; *dotted line*, control; *hatched area*, distance between the lower and upper confidence limits of threshold inhibition. (After Gizatullina, 1971.)

blood at the end of the experiment was higher in test animals than in the control. Krasovsky et al. (1970a) found the blood level of cholinesterase to have decreased after the first three to five exposures and to remain constant thereafter despite continued administration of organophosphorus compounds.

As regards the two organochlorine compounds (carbon tetrachloride and hexachloran), Gizatullina found the cumulation coefficient to be lowest with the smallest daily dose (0.25 $D_{min\ 50}$) and highest with the escalating dose schedule. No signs of habituation were evident in the course of 10 exposures to carbon tetrachloride or hexachloran, but continued administration of hexachloran (up to 20 exposures) led to restoration of the summated threshold index in both treatments with the constant doses.

Liver weight after 20 hexachloran exposures was increased 5-fold in mice on the increasing dose schedule, 2.5-fold in those given 0.5 $D_{min\ 50}$, and 1.5-fold in those given 0.25 $D_{min\ 50}$, as compared to the control. In the treatments with 0.5 and 0.25 $D_{\text{min }50}$ the summated threshold index was changed only insignificantly after the last exposure. Beginning with the 11th exposure, the average body weight in both these groups was 2 or more grams less than in the control.

It follows from the above studies that, while the direction of changes in cumulation coefficients on passing from one daily dose to another is generally the same at the threshold and lethal levels, habituation tends to develop when exposure to constant doses is continued at the threshold level. Thus the administration both of organophosphorus and of organochlorine compounds led to habituation when the experiment was continued after sufficient changes had occurred to permit the calculation of $K_{\text{cum min}}$. Along with a decrease in, or even the disappearance of, some specific response to the administered substance, a significant change in a nonspecific response may be detected.

The foregoing results remind us once again of possible different effects of the same substance on different functions and organs, especially when the functional state of the organism has been altered as the result of continued administration of the substance. Adaptation to the specific action of a poison may occur in the presence and at the expense of considerable alterations in other, often nonspecific, responses. The well-known fact that the initial symptoms of chronic poisoning caused by different poisons tend to be similar, especially as regards the autonomic and central nervous systems, makes it necessary for the toxicologist to pay special attention to the nonspecific indices of nervous activity.

In our view the study of cumulation at the threshold level should not be confined to the period necessary to calculate $K_{\text{cum min}}$ using two or more fractions of the D_{min}. Rather, the experiment should be extended up to 4 weeks so as to be able to detect habituation and, more important, to reveal any significant unfavorable alterations which may occur, in the course of habituation, in other indices, both specific and nonspecific. It is particularly important to estimate the magnitude of the critical dose, that is, the maximal dose which does not yet cause any significant change in a given index in the course of the experiment.

At present, habituation to a harmful substance is usually interpreted as an indication of a considerable effect exerted by the substance, while the degree to which the compensatory mechanisms are involved is assessed from changes in nonspecific indices or from functional stress tests.

It should be noted that habituation per se is indicative of cumulation, for habituation develops because traces of the poison are present in the body, and these traces may result in significant alterations which actuate defense mechanisms.

The smallest adverse effects are usually produced by the doses or concentrations of a harmful substance which are capable of bringing about sustained fluctuations in particular responses as the state of nonspecific resistance persists in the organism (Lazarev et al., 1959; Lazarev and Rozin, 1960; Liublina et al., 1971).

The results of studies on the determination of $K_{cum\ min}$ described here and elsewhere (e.g., Krasovsky et al., 1970a, b; Krasovsky et al., 1971) make it possible to formulate some recommendations to help resolve or obviate the above-mentioned difficulties encountered in staging experiments at the threshold level.

As concerns the choice of tests, it seems advisable to employ not one but several different tests, in particular, to use a specific test in conjunction with nonspecific ones when the mechanism of action of the substance is known. It appears that one of the methods available for the study of effects of poisons on the nervous system must be included as a nonspecific test in any case, since the nervous system is always affected by a harmful substance, even though the changes may be secondary. A variety of such tests are available, including, among others, those for conditioned reflex activity, unconditioned motor reflexes, summation of subthreshold impulses, and determination of the summated threshold index (Speransky, 1965). Of the nonspecific tests the following three may usually be employed: muscle strength (for mice and rats), motor activity, and measurement of the time taken to restore a function after a specified amount of exercise. The most convenient test appears to be the determination of summated threshold index. As for exposure regimens, Krasovsky et al. (1970a) advise using at least two or three doses differing by a factor of 5 to 10, while Ulanova (1970) prefers Lim's method (see above). Tests by Gizatullina (1970) have indicated that a daily dose equal to 0.1 of the $D_{min\ 50}$ is too small for use in an experiment lasting 2 to 4 weeks and that such large differences (5- to 10-fold) between daily doses are inadvisable. Krasovsky and Shigan (1971) have advocated the use of the smallest dose whose effect disappears within 24 hr in half of the animals (ED_{50}). This ED_{50} is estimated on a quantal basis so that probit analysis can be used in the calculations. Also, the response is measured several times postadministration (after 1, 2, 3, ... hr), and hourly dose-response curves are plotted.

In our judgment there is no need to measure hourly changes or to administer the whole ED_{50}. As a rule the $D_{min\ 50}$ should be smaller than the ED_{50}, and experience shows that $K_{cum\ min}$ can be determined after only half of the $D_{min\ 50}$ has been administered. In estimating the cumulation, it is convenient to start with low doses that produce no effect on single exposure. It is more economical to employ daily doses amounting to 0.5 and 0.25 of the $D_{min\ 50}$, making use, in rare cases, of 0.125 of the $D_{min\ 50}$ as well. Experiments with escalating doses, such as those used in Lim's method, are not advisable in view of the likelihood of provoking enhanced adaptation and thus of underestimating the degree of cumulation.

The probit method of analysis is not suitable for estimating the probable accuracy of the threshold dose from graded response data: it is necessary first to convert the results to the quantal form. To do this, the mean and the confidence limits of the response under study are first determined from data on its variations in the control group (at least 20 animals). Then, in the course of the experiment on the determination of the $D_{min\ 50}$, each individual response is measured quantally, depending on whether or not its value exceeds the confidence limit.

If a given selected response (index) tends to show phasic changes (as is usually the case when neural elements are acted upon by progressively increasing doses or concentrations), and, especially, if the direction of the changes reverses on passing from one phase to another, a more reliable result can be obtained by determining the threshold and subthreshold doses for each individual animal. After data on individual threshold doses have been obtained, probit analysis can be employed (e.g., according to Prozorovsky, 1967), supposing that all the doses have been tested on each animal and that every animal has responded not only to its threshold dose but also to all higher doses and has not responded to lower ones.

When the experiment is continued after all the data necessary for the calculation of $K_{cum\ min}$ have been collected, habituation is often observed to occur: some or all of the responses studied begin to change in the direction of the control values (see Figure 33). The point where an inflection appears in the dose-response curve can apparently be defined by the same ratio as the $K_{cum\ min}$, but the summative dose will now show the value of this coefficient at the point of inflection; the latter coefficient may be termed a coefficient of primary habituation. A similar coefficient, but calculated from the total dose received by the animals by the time that the response under study returned to baseline level (if such a return occurred), may be called a coefficient of complete primary habituation for the given dosage level. By comparing these three coefficients (other coefficients can also be calculated, e.g., a coefficient corresponding to the time at which secondary changes begin to occur) and the fractional daily doses for which they have been obtained, important tentative conclusions can be derived as regards both cumulation and adaptation in response to a given poison in the course of its repeated administration; hence an approximate concept of the $D_{min\ chr}$ and of the MAC may be gained.

It is possible to approach the MAC even more closely by determining the critical dose, that is, the highest dose that can be administered (say, five times per week for a period of 4 weeks) without observing any cumulative effect. Additional physical stress tests are required, however, before one can be sure that no cumulation has occurred. One example is provided by our experiments with norbornanes (Dobrynina and Liublina, 1974), in which 11 intraperitoneal injections of a norbornane were given to mice in the course of 15 days in daily doses of 0.25 or 0.5 of the threshold dose for 50% of mice, the threshold being determined from changes in the summated threshold index. Neither the weight of the animals nor the index measured before and 10 min after each injection showed any significant differences from the control. However, when the mice were made to swim, both test groups differed significantly from the control: the control mice were able to swim twice as long.

Evaluation of the cumulative properties of harmful substances was the subject of many of the papers presented to the First Symposium on the Application of Mathematical Methods in the Evaluation and Prediction of Hazards from the Accumulation of Pesticides in the Environment and in the Organism (Kiev, 1971). Mathematical expertise is now increasingly relied upon for the calculation of accumulation of poisons in the body, and successful attempts are being made to estimate quantitatively the processes of absorption, distribution, detoxication, and elimination of poisons with the aid of mathematical models of varying degrees of complexity. Models can also be developed, of course, for the study of cumulation. One such model, which simulates the inhibition of a vitally important biochemical function and the concurrent enzymic process of detoxication, was described by Khokhlov add Broitman (1971). These authors determined the ratios of parameters for which the effect produced by a poison is additive with respect to the doses as well as those for which the effect strongly departs from additivity and shows an undulating pattern, with fluctuations gradually dying down as the dose is decreased. In future, mathematical models should be expected to be used on an ever larger scale in quantitative toxicology, including cumulation and adaptation studies.

Research on the cumulative action of harmful substances at the threshold level is still at the incipient stage, and continued efforts by toxicologists along this line should provide further insights into the cumulation of various poisons, better methods for its study, and a clearer interpretation of both cumulation and adaptation.

ADDENDUM: SOME FURTHER ASPECTS OF CUMULATION

Mention should be made of a paper by Kagan (1975) which surveys the methodology of cumulative action studies and discusses criteria for assessing cumulative effects, the relationship between cumulation and adaptation, and the use of data on cumulation and adaptation in the development of hygienic standards.

A1. THREE TYPES OF CUMULATIVE ACTION

Kagan and Shtabsky (1974), in their theoretical study on the molecular mechanisms of cumulation have clearly demonstrated the need to distinguish between at least three types of cumulative action rather than between two (i.e., material and functional cumulation).

In the case of material cumulation the molecules of a substance S are released from the receptor site in chemically unchanged form after contact with the appropriate receptor R. This receptor then returns to its normal state and is again capable of performing its physiological functions. The duration of the primary cumulative effect depends on the time of existence of the receptor-substance complex RS $(R + S \rightleftharpoons RS)$ and may be characterized by the half-life of the effect T, which coincides with the half-life T_S of the substance itself.

In the event of functional cumulation, the substance is released from the receptor site during or shortly after its interaction with the receptor, but the latter remains in a state of denaturation of one degree or another: $R + S \rightarrow R' + S$, where R' is the changed receptor. The half-life of the effect is now of course longer than that of the substance in the critical organ $(T > T_S)$.

However, one cannot ignore cases of cumulation of a mixed type, in which $R + S \rightarrow RS' + S''$, where S' and S'' are fractions of the original molecule of substance. Here, as in functional cumulation, $T > T_S$, but, as in material cumulation, the primary cumulative effect depends for its duration on the receptor-bound fraction of the substance.

An example of material cumulation without functional cumulation is the accumulation of a poisonous metal in the body up to the point when signs and symptoms appear to indicate that the poison has produced an effect. Examples of purely functional cumulation are cases of chronic poisoning with nonelectrolytes which are narcotics of type II (see Chapter 7, p. 317) and so are rapidly eliminated from the body in expired air. Mixed cumulation occurs in all instances of chronic poisoning involving accumulation of the substance responsible for the poisoning. Kagan and Shtabsky adduce as examples of mixed cumulation the reactions of protein acylation—in particular, the phosphorylation and carbamoylation of esterases. The phosphorylated cholinesterase remains inactive much longer than the carbamoylated one, even though a reversible intermediate complex forms in both cases. The duration of cumulative action depends on the rate of enzyme release from the enzyme-inhibitor complex, being the longer the slower this rate. The original molecule of the inhibitor is not restored in this case. Enzyme activity is half restored after 25 to 27 min for derivatives of dimethylcarbamic acid, after 37 to 39 min for methylcarbamic acid derivatives, and after 1400 min for bis-quaternary carbamates (Golikov and Rozengart, 1964). It follows, then, that the cumulative action of a poison can be predicted by determining the time taken to restore the activities of enzymes and other protein structures interacting with the poison.

Thus it appears that the type of cumulation can already be determined in an acute test and that data on the half-lives of substances and on primary cumulative effects may be of use in developing exposure tests and in establishing hygienic standards for harmful substances.

A2. STANDARDIZATION OF CUMULATION COEFFICIENTS

Shtabsky and Kagan (1974) have proposed that all toxic substances be divided into two groups: those which kill test animals over a protracted period of time (Group 1), and those which kill them rapidly, after a single dose (Group 2). Also, they have introduced the concept of a single dose D_1 that kills 50% of tests animals within the first 24 hr after administration and of a single dose D_2 that does so within a fortnight. If deaths occur over a period of time, $D_1 > D_2$; if they occur rapidly, $D_1 = D_2$. Late deaths after a single dose indicate a slow development of the toxic effect in the organ responsible for the lethal outcome. This means that the cumulative properties of substances from Group 1 are superior to those of substances from Group 2. One can therefore gain a concept of cumulative properties from the results of an acute test using the cumulation index $I_{cum} = 1 - (D_2/D_1)$. For substances of Group 2 this index is zero, while for those of Group 1 it is the higher the more strongly marked the cumulative properties of the substance.

When cumulation is assessed from an acute or a subacute test (involving repeated administration of fractional doses), the results obtained for a substance of Group 1 cannot in fact be compared with those obtained for a Group 2 substance because the doses used in the former case are fractions of the D_1, while in the latter case they are fractions of the D_2. To assure comparability of the results, Shtabsky and Kagan (1974) have proposed expressing repeated doses as fractions of the D_1 and using what they call the standardized cumulation coefficient, defined as $K_{cum}^{stand} = \sum D_n/D_1 = D_2/D_1 \cdot K_{cum}$. where $\sum D_n$ is the summated median lethal dose. The nonstandardized cumulation coefficient K_{cum} (as defined by the equation shown on p. 253) is as many times greater than the standardized coefficient as the D_1 is greater than the D_2. Having determined the D_1 experimentally, one can convert K_{cum} to K_{cum}^{stand} by multiplying it by the ratio D_2/D_1. In this way comparable cumulation coefficients can be obtained. Kagan and Stankevich's method (described on p. 253) now makes it possible to obtain comparable estimates of cumulative properties of different substances (irrespective of whether the cumulation is material, functional, or both), even from acute exposure results, and to express K_{cum}^{stand} in probabilistic terms, since K_{cum} is calculated with its confidence limits in this method.

The utility of cumulation coefficients thus standardized is obvious, and their use is continually expanding.

A3.   QUANTITATIVE ASSESSMENT OF ADAPTATION TO POISONS

Popov et al. (1976) suggested that the magnitude of adaptation be measured in dimensionless relative units. To determine adaptation, they subtracted the experimental values of cumulative effect (ECE) from a curve of theoretical cumulative effect (TCE), constructed from a mathematical model relating single dose and dynamic effect, and divided the difference by TCE:

$$\text{Adaptation (rel. units)} = \frac{\text{TCE} - \text{ECE}}{\text{TCE}} \qquad (A1)$$

This equation was used to construct a mathematical model for adaptation from data on certain liver function indices as measured in tests with repeated administration (for 2 months) of carbon tetrachloride in small doses. All the adaptation curves plotted according to (A1) for particular indices had an oscillating course and damped out with time. Equations were then derived from the adaptation curves for individual indices of liver function.

ADDENDUM REFERENCES

Golikov, S. N., and V. I. Rozengart, *Kholinesterazy i Antikholinesterazniye Veshchestva* [*Cholinesterases and Anticholinesterase Substances*], Meditsina, Leningrad, 1964.

Kagan, Yu. S., Accumulation and adaptation processes in the action of chemical agents in the environment, in *Methods Used in the USSR for Establishing Biologically Safe Levels of Toxic Substances*, World Health Organization, Geneva, 1975.

Kagan, Yu, S., and B. M. Shtabsky, On molecular mechanisms of cumulation: three types of cumulative action by toxic substances, *Gig. Sanit.*, **11**, 69–73 (1974).

Popov, T. A., Yu. G. Antomonov, and A. B. Kotova, A mathematical model for the adaptation to hepatotropic poisons, in *Primeneniye Metematicheskikh Metodov dlya Otsenki i Prognozirovaniya Realnoi Opasnosti Nakopleniya Pestitsidov vo Vneshnei Srede i Organizme. Materialy Vtorogo Simpoziuma*, pp. 42–44, Institut Gigiyeny i Toksikologii Pestitsidov, Polimernykh i Plasticheskikh Mass, Kiev, 1976.

Shtabsky, B. M., and Yu. S. Kagan, Estimating the cumulative properties of chemicals from the cumulation index and standardized cumulation coefficient, *Gig. Sanit.*, **3**, 65–67 (1974).

6

QUANTITATIVE EVALUATION OF THE TOXIC EFFECT FROM POISONS ACTING JOINTLY

1. INTRODUCTION (AND SOME ASPECTS OF TERMINOLOGY)

In the USSR the question of the combined actions of poisons is given high priority in publications concerned with the establishment of hygienic standards for harmful substances in the environment, or the current status of and prospects for the development of toxicology and hygiene (e.g., Letavet, 1962; Kagan, 1963b; Korbakova, 1964; Korbakova et al., 1970; Marchenko and Zapalkevich, 1965; Volkova et al., 1969; Sanotsky, 1969; Cherkinsky, 1969; Krotkov and Sidorenko, 1970; Gusev, 1970). This is understandable, since in practice it is only on rare occasions that industrial, communal, or agricultural toxicologists have to deal with the toxic effects produced by a single substance. In real life man is, in most situations, exposed to a combination of toxic agents.

The problem of the combined effects of harmful agents is vast and multidimensional, encompassing, as it does, a wide range of activities all the way from the development of various experimental procedures and of methods for studying the mechanism of toxic action, to questions of health legislation. The scope of this chapter allows us to consider briefly only one aspect of this problem, namely, the quantitative estimation of the toxic effect resulting from simultaneous joint action of two or more toxic substances. Other aspects such as successive exposure to different toxic substances will not be discussed here.

Although the various questions involved in quantitative evaluation of the combined action of toxic substances are of particular interest to industrial toxicologists and have been dealt with in greater detail by them, it should be noted that much credit for the progress made in this field is due to pharmacologists.

270

As was noted by Moshkovsky in 1943, there exist a very large number of terms for designating various kinds of combined effect. Many of them are not clearly defined and some are ambiguous, the same terms being used with different, sometimes even opposite, meanings by different authors. One example is the term "potentiation," introduced by Bürgi (cited in Moshkovsky, 1943) to denote a combined effect which is greater than the sum of the individual effects produced by the substances when applied separately. Straub (cited in Moshkovsky, 1943) proposed to replace it by "multiplication." Subsequently, the terms "summation," "augmentation." and "synergism" were variously used to refer to a combined effect greater than the sum of the individual effects. Loewe, an acknowledged authority in the field of quantitative pharmacology, used "potentiation" to mean the highest degree of antagonism in the action of drugs, that is, in a sense opposite to that employed by Bürgi. Much the same can be said about the term "synergism," which has been used to denote both enhancement and weakening of the combined effect. By way of illustration two systems of designations proposed for combined effects are given in Tables 22 and 23 (reproduced from Moshkovsky, 1943).

Moshkovsky (1943) listed a number of other terms used with different meanings to designate combined effects ("coagitation," "superadditivity," "isoadditivity," "heteroadditivity," "cooperation," "negative potentiation," "depotentiation," "potentiated antagonism," and "isodynamic," "meiodynamic," and "pleiodynamic" actions). He also proposed his own nomenclature (Table 24).

All three systems shown in the tables were devised for drugs, but many of the terms listed there and their various combinations have been widely used in toxicology as well as pharmacology. In toxicology, however, many

Table 22.   The Nomenclature of Combined Effects Proposed by Rentz

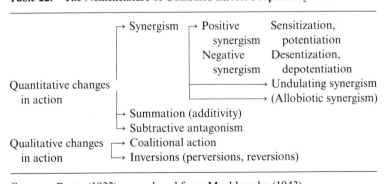

Source.   Rentz (1932), reproduced from Moshkovsky (1943).

Table 23.   The Nomenclature of Combined Effects Proposed by Bürgi

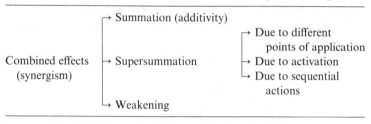

Source.   Bürgi (1938), reproduced from Moshkovsky (1943).

researchers give preference to the system of terms originally proposed by Bliss (1939) and later given modified definitions by Finney (1952) and Ball (1959). In this system distinction is made between three types of joint action, defined as follows:

1. *Similar joint action*, in which toxic substances applied jointly in a mixture are assumed to act upon the same system of receptors within the test animal, so that one can be substituted for another without changing the toxicity of the mixture.
2. *Independent joint action*, in which the toxic components of a mixture are assumed to act at different sites in the body, so that the effects produced are unrelated and the test animal dies from the effect produced by only one component rather than from the combined effect of the poisons.
3. *Synergistic* or *antagonistic joint action*, in which the effectiveness of the mixture cannot be assessed from that of the individual components but depends upon a knowledge of their combined toxicity.

As regards the nomenclature used to describe joint actions, it appears that a distinction should be drawn between terms describing the mechanism of action and those used to describe the toxic effect itself. Some authors do not make such a distinction, and this adds to the terminological confusion which still persists. For example, the terms "similar," "independent," and "synergistic (antagonistic) joint action " as defined above relate to the mechanism of joint action. The same is probably true, in general, of the terms "antagonism " and "synergism." These are often used to describe the mechanism of action not only of jointly acting substances, but also of individual poisons (e.g., with reference to their ability to inhibit or stimulate the same functions, to produce similar or opposite actions). All the terms listed above are, however, also used in evaluating combined effects as such.

Without going into a discussion of the "optimality" of the various terms employed in joint-action studies, it should merely be noted that, because of their ambiguity, the above-mentioned terms are not very convenient for the

Table 24.   The Nomenclature and Quantitative Characteristics[a] of Combined Effects Proposed by Moshkovsky

1	Interference	Complete	$(A + \alpha) = 0$	The effect is abolished by an ineffective substance
2			$(A + B) = 0$	The effect is abolished by another effective substance
3		Partial	$(A) > (A + \alpha) > 0$	The effect is weakened by adding an ineffective substance
4			$(A) > (A + B) > 0$	The effect is weakened by adding an effective substance
5	Masking		$(A + B) = (A)$	The effect is not changed when another effective substance is added
6	Additivity	Partial	$(A) < (A + B) < (A_S)$	The combined effect is greater than the uncombined effect but not greater than the summative effect
7		Complete	$(A + B) = (A_S)$	
8	Potentiation		$(A + B) > (A_S)$	The combined effect is greater than the summative effect
9			$(A + \alpha) > (A)$	The effect is enhanced by an ineffective substance

Source.   Moshkovsky (1943).

[a] A and B = effective substances; (A) and (B) = effects produced by A and B in doses a and b; α = substance ineffective in respect to the parameter(s) studied; $(A + B)$ = combined effect; (A_S) = summative effect, that is, the one exerted by substance A in dose $a + a_b$, where a_b is the dose equipotent with dose b of substance B.

quantitative description of combined toxic effects. For this purpose it seems advisable to use only one term, "additivity" ("additive"). Accordingly, a combined effect should be referred to as "additive," "more than additive," or "less than additive," depending on whether it is equal to, more than, or less than the sum of the individual effects produced by the substances concerned.

2. GRAPHIC METHODS

Much of the progress made in the study of the joint action of poisons has been associated with the work of Loewe. In the USSR Loewe's method for the graphic study of pharmacological or toxic effects produced by a combination of drugs or poisons became known, and has been rather extensively used, because of Lazarev (1938) and Moshkovsky (1943). Subsequent authors (e.g., Kudrin and Ponomareva, 1967) have relied mainly on Lazarev's monograph for their descriptions of this method. The following account of Loewe's method (see p. 278) is likewise taken from Lazarev's book.

As was stated in Chapter 2, the relationship between effect (response), dose, and time can be described by three sets of curves: dose-response, dose-time, and time-response. According to Loewe, any curve relating the effect to some characteristic of the stimulus (dose, concentration, duration of action) is a "bologram" (*Bologramme*), while a curve describing the relation between two variables at a fixed value of the third was termed by Loewe an "isobol" (*Isobolen*). In the case of two poisons acting jointly, an isobol is a graphic representation of the relation between the doses or concentrations of the poisons eliciting the same selected response (narcosis, 50% decline in hemoglobin level, etc.).

For the graphic representation of experimental results obtained in joint-action studies, Loewe's method has been used more frequently than any other, although alternative procedures are available. One of these, called the "deviation from additivity" method (Ermakov, 1943), will be described first, followed by a description Loewe's method.

2.1. The Deviation from Additivity Method

Essentially this method consists in measuring the difference between the observed effect from combinations of two or more substances in different ratios and the effect theoretically expected on the assumption that the combined effect is simply the sum of the individual effects produced by each substance when applied separately. This method is considered here using two figures (Figures 34 and 35) from Ermakov's paper (1943), which describes a study on the larvicidal properties of some film-forming agents and their binary mixtures used to control mosquito larvae.

In Figure 34 the two lower curves are concentration-response curves plotted from experimental data for a polymer (an intermediate product of petroleum cracking) and a soap-oil emulsion when applied separately in a neutral medium at different concentrations at the rate of 40 kg/ha. The concentrations killing 60% and 20% of mosquito larvae within 24 hrs were taken

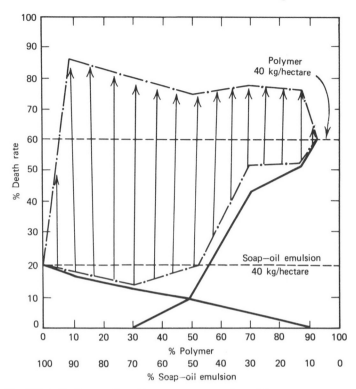

Figure 34. Effect of mixtures of a polymer and a soap-oil emulsion on mosquito larvae. See text for explanation. (From Ermakov, 1943.)

as the 100% response levels for the polymer and the soap-oil emulsion, respectively; these levels are shown in the figure by dotted straight lines. The two other curves describe the responses to mixtures of the two agents in various ratios (10 and 90%, 20 and 80%, 30 and 70%, etc.), also applied at the rate of 40 kg/ha. The lower of these curves was plotted from theoretical considerations assuming that the effect is additive, while the upper curve was plotted from experimental data. The area between these two curves is crossed by arrows pointing upward to indicate that the observed effect is more than additive, that is, is greater than expected.

The theoretical curve is constructed by adding together the percent responses to each constituent for the corresponding ratio. For example, the concentration of the polymer equal to 70% of the 100%-response concentration (i.e., the one killing 60% of mosquito larvae) kills 45% of larvae, while the concentration of the soap-oil emulsion equal to 30% of its 100%-response

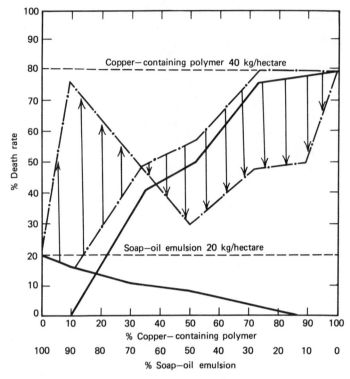

Figure 35. Effect of mixtures of a copper-containing polymer and a soap-oil emulsion on mosquito larvae. See text for explanation. (From Ermakov, 1943.)

concentration (i.e., the one killing 20% of larvae) kills 5% of larvae; therefore the expected response to the mixture is the 50% kill. This value is plotted on an imaginary perpendicular erected from the point on the horizontal axis which corresponds to the 70:30% ratio. The other points are obtained in the same way.

As can be seen from the figure, the actual percent response to the mixture was greater than additive for all the ratios used (e.g., 85% for 10 and 90%, 80% for 30 and 70%, 75% for 50 and 50%, 80% for 70 and 30%, 80% for 90 and 10%).

A different situation is seen in Figure 35, which shows curves that are similar but are plotted for the same soap-oil emulsion and a more toxic agent referred to by the author as the "cupropolymer" (a saturated solution of copper salts of fatty acids in the polymer). When the proportion of the cupropolymer in the mixture was low (10 to 30%), the larvicidal effect from the mixture was much more than additive (the arrows point upward); as its proportion was raised further, the effect decreased to become less than additive (the arrows point downward). Ermakov examined in detail the sharp differences observed in the direction of changes in combined toxicity at different ratios of the components and explained the reasons for this phenomenon.

When applying this method it is important that the highest dose or concentration of each substance be lower than the one causing the extreme effect (e.g., narcosis or death of all animals). Otherwise it may be difficult to evaluate correctly the effect produced by the combination of substances. The most suitable dose or concentration of each substance appears to be the one that produces the selected effect in approximately 50% of cases (in quantal response tests) or causes a 50% change in some response (in graded-response testing).

A major limitation of the method just described is that neither the empirical dose-response curves for the separate substances (and, consequently, the calculated curve for their mixture) nor the actual dose-response curve for their combined action will be the most probable ones. If the experiment is repeated under identical conditions, the toxic effect may be rather different because of individual variations in the sensitivity of biological test objects and of other factors discussed in Chapter 1. Another limitation, closely associated with the first one, is that it is not possible to assess, in terms of probability, by how much the empirical combined action curve will deviate from the curve constructed on the assumption that the effect is additive.

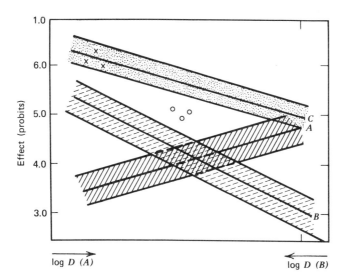

Figure 36. The zone of additivity of effect plotted on a logarithmic-probit grid. See text for explanation.

These limitations can be overcome to a large extent by constructing the curves on a logarithmic-probit grid rather than on an ordinary arithmetic grid. The dose-response curve for each toxic agent can then be obtained, together with its confidence limits, from an equation of a straight line giving the regression of response on dose. The theoretical dose-response line thus obtained for the mixture will apparently be the most probable one. As a first approximation the confidence limits for this calculated additivity line can be taken as equal to the half sum of the confidence limits of the regression lines for the individual constituents. Figure 36 shows empirical regression lines for hypothetical substances A and B and a theoretical line C for their combined effect, with the corresponding confidence limits. If joint-action data points lie within the confidence limits (these points are shown by crosses), this will indicate that the difference between the observed and predicted effects is not significant; in other words, it can be concluded that the combined effect is just additive. If the points fall outside the confidence interval (circles in Figure 36), the difference is to be considered as significant.

2.2. Loewe's Method

The toxicity of a binary mixture can be studied on an arithmetic grid by a method somewhat different from that described above. Thus the dose or concentration of one constituent causing a selected effect (e.g., narcosis, a specified decrease of some physiological, biochemical, or other index) may be plotted against the dose or concentration of the other constituent producing the same effect. The curve thus obtained will be what Loewe called an isobolic diagram (*Isobolen-Diagramme*). If the two substances act in a purely additive manner, this graph will show in what ratios of doses or concentrations the substances produce the same selected effect. However, as pointed out by Loewe (cited in Lazarev, 1938), such a graph may be found inconvenient to use when, for example, the dose of one constituent producing the selected response is much greater (e.g., several dozens of times) than the corresponding dose of the other: if the scale of the coordinate grid is too small, the curve cannot be drawn accurately enough; and if it is sufficiently large, the axis along which the dose of the less toxic substance is to be plotted will be too long for an ordinary sheet of paper.

To obviate this difficulty Loewe proposed plotting not the minimal doses or concentrations causing the selected response, but rather their fractions (percentages). This is illustrated in Figure 37, where the points n and m are the minimal doses (or concentrations) of two substances producing the same selected effect when applied separately, these points being placed at equal distances from the origin. In this way one obtains what Loewe termed an

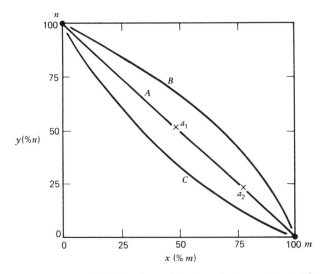

Figure 37. Different types of isobols on Loewe's isodynamic diagram. See text for explanation.

"isodynamic diagram," which, unlike the isobolic diagram described above, will always be symmetrical, since not the absolute doses or concentrations (g, mg/liter, etc.) but rather the relative values are plotted, that is, equal percentages of the equipotent doses or concentrations (Figure 37).

The straight line A connecting points n and m in Figure 37 is an isobol. If the toxic effect is additive, this line would be expected to characterize a binary mixture in which the sum of concentrations of the two constituents, expressed in percentages of their minimal concentrations producing the selected effect (n and m in Figure 37), is equal to 100%. For example, point a_1 on line A corresponds to a mixture containing 50% of the concentration (m) of one constituent and 50% of the concentration (n) of the other, while point a_2 corresponds to 75% of m and 25% of n.

Line A in Figure 37 is thus a theoretical line of complete additivity. If the experimentally found points corresponding to the different ratios of the constituents (10 and 90%, 50 and 50%, 70 and 30%, etc.) lie on the theoretical line, one constituent can be substituted pro rata for the other without changing the combined effect, that is to say, the effect will just be additive.

With this approach any empirical line (isobol) connecting points m and n and lying to the left of the theoretical line A (line C in Figure 37) will suggest that the effect is less than additive, while any isobol lying to the right of line A (line B in Figure 37) will indicate that the effect is more than additive.

However, as pointed out by Lazarev (1938), the straight line A is not, as a matter of fact, the only possible isobol of simple summation. A concave (C) or

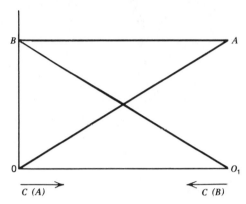

Figure 38. Summation of linear bolograms for two poisons. (From Lazarev, 1938.)

a convex (B) line can also be obtained even in cases of simple additivity. This is possible when the toxic effect produced by the binary mixture is measured, not for some fixed level of response, but taking into account the dose-response curves for each constituent, that is, when not fractions of the equally effective doses of each substance, but rather magnitudes of the individual effects, are summed up, as, for instance, in the deviation from additivity method. This situation is illustrated by the graphs of Figures 38 to 41, which are analogous in essence to Figures 34 and 35 discussed above.

Line AB in Figure 38 is analogous to line A in Figure 37. The concentration of substance A increases from 0 to 0_1, being equal at 0_1 to 100% of the concentration which brings about the selected effect. The concentration of

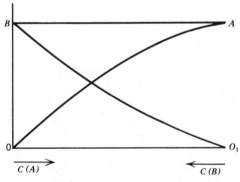

Figure 39. Summation of bolograms for two different poisons. The bolograms are mirror images of each other. (From Lazarev, 1938.)

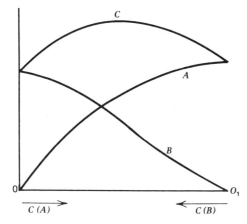

Figure 40. Summation of bolograms for two poisons. See text for explanation.

substance B increases in the opposite direction, from 0_1 to 0. Line AB is a bologram describing the effect of a mixture for the situation in which the effect remains unchanged when a given amount of one constituent is substituted at a constant proportion for an equal amount of the other.

Clearly, the situation where line AB is straight and parallel to the abscissa will be infrequent at best. In fact, it can be straight in only two cases: (1) when the dose-response relationships of both constituents are strictly linear, as is

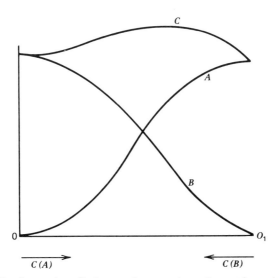

Figure 41. Summation of bolograms for two poisons. See text for explanation.

shown in Figure 38, and (2) when their dose-response curves are mirror images of each other, as shown in Figure 39. In all other cases the dose-response curves for binary mixtures will be concave or even wavy (undulating), as shown in Figures 40 and 41.

It follows from the foregoing consideration of Loewe's method that the joint action of poisons cannot be studied graphically on an isodynamic arithmetic grid unless the dose-response curves of the constituents are taken into account. This is so because these curves are not straight lines. If, for example, dose a of a substance A causes a given toxic effect, taken as 100%, a dose equal to one tenth of a will be unlikely to produce an effect equal to 10% of the first one. Such a situation is illustrated in Figure 42, which shows one of the most common dose-response curves. It can be seen that, while a dose equal to 40 (arbitrary) units causes 50% mortality, a 20-unit dose will kill not 25%, but about 10%, of test animals, that is, will produce an effect about one fifth of that from the first dose. A dose of 60 units, on the other hand, will be much more effective than one would expect on the assumption that the dose-response relationship is linear (95% rather than 75% kill in the hypothetical example shown in the figure).

It may be added that the nonlinear nature of dose-response relationships must of course be taken into consideration not only in joint-action studies but also in studying, for example, the cumulative properties of individual harmful substances. The effect produced by a given dose of poison administered on a single occasion and that exerted by the same dose repeatedly administered in fractional doses equal, say, to one tenth of the full dose, are unlikely to be commensurable.

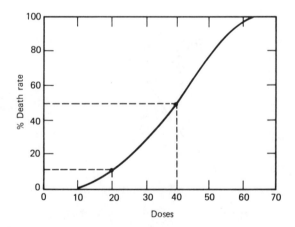

Figure 42. A dose-response curve in arithmetic coordinates. See text for explanation.

In conclusion, it should be noted that, if the dose-response curves of the constituents of the mixture are considered, Loewe's method will not differ in any way from the deviation from additivity method described above. It seems that the combined effect from a mixture of poisons can be best evaluated, not on the basis of the isodynamic amounts of the constituents, but by considering the dose-response curves of these constituents, that is, by taking into account their actual rather than calculated toxicities. In other words, in constructing the bolograms for the combined effect expected to occur on the assumption of simple additivity, not the doses or concentrations, but rather the magnitudes of the toxic effects should be summed up, using a probit-log dose grid as shown, for example, in Figure 36.

3. ANALYTIC METHODS

Graphic methods for the evaluation of joint action have been widely used mainly because the data can be represented and analyzed in a simple, clear way. Unfortunately graphic methods (especially the one of Loewe) can be applied only to binary and ternary mixtures, although in the latter case the graphic representation loses much of its clarity and simplicity. For this reason and also because of the well-known advantages of analytic methods* over graphic ones, attempts have been made, beginning with Bliss (1939), to apply the former to the analysis and evaluation of the toxicity of poisons acting jointly (e.g., Finney, 1952, 1971; Ball, 1959, Renzetti, 1961). These methods have been particularly employed by entomologists in predicting the effectiveness of mixtures of insecticides. As regards toxicology, they have so far been used to a limited extent and will not be described here. For a detailed acquaintance reference may be made to the works mentioned above, particularly to Finney's book (1971), where many ingenious mathematical procedures are detailed and a separate chapter is devoted to the estimation of toxicity of mixtures. Here only two limitations of analytic techniques based on regression analysis will be mentioned.

First, based as they are on the theory developed by Bliss (other authors have only refined it and still rely on regression analysis), these techniques can be applied only in cases where the dose-response relationships are linear in a probit-log grid, where the dose-response lines of the individual ingredients of a mixture are parallel, and, finally, where these ingredients have the same or very similar mechanisms of action.

---

* Equations or some of their coefficients may sometimes themselves constitute an important object of study: equations can be used for differentiation, integration, and interpolation; they have the advantage of being compact and can serve to describe the combined effect of any number of constituents in a mixture.

Second, the inferences drawn from a multiple regression equation are often valid only for a particular mixture and cannot be extended to other cases, including those where the same constituents are present in a different ratio. This is a serious limitation in view of the time-consuming nature of the work involved in computing a multiple regression equation.

There can be no doubt, however, that the rapid advances in the field of experimental design and, in particular, in the development of methods for the analysis of variance and for factor, multiple correlation, and especially discriminant analyses, as well as of mathematical modeling and computer applications, will stimulate the development of new approaches to the analytical evaluation of combined effects.

4. MAXIMUM PERMISSIBLE LEVELS OF HARMFUL SUBSTANCES JOINTLY PRESENT IN THE ENVIRONMENT

As early as 1938, Lazarev, in considering graphic methods for joint-action studies, made several recommendations relating to the establishment of hygienic standards for multiple contaminants of the work environment. Thus, with respect to airborne narcotic substances producing no "serious post-effects," he proposed the following rules:

> The sum of concentrations of narcotics present in the air expressed as percentages of the maximum allowable concentration for each of these narcotics separately, must not exceed 100% (Lazarev, 1938, p. 346). . . .
> [But if] we have in industry a mixture comprising a narcotic with specific action and several pure narcotics, we can justly apply the following rule: the sum of concentrations of all narcotic substances, expressed as percentages of the respective maximum allowable concentrations for each individual substance, must not exceed 100%; the concentration of the specifically acting substance (e.g., benzene) must not exceed the maximum allowable value established for it (*ibid.*, p. 347).

The last clause (after the semicolon) is formulated with insufficient clarity. Indeed, not only the concentration of any specifically acting substance,* but

---

* *Specifically* acting substances are defined as those producing specific, selective effects. For example, cholinesterase inhibition is a specific effect of organophosphorus compounds (in other words, organophosphorus poisons act specifically on cholinesterase activity); impairment of hematopoiesis is a specific effect of benzene; disturbance of porphyrin metabolism is a specific effect of lead. *Nonspecifically* acting substances are taken to be those adversely affecting the general state of the organism, as manifested in various functional alterations (narcosis, changes in indices of the higher nervous activity, etc.). Typical nonspecifically acting substances are such narcotics as ethanol and chloroform, as well as many other poisons that are nonelectrolytes. Clearly the separation of harmful substances into specifically and nonspecifically acting is somewhat artificial or arbitrary.

also that of each "pure" narcotic must not exceed the maximum allowable values if the above 100 % rule is to be observed. Generally, however, Lazarev's recommendations, made in 1938 with regard to narcotics, are still relevant today and have been applied by Soviet toxicologists to a wide variety of harmful substances.

Averianov (1957) proposed the following formula, to be used in calculating the required ventilation for workrooms containing multiple air contaminants:

$$\frac{a_1}{x_1} + \frac{a_2}{x_2} + \cdots \frac{a_n}{x_n} \leq 1$$

where $a_1, a_2, \ldots, a_n$ are the actual concentrations of harmful substances in the workroom air, and $x_1, x_2, \ldots, x_n$ are their maximum allowable concentrations. This formula for simple additive effects is of course a mathematical expression of the above rule formulated by Lazarev, and it has been widely used in the USSR and even incorporated into one of the sanitary standards (CH-245-71).

Experience has shown, however, that this equation is inapplicable to a number of combinations of airborne substances unless correction factors are used. One such correction factor, which allows for the enhancement of the effect from carbon monoxide and oxides of nitrogen acting jointly, was proposed, for example, by Kustov and Tiunov (1960).

The above formula is also a mathematical expression of the requirements of Loewe's isodynamic diagram, discussed in Section 2. In the case of binary mixtures this formula corresponds to the situation described by line A in Figure 37. As suggested on p. 281, such a situation appears to be an exception rather than the rule. The same is probably true of the level of maximum permissible values. For the latter level, however, dose-effect data are practically nonexistent (if one can speak of effect at this level at all). In the absence of relevant information confirmed experimentally it is not possible to say anything definite concerning the nature of additivity at the maximum permissible level. For this reason the use of a formula of simple summation as a basis for setting up standards for multiple air contaminants does not seem to be justified.

Although, as already stated, there are no data on the joint action of harmful substances at the maximum permissible level, such data are available for the higher level of threshold values. As far as additivity is concerned, the experience gained so far may be summarized as follows: chronic threshold toxicity data for mixtures are sometimes quite different from acute toxicity data (e.g., Volkova et al., 1969; Korbakova, 1964; Korbakova et al., 1969, 1970). Thus, whereas in acute tests the toxic effects from mixtures were in some cases more than additive, at the threshold level of chronic action these effects were often found to be additive or even less than additive (Sanotsky, 1969; Ulanova, 1969).

These and many other similar results have led workers of the Institute of Industrial Hygiene and Occupational Diseases, USSR Academy of Medical Sciences (Moscow), to adopt a novel approach to the problem of establishing standards for mixtures of gases and vapors of chemicals occurring in mixtures of relatively constant composition (studies in this institute have shown that the ratios of the leading components of vapor-gas and vapor-gas-aerosol mixtures are very often relatively constant). It has been recommended, in particular, that:

> ... The hygienic standards for relatively constant mixtures whose composition is not fully known should be established on the basis of the leading component that determines the clinical signs resulting from exposure to the mixture as a whole. At the same time attention should be called to the need for setting up a standard for the most typical component that characterizes the source of pollution (Sanotsky, 1969).

This approach may be tentatively called qualitative in contrast to the quantitative approach based on the principle of additivity.

Discussion of the problem of establishing maximum allowable concentrations for toxic substances acting jointly lies outside the scope of this chapter. Some aspects of this problem have been touched upon only in view of the fact that the use of certain quantitative approaches to the evaluation of combined effects at the level of effective doses and concentrations is still extended to the area of maximum permissible values, although without sufficient theoretical and experimental grounds.

ADDENDUM 1: TOXIC EFFECTS FROM EXPOSURE TO A COMBINATION OF CHEMICALS AND FROM EXPOSURE TO CHEMICAL AND PHYSICAL AGENTS

In the past few years the effects of exposure to combined environmental stresses have been causing increasing concern, and this topic is alotted more and more space in journals and books devoted to environmental health. As far as toxicology is concerned, the problem of combined exposure is becoming one of central importance. Workers, as well as the general population, are ever more frequently and severely exposed to a variety of environmental stresses. A good demonstration of the importance now attached to this subject are the Soviet-American Symposia on the Comprehensive Analysis of the Environment, referred to in the Preface to this book.

Over the last decade or so a large body of information about the combined effects of harmful substances has been amassed, especially in the field of industrial toxicology. In the USSR several books have been published, of which two deserve special mention: a collection of papers entitled *Combined Action of Chemical and Physical Agents in the Industrial Environment* (1972), and a monograph, *Combined Action of Industrial Poisons*, by Kustov et al. (1975).*

This section contains examples of toxic effects produced by a combination of harmful substances, by gas-vapor-aerosol mixtures, as well as those resulting from combined exposure to poisons and some physical environmental factors. The combined effects are assessed using the "additivity scale" referred to on p. 273, that is, a given effect is described either as "additive" (simple summation), "less than additive," or "more than additive." In some instances the possible reasons for observed deviations from additivity are briefly discussed.

A.1.1. SINGLE (ACUTE) EXPOSURE

Most of the studies carried out so far have been concerned with acute exposures, that is, have used doses or concentrations of several (more often two) substances much higher than threshold values.

The first major survey of combined effects, mainly of hydrocarbons, was that contained in Lazarev's (1938) book. Purified gasolines and their ingredients, as well as other hydrocarbons with narcotic actions, were shown to produce simple additive effects when acting jointly. However, when the death of animals was used as the criterion of toxicity, or if the individual components (of binary mixtures in most cases) also produced specific effects in addition to narcotic ones, the overall effect was sometimes less than additive. In one of his last publications Lazarev (1967) showed that a summation of effects occurs only on combined exposure to similar narcotics (nonelectrolytes), whereas a combination of narcotics belonging to the extreme groups of Lazarev's system of nonelectrolytes (see Chapter 7, p. 329) produces a weaker narcotic effect.

Kustov et al. (1975) have undertaken a series of investigations into the combined effects of aromatic hydrocarbons, including benzene and toluene, toluene and xylol, and benzene and xylol. Additive effects in white rats, for example, were recorded only in oral studies, and in mice only in inhalation studies. In general, most investigators have found jointly acting hydrocarbons with narcotic actions to produce just additive effects in most cases. Examples are the effects of styrene, benzene, and Nekal (sodium dibutylnaphthalene

---

* Many of the examples given below are taken from this monograph.

sulfonate) in rats and fishes; benzene and acetone in pigeons; α-methyl-styrene and acetophenone in rats and mice; and tetrachloropropane, tetra-chloropentane, and tetrachloroheptane in rats and guinea pigs.

Additive effects have been recorded by many authors in human experiments where odor perception threshold or change in dark adaptation of the eye was used as the criterion. Examples are combinations of benzene and iso-propylbenzene; propylene, ethylene, and butylene; styrene and Nekal; acetone and phenol; cyclohexane and benzene; phenol and acetophenone.

It should be underlined that the combined effect of narcotics depends primarily on their type (i.e., whether they are of type I or type II; see Chapter 7, p. 317), their concentrations, and the phase of a given response elicited by each narcotic. If, for example, both narcotics of a binary mixture elicit the same phase of response, their combined effect will be just additive or more than additive. With low concentrations a simple summation is seen for most combinations of various narcotics (Kagan et al., 1967).

Additive effects are also typical for binary mixtures of irritant gases such as chlorine and oxides of nitrogen, oxides of nitrogen and sulfur dioxide, sulfur dioxide and sulfuric acid aerosols, and maleic anhydride and dinyl. Gusev (1970) has concluded that most combinations of irritant and foul-smelling substances also tend to exert just additive effects.

The situation is less clear with substances other than narcotics and irritants. Additive and more than additive actions are encountered with almost equal frequencies. Simple summation has been reported for trichlorfon and Thiophos (parathion), trichlorfon and phosphamide, and some other organophosphorus compounds.

In the case of substances with different sites of action in the body, simple summation is seen less commonly but has been reported to occur with Sevin (Arylam) and cyanamide, Sevin and Butyphos (tributyl phosphate), hydrogen sulfide and phenol, hydrogen sulfide and carbon monoxide, carbon monoxide and Freon-12, carbon monoxide and triethylamine, carbon monoxide and furfural, and some other combinations.

Kustov et al. (1975) studied the possible mechanisms of additive action shown by the above-mentioned and other binary combinations and concluded that, when a summation effect is seen in the case of two substances with a well-known and an unknown mode of action, respectively, these substances are likely to have similar pathogenetic mechanisms (e.g., a hypoxic mechanism in the case of carbon monoxide and Freon-12).

In summary, simple summation of individual effects appears to be the most frequent type of combined effect with single (acute) exposures. Such situations are relatively simple to analyze and evaluate quantitatively in order to determine the hazards presented by mixtures with varying proportions of ingredients. Not uncommonly, however, practical toxicologists have to deal with substances whose combined effects are more than additive.

The causes of *more than additive effects* are varied. The most obvious cause may be the suppression by one substance of the biotransformations undergone by another, for example inhibition of the enzyme system responsible for its detoxication. Thus urethane is known to enhance the effect of eserine by inhibiting cholinesterase. The combined action of histamine and hydroxylamine, aminoguanidine, cadaverine, or guanidine is more than additive because of the inhibition of diamine oxidase by these substances. The toxic effect was found to be more than additive with many binary combinations of organophosphorus compounds (cholinesterase depression by one substance with resultant suppression of detoxication of the other). For example, trichlorfon and Malathion, trichlorfon and metaphos (methyl parathion), Malathion and Thiophos, Sesamex* and vinyl phosphate all produced more than additive effects when acting jointly.

Similar effects are often produced by combinations of chlorinated hydrocarbons. In this case the more than additive effect observed may be explained by depression of microsomal enzymes that metabolize foreign substances, as has been shown, for example, for mixtures of carbon tetrachloride and ethylene dichloride and of carbon monoxide and benzene.

The combined actions of carbon monoxide and one or more other poisons have been the object of more research in toxicology than any other combinations. More than additive effects are known to result, for example, from concomitant administration of carbon monoxide and tetraethyl lead, epinephrine, cyanides, or ethanol.

Combined effects greater than the sum of individual effects have been recorded for combinations of ozone with some industrial poisons, for instance, sulfuric acid aerosol or oxides of nitrogen.

Combined effects of carbon monoxide and nitrogen oxides have been studied by many researchers. (As is known, such combinations often occur in arc welding and in blasting, as well as in internal combustion engines.) The majority of authors have reported more than additive effects for these widespread air pollutants.

While more than additive effects are of greatest interest to practical toxicologists, there are many situations where the combined effect is actually less than would be expected on the assumption that the individual effects are just summated. Such *less than additive effects* occur, for example, with sulfur dioxide and chlorine, sulfur dioxide and ammonia, and ammonia and carbon dioxide. In these and similar instances the smaller than additive effect is accounted for by the interaction of the substances to form less toxic compounds.

Less than additive effects may have a physiological, rather than a chemical, mechanism. Examples include sympathomimetics and sympatholytics,

---

* [1-(3,4-Methylenedioxyphenoxy)ethyl-1]ethylcarbitol.

soporifics and nervous system stimulants, hypertensive and hypotensive drugs. Similar actions are known for industrial poisons. Thus less than additive effects are produced by chlorinated hydrocarbons in combination with organophosphorus compounds, in particular, those whose hydrolytic products are less toxic than is the parent compound (e.g., aldrin and parathion; aldrin and tetraethyl pyrophosphate).

A knowledge of the mechanisms underlying such effects may sometimes help in developing methods of treating intoxications. For instance, when the mechanism of competitive relationships between ethanol and methanol in the body became known, an effective method of treating poisoning with methanol or ethylene glycol by using ethyl alcohol was proposed.

Less than additive effects are known for many combinations of industrial poisons, including nitrogen oxides and sulfurous anhydride; mixtures of DDT plus hexachloran and mercaptophos, Ekatine, or parathion; dimethylamide and formic acid; methane and carbon monoxide; styrene and formaldehyde; carbon monoxide and toluene.

Evidently the main practical application of acute single-exposure data is to assess or predict human health hazards in emergency situations. As for the hygienic aspects, that is, the evaluation of hazards from prolonged exposures to low concentrations or doses, of much greater relevance, of course, are chronic tests.

A.1.2. CHRONIC EXPOSURE

Although it has been repeatedly stated in the literature that the combined effects of two or more poisons in low doses or concentrations are no more than additive in a vast majority of cases, both in chronic tests and in real-life situations, this view, which is based on combined effect studies using substances having relatively simple chemical structures and more or less similar mechanisms of action, does not seem to be well validated.

The available chronic exposure data on combined effects are far less extensive than acute exposure data for the obvious reason that a chronic experiment is more complicated, costly, laborious, and time-consuming, and its results are much more difficult to assess quantitatively.

As in the preceding section, examples of additive actions will be given first. Such actions have been reported for carbon monoxide and Freon-12 and for carbon monoxide and triethylamine from continuous experiments of 40 days each, using near-threshold concentrations. Another example is the combined effects of four compounds—aniline, furfural, epichlorohydrin, and carbon monoxide—seen at the levels of threshold and maximum allowable concentrations in tests with continuous 90-day exposure. Kustov et al. (1975) have concluded that it is desirable to employ effective doses or concentrations in chronic exposure studies of combined effects.

More than additive effects of combinations of industrial poisons have been reported relatively seldom from chronic exposure studies. Such effects were found to be produced, for example, by dialkylphenyl phosphate, dibutyl-phthalate, and polyvinyl chloride at the level of tentative MACs. Another example is the effect of mixtures of DDT and ethanol and of manganese compounds and fluorine. A similar effect was recorded in experiments with long-term intragastric administration of γ-hexachlorocyclohexane and tetra-methylthiuram disulfide (TMTD) and of Sevin and Butyphos.

Further examples are the combined effects, with 60-day continuous exposure, of four substances: furfural, aniline, epichlorohydrin, and carbon monoxide; 200-day and 104-day exposures, 5 to 6 hr per day, for 6 days per week, to carbon monoxide and nitrogen oxides; and 85-day continuous exposures to ethanol and arsenic, ethanol and thiuram disulfide, and ozone and sulfuric acid aerosol.

Table A1 presents interesting data of Genin et al. (1975) on enhanced carcinogenicity resulting from concomitant administration of hydrazoben-zene and benzidine sulfate. The authors rightly believe that under current conditions of benzidine sulfate manufacture the occupational risk of urinary bladder tumors greatly increases as a result of contact with hydrazobenzene and benzidine sulfate.

Lastly, there is an example of an apparently more than additive effect from a combination of benzine and dichloroethane (Vozovaya, 1975). Long-term health monitoring of women workers in a rubber goods factory revealed an appreciable deterioration of the reproductive performance in cases of con-cominant exposure to benzine and chlorinated hydrocarbons. This observation and also the fact that these chemicals are very common industrial poisons prompted a special experiment wherein two series of female rats were exposed for 6 and 9 months, respectively, to the action of benzine, dichloroethane, or a combination of these. In rats exposed to benzine (1783 mg/m^3, 4 hr daily) the reproductive capacity remained unchanged, and the only difference from the control was an insignificant reduction in the birth weight of the offspring. Exposure to dichloroethane (57 mg/m^3, 4 hr daily) resulted in reduced fertility (fertility being defined by the author as the number of newborn rats per female), increased rate of stillbirths, and reduced birth weight. Combined exposure to lower levels of benzine and dichloroethane led to a similar reduc-tion in birth weight, a greater decrease in fertility, as well as a strikingly reduced parturition rate; parturition occurred in only 35.7% of the rats against 88.3% in the control group.

Here are some instances of *less than additive* effects. Cases are known where less than additive effects seen in acute tests occur also in chronic tests. Two

Table A1. Carcinogenic Activity of a Combination of Benzidine Sulfate and Hydrazobenzene

| Treatment | Number of Rats | | | Percent of Rats with Tumors | Mean Latent Period of Tumor Development (days) |
	Total	Survived till Onset of First Tumors	With Tumors		
1. Benzidine sulfate plus hydrazobenzene	50	14	10	71.4	506 ± 14.9
2. Benzidine sulfate	50	14	5	35.7	599 ± 39.2
3. Hydrazobenzene	50	19	4	21.0	603 ± 44.9
4. Control	50	36	1	2.6	630

Source. Genin et al. (1975).

examples are shown in Tables A2 and A3. Other examples include combinations of sulfur dioxide and nitrogen dioxide; DDT and hexachloran in combination with mercaptophos, Ekatine, or parathion; nitrogen dioxide and carbon tetrachloride; tetrachloroheptane and chloroenanthic acid; α-naphthoquinone and maleic anhydride; and oxides of nitrogen and of copper. In general, less than additive effects with combined exposure to industrial poisons are rather common, especially at low levels of doses or concentrations.

Table A2. Combined Effect of Carbon Monoxide and Toluene on Mice (exposure time = 2 hr; concentrations in mg/liter)

Toluene Concentration	Carbon Monoxide Concentration	Number of Animals Died	Number of Animals Survived	Mortality (%)
45	—	9	1	90
39	—	7	3	70
35	—	6	4	60
31	—	5	5	50
28	—	4	6	40
22	—	3	7	30
15	—	1	9	10
15	—	1	9	10
—	5.6	8	2	80
—	5.0	6	4	60
—	5.0	5	5	50
—	4.5	5	5	50
—	4.0	5	5	50
—	3.0	4	6	40
—	2.6	3	7	30
—	2.4	3	7	30
—	1.8	1	9	10
—	1.7	0	10	0
45	4.0	10	0	100
45	2.4	6	4	60
39	5.0	8	2	80
35	1.8	4	6	40
31	2.6	4	6	40
22	5.6	6	4	60
15	3.0	0	10	0
15	1.75	0	10	0

Source. Kustov et al. (1975).

Table A3.   Responses of Mice to Chronic (30-Day) Continuous Exposure to Carbon Monoxide, Toluene, and Their Combination

Treatment	Concentration (mg/liter)	Number of Animals Died	Survived	Mortality (%)
Control		0	25	0
Carbon monoxide	0.05	1	24	4
Toluene	0.6	24	1	96
Carbon monoxide + toluene	0.05 0.6	13	12	52

Source.   Kustov et al. (1975).

Two or more harmful substances sometimes enter the organism not simultaneously, but consecutively. This may happen in certain occupational exposures, notably in agriculture. By way of example let us consider the results of a study (Dmitriyeva, 1974) carried out on 133 persons occupationally exposed to fungicides (one season) and then to horticultural pesticides (another season) in the course of one agricultural year. The additional contact with a set of pesticides was found to have aggravated the effect of fungicides (as judged by comparing the blood levels of SH groups, cholinesterase, and lactate dehydrogenase in the test group with those in the control, consisting of 24 persons without a history of contact with horticultural pesticides). Similar results were obtained by the author in an experiment where rats were consecutively administered Granozan (seed disinfectant) and Anthio (pesticide) in doses of 0.05 LD_{50} for 15 days each.

A.1.3.   EFFECT OF VAPOR-GAS-AEROSOL MIXTURES

Combined effects from gas-aerosol or vapor-gas-aerosol mixtures is a comparatively new area of research in toxicology. The first detailed account of such effects appears to be contained in the monograph by Kustov et al. (1975).

As is well known, the air of a work environment is rarely polluted by some one substance, the workers being almost invariably exposed to a complex combination of industrial poisons. It is also known that the composition of harmful mixtures is relatively constant in most industrial enterprises because of the constancy of technological processes.*

---

* A vapor-gas-aerosol mixture is considered to be relatively constant when its qualitative composition remains unchanged and the concentrations of its components vary within relatively narrow limits (one order of magnitude).

Thus, in vinyl chloride manufacture, dichloroethane, methanol, and vinyl chloride are released to the air during both the synthesis and the rectification stages; in Freon production, the air is contaminated with hydrogen sulfide, hydrogen fluoride, and organofluoric compounds throughout the manufacturing process; and so on. The list of such substances remains practically constant. For this reason workers at the Institute of Industrial Hygiene and Occupational Diseases under the USSR Academy of Medical Sciences (Moscow) have found it possible to classify the more common mixtures into four groups.

Group 1: mixtures consisting of the starting, intermediate, and final materials of a production process.

Group 2: mixtures comprising the compounds contaminating the starting material, the raw materials that have not reacted completely during the production process, and waste products.

Group 3: mixtures of compounds resulting from thermo-oxidative degradation of synthetic polymeric materials or from hydrolytic breakdown of the main product under manufacture, as well as mixtures formed in chemical reactions in the air between the substances contaminating the main product.

Group 4: mixtures of compounds of similar or identical chemical compositions. Examples are gasolines, kerosenes, and white spirits (complex mixtures of aliphatic and aromatic hydrocarbons); a mixture of nitrogen oxides; dinyl (25% diphenyl + 75% diphenyl oxide); and titanium tetrachloride (solid hydrolytic products + orthotitanic acid + hydrochloric acid).

This classification is based on the premise that, for each of the four groups, it is possible to work out common approaches to the establishment of hygienic standards for the content of the mixtures in the air of the work environment. Clearly, the validity of these approaches and, consequently, the reliability of the classification itself depend significantly on the extent to which the combined effects of particular vapor-gas or vapor-gas-aerosol mixtures are known.

Some authors recommend that, when evaluating the toxicity of a complex mixture, priority be given to the most toxic component. If the mixture contains two or more components of more or less equal toxicities, the prime consideration should be the component whose content is tenfold or more higher than that of the other component or components having the same toxicity. This approach, however, raises well-grounded objections. For one thing, some low-toxic components when acting jointly with other components may produce more than additive effects, and, on the contrary, very toxic ingredients may fail to reveal their individual toxicities. For another, components present in relatively low concentrations may nevertheless significantly contribute to the toxicity of the mixture as a whole and thus to the overall toxic effect. A good illustration of this comes from a study on the toxicity of a mixture of volatile products of the thermo-oxidative destruction of the lubricating oil B-3V (State Standard 5.556.70); the results are shown in Table A4.

Analysis revealed that the components determining the magnitude and pattern of the toxic effect produced by the mixture at the lethal level were carbon monoxide and organic acids, and these are ascribed ranks 1 and 2, respectively, in Table A4. At the same time they rank last in terms of percentage content in the mixture. It may be added that carbon monoxide has been shown to be an important determinant of the toxicity of many other complex mixtures containing thermo-oxidation breakdown products of a copolymer of ethylene and propylene, of foam plastic, of low-pressure polyethylene, and of other synthetic polymers. The contribution of carbon monoxide to the toxicity of breakdown products of oil B-3V was, however, much smaller at the threshold level of exposure, where the main determinants of toxicity were found to be the organic acids and ketones.

As can be seen from Table A4, the oil aerosol did not make a significant contribution to the toxicity of the mixture. Sometimes oil aerosols may play much more active, or even decisive, roles in toxic effect development. Unfortunately the mechanisms by which this occurs remain largely unknown, although some attempts to elucidate them have been made. For example,

Table A4.   Volatile Breakdown Products of Thermal Oxidation (at 250°C) of the Synthetic Oil B-3V and Their Percentage Contents in Vapor-Gas-Aerosol Mixture

Components	Rank in Terms of Contribution to Overall Toxicity[a]	Proportion in Mixture	
		%	Rank
Carbon monoxide	1	1.1– 2.7	5
Organic acids (calculated as acetic acid)	2	0.9– 1.7	6
Aldehydes (calculated as formaldehyde)	3	8.3–27.4	4
Oil aerosol	4	11.5–40.0	2.5
Ketones (calculated as acetone)	5	16.4–55.8	1
Oil vapor	6	11.9–38.6	2.5

Source.   Kustov et al. (1975).
[a] Ranks assigned on the basis of absolute regression coefficients.

Litau and Soloviyev (1973) studied the toxicity for rats of a mixture of volatile products of the thermo-oxidative degradation of a lubricant based on adipic acid esters and found that the oil aerosol greatly increased the toxic effect of the mixture. The authors found it difficult to account for this increase solely by a deeper penetration of the components of the mixture into the lungs or by their sorption and desorption processes on aerosol particles (the explanations often offered in such cases). They have suggested that oil aerosols act directly on the phospholipid boundary layer (surfactant) of the respiratory airways to assure the penetration of larger quantities of the mixture.

Instances are known where aerosols diminish rather than enhance the toxicity of mixtures. Some examples are shown in Table A5.

In some cases of chemical or physical interaction between the components of mixtures, the mechanism of toxicity alteration is fairly simple. Thus the chemical interaction between hydrogen chloride gas and sodium hydroxide aerosol that occurs in the mixture reduces the latter's toxicity because of the formation of common salt and water. Tiunov and Savateyev (1962), from their study of physical interactions between the components of mixtures, formulated the rule that, if an oil aerosol penetrates the airways to a greater depth than the other component of a binary mixture, the toxicity is enhanced; otherwise it is reduced. If both components penetrate the airway to the same extent, the toxicity remains unchanged (e.g., the effect of aerosol and acrolein is just additive).

The toxic effect of a gas-aerosol mixture also depends, of course, on the amount and properties of the aerosol. Sulfur dioxide, for example, produces a more severe effect in the presence of a highly dispersed aerosol of potassium chloride or manganese chloride (particle size about 1μ) than in the presence of common salt aerosol. Generally, the smaller the particle size, the more effective is the aerosol. Another important factor is considered to be aerosol concentration; for example, the higher the concentration, the greater is the toxic effect of irritant gases, as a rule.

The above considerations apply, in the main, to more complex gas-vapor-aerosol mixtures whose toxic effect likewise depends to a large extent on chemical properties, particle size, and concentration of the aerosol and on its physicochemical interactions with the other components.

As regards gaseous components, their impact on aerosol toxicity is much less clear. Most of the available data come from studies concerned with elucidating the role of certain gases in the development of silicosis. Some gases were shown to accelerate the silicotic process; others, to inhibit it. The former include, among others, explosive gases, sulfur dioxide, exhaust gases of diesel engines, and mercury vapors. One example of the latter is nitrogen oxides, which were found to slow the development of silicosis caused by intratracheal introduction of tridymite dust or of copper oxide aerosol. Some gaseous

Table A5. Toxic Effects of Various Gas-Aerosol Mixtures

Enhanced Toxic Effect	"Independent" Actions of Mixture Components	Weakened Toxic Effect
SO_2 + sodium chloride aerosol (particle size less than 1μ)	SO_2 + sodium chloride aerosol (particle size about 2μ)	Mineral oil aerosol + nitric acid fume
SO_2 + aerosol of zinc ammonium sulfate	Acrolein + mineral oil aerosol	Acrolein + kerosene fume
SO_2 + potassium chloride aerosol		Hydrochloric acid + alkali aerosol
SO_2 + manganese chloride aerosol	Acrolein + kerosene fume	SO_2 + alkali aerosol
SO_2 + bacterial aerosol	SO_2 + sodium chloride aerosol (human volunteers)	
SO_2 + coal dust	SO_2 + graphite dust	
SO_2 + kerosene fume		
SO_2 + ammonium + oxides of nitrogen + sulfuric acid aerosol		
SO_2 + sulfuric acid mist		
SO_2 + sulfuric acid aerosol		
Ozone + sulfuric acid aerosol		
Kerosene fume + sulfuric acid mist		
Ozone + mineral oil aerosol		
Nitrogen dioxide + mineral oil aerosol		

Formaldehyde vapor + mineral oil aerosol

Formaldehyde vapor + sodium chloride aerosol

Formaldehyde vapor + aerosol of silicon salts

Formaldehyde vapor + aluminum oxide aerosol

Acetaldehyde + kerosene fume

3,4-Benzpyrene + channel black

Ammonium + coal dust

Source. Kustov et al. (1975).

substances do not affect the silicotic process at all. It should be noted that all these findings have been reported both from animal experiments and from clinical studies of occupationally exposed workers.

The mechanisms by which toxic gaseous components aggravate or alleviate silicosis appear to be very complex and have not been adequately studied. Progress made in this area and some of the current concepts regarding the mechanisms of combined effects relevant to the etiology and pathogenesis of silicosis have been summarized by Katsnelson (1972).

Returning now to the classification of vapor-gas and vapor-gas-aerosol mixtures and the development of regulations for the levels of such mixtures in the work environment (see p. 295), let us consider briefly some of the pertinent recommendations.

For mixtures of Groups 1 and 2, it has been recommended that standards (MACs) be set for at least two components of each mixture. One of these, called the *critical* ("leading") component, determines the nature of the toxic effect produced by the mixture as a whole; the other, termed *characteristic*, is indicative of the source of mixture formation. For example, the characteristic components for breakdown products of organosilicon compounds, titanium tetrachloride, and isopropylboron are, respectively, silicon-containing compounds, titanium ion, and boric acid. On the other hand, the critical components are, for example, hydrogen chloride for titanium tetrachloride and carbon monoxide for isopropylboron.

The MAC for a compound considered to be the critical component of a mixture may differ greatly from that established for the same compound when it acts alone. For instance, the MAC for the hydrochloric acid resulting from titanium tetrachloride breakdown should be five times smaller than that for hydrochloric acid as such (Sanotsky, 1969).

For mixtures of Group 3 it is recommended that the prime consideration in the establishment of MACs be the breakdown products that specifically characterize the parent compound.

For mixtures of Group 4 MACs should be based on measuring the total content of mixture components in the work environment. Thus the MACs for vapors of gasoline, kerosene, and other mixtures of hydrocarbons are expressed in terms of total carbon; the MAC for mixtures of oxides of nitrogen is stated in terms of NO_2.

A.14. EXPOSURE TO CHEMICAL AND PHYSICAL AGENTS

It is only on rare occasions that human exposure to toxic substances is not accompanied by exposure to other unfavorable factors such as high or low temperature, increased or decreased humidity, vibration and noise, or various kinds of radiation. The effect of mixed exposure to chemical and physical factors may be different quantitatively than that of isolated exposure to chemical or to physical agents.

Temperature

Effects of altered environmental temperature (especially heat) on the toxicities of chemicals have been studied much more extensively than those of any other physical factor. Kustov et al. (1975) have collected much of the relevant information scattered in the literature and have prepared an interesting table, 20 pages long, entitled "Combined Action of Industrial Poisons and Elevated Ambient Temperature," which lists substances, temperatures, animal species, avenues of absorption, exposure durations, concentrations or doses, criteria and types of effect, and sources from which the data were taken.

The most general conclusion one can make is that elevated temperature as a rule enhances the toxic effect and accelerates its onset. Among exceptions to this rule is alleviation of the silicosis caused by quartz dust inhalation, as observed by Katsnelson et al. (1967), under elevated ambient temperatures in rabbits (30 to 32°C) and rats (38 to 40°C).

As might be expected, the magnitude of the effect from concomitant exposure to toxic chemicals and heat varied with temperature, animal species, route of entry, duration and regimen of exposure, and concentration or dose of the poison. Thus exposures to 35°, 40°, 45°, and 50°C were found to increase the toxic effect of aniline in rats but not in dogs. One-hour exposure of guinea pigs and rabbits to carbon monoxide in concentrations of 0.23, 0.75, or 1.5 mg/liter was less effective at 29 to 32°C than at lower ambient temperatures; in contrast, 1-hr exposure of rats and rabbits to higher carbon monoxide concentrations (2 to 8 mg/liter) at practically the same temperature (32 to 34°C) resulted in a much more severe toxic effect. At still higher temperatures the toxic effect of carbon monoxide was invariably increased. Generally, chronic exposure to carbon monoxide and heat was more effective than short-term exposure under similar conditions.

It should be noted that, in common with most other physical environmental factors, the "temperature component" of the environment modifies the toxic effect mainly in an indirect way, by altering the functional state of the organism. Thus exposure to heat may impair thermoregulation, resulting in water loss and in higher breathing and blood flow rates (so that more of the poison can enter the body and various tissues for a given period), and it may increase the rates of many biochemical processes and alter metabolic activities. On the other hand, the interaction between the poison and the organism tends to reduce the latter's tolerance to heat and thus adversely affect the thermoregulatory processes. Concomitant exposure to a toxic substance and heat may therefore lead to a summation of their biological effects, producing a so-called mutual aggravation syndrome (Fridliand, 1966). Evidently, both the temperature and the dose or concentration of the poison must be high enough for this syndrome to arise.

The temperature factor should be an important consideration when setting standards for harmful substances. Some authors have not only recommended taking into account the mutual aggravation syndrome mentioned above but also proposed correction factors to reduce the MACs for exposures involving increased temperatures. For example, Demidenko and Mirgiyazova (1974) have concluded from their study, where the combined effect of high temperature (36 to 40°C) and the organophosphorus pesticide Anthio was found to be more than additive, that the MACs for pesticides should be reduced by a factor of 5 to 10 in hot climates.

Information about combined exposure to cold and toxic substances is much more limited, but the overall pattern is the same: reduced temperatures tend to increase the toxic effect of most substances (e.g., carbon monoxide, gasoline, benzene, hydrogen sulfide, trichloroethylene, aniline, nitrogen oxides), although here, too, much depends on, among other things, the concentration or dose of poison, the duration and regimen of exposure, and the degree of temperature reduction. For a number of industrial poisons temperature ranges are known within which the toxic effect is reduced (e.g., 21 to 10°C for the gasoline *Kalosha*, about 12°C for trichlorfon, 22 to 15°C for oxides of nitrogen.)

In conclusion it should be added that physicochemical properties are particularly important for poisons which are nonelectrolytes. Thus the toxicity of type II narcotics (see Chapter 7, p. 317) increases, while that of type I narcotics decreases, at low temperatures. Conversely, type I narcotics are more effective, and most (but not all) type II narcotics are less effective, at high temperatures.

Air Humidity

There are relatively few published studies specifically concerned with the toxic effects of industrial poisons under conditions of increased air humidity. The effect can be predicted to a certain extent for poisons that interact with the moisture contained in the air and in the respiratory tract. For example, the irritant action of nitrogen oxides is known to increase because of the formation of drops of nitric and nitrous acids. The toxicities of some readily hydrolyzed chlorine-containing compounds can be significantly modified as a result of the formation of hydrochloric acid.

For substances that do not interact with air moisture, the mechanism of toxic effect is complex and uncertain, but in some cases increased air humidity is presumed to increase bodily susceptibility to the poison by impairing heat regulation and thus leading to overheating.

Barometric Pressure

The impact of altered barometric pressure on the toxic action of poisons remains a largely unexplored field of study. While data on toxic effects under low pressure are published from time to time, mainly in connection with research on hypoxia, not much is known about the influence of high barometric pressure, and very little relevant information can be given in addition to that contained in N. V. Lazarev's book *The Biological Action of Gases under Pressure* (1941), already referred to in Chapter 1. What is clear is that increased pressure (hyperbarism), which is known to alter many physiologic functions, should also be expected to modify the effect of poison-body interaction and to result in a kind of "mutual aggravation syndrome." Anyway, there appear to be no indications to suggest that the toxic effect may decrease under raised barometric pressure.

Hypoxia

Carbon monoxide, alcohol, benzene, nitrogen oxides, and carbon tetrachloride have all been shown to exert much more severe effects in conditions of hypoxic hypoxia. In an experiment on mice and rats Yusupov (1975) has found both the toxicity and the cumulative properties of several pesticides to be more marked in the mountains (3640 m above sea level); he has also suggested that administration of pesticides at high altitudes aggravates hypoxia.

There are, however, indications in the literature that some poisons show lower toxicity under reduced pressure. This is true, for example, of nitrogen dioxide and ozone (Kustov et al., 1975).

Noise and Vibration

It is generally recognized that occupational noise enhances toxic effect and hastens its onset. This has been demonstrated for carbon monoxide, styrene, alkyl nitrite, oil gases, boric acid aerosol, and a number of other poisons. The majority of authors feel it necessary to set more rigid standards for permissible levels of both airborne occupational pollutants and industrial noise when these occur in combination in the work environment.

Much the same can be said about vibration. Although the impact of vibration on toxicity has been studied less than that of noise, it is generally agreed that vibration enhances the effects of cobalt dust, silicon dust, dichloroethane, carbon monoxide, and some other substances. Bokov et al. (1975) have found this to be true also for volatile components of epoxy resins.

Ultrasound

There is still much to be learned about combined effects of ultrasonic waves and toxic substances. Shchipacheva (1970), for example, found that concomitant exposure to ethanol and ultrasound (100 and 130 dB and 54 and 50 kHz, respectively) had a stronger adverse effect on the central nervous system function of rats than did exposure to vibration or ethanol alone. However, when the intensity of ultrasound was reduced by 15 dB by screening the rat's body, the effect of ethanol given in the same concentration as before was similar to that in the control rats not exposed to vibration.

Radiant Energy

Here, too, not much is known about combined exposure effects. In 1938 N. V. Lazarev wrote that ultraviolet radiation may reduce the sensitivity of white mice to ethanol by intensifying oxidative processes, with resulting more rapid detoxication of the poison. The toxic effect of carbon monoxide is known to be decreased in conditions of UV radiation because of accelerated dissociation of carboxyhemoglobin and more rapid elimination of carbon monoxide from the body.

Gabovich et al. (1973) have studied the deposition of lead in rats, using various regimens of UV irradiation, and have found that in conditions of UV deficiency the content of lead in bony tissue is increased 2- to 2.5-fold with a lead dose of 2 mg/kg and more than 10-fold with a lead dose of 20 mg/kg (as compared with the control, given the same amounts of lead under normal UV radiation conditions); the lead content was increased 2- to 4-fold in the spleen, lungs, and heart and 1.1- to 2-fold in the liver, brain, and skeletal muscle. Combined exposure to lead and UV radiation resulted in reduced accumulation of lead in organs and tissues and in its more rapid excretion in the feces and urine. The bone of irradiated rats contained only half the amount of lead found in nonirradiated animals; much less lead also was present in teeth, spleen, lungs, and brain.

In another study Gabovich et al. (1975) have found the susceptibility of rats to hexachlorobenzene to be appreciably increased in UV insufficiency, during overheating, and on combined exposure to UV and heat. Ultraviolet irradiation increased the tolerance to hexachlorobenzene when given in doses close to the optimum one (half of the erythema dose) and reduced it when given in higher doses. The untoward effect of large UV doses increased when UV irradiation was combined with exposure to heat. Elevated temperature is believed by the authors to reduce the protective action of optimal UV irradiation.

The problem of UV radiation is recognized as one of major significance for toxicology. The growing pollution of the atmosphere in big cities by various harmful emissions leads to reduced natural UV radiation, thereby becoming even more hazardous for the population. This emphasizes the importance of research on the combined action of toxic substances and UV radiation from the general hygienic, the ecologic, and the socioeconomic points of view.

Ionizing Radiation

The increasing use of nuclear energy calls for research on combined exposure to poisons and ionizing radiation, and this subject is receiving more and more attention from radiologists and toxicologists. One of the best reviews of the pertinent literature appears to be a long chapter in the monograph by Kustov et al. (1975).

Most of the available data concerns single, acute exposures. It has been found, for example, that acute exposure to a hypoxia-producing poison, combined with concomitant or consecutive exposure to ionizing radiation, tends to lessen the radiation injury. Such poisons include, among others, carbon monoxide, sodium nitrite, aniline and its derivatives, cyanides, nitriles, and azides. In contrast, combined exposure to radiation and sulfhydryl poisons results in enhanced radiobiologic effects. Radiosensitizing poisons include mercury and its compounds, methyl ethyl ketone peroxide, formaldehyde, acrylic acid, and a number of other substances with unsaturated bonds.

It must be recognized that, so far, only a few qualitative relationships have been established in this important area of industrial toxicology. Since, in combined exposure studies, ionizing radiation doses, as well as doses and concentrations of toxic substances, have not been selected in a systematic way, it does not seem possible at this stage to detect any sustained quantitative relationships.

ADDENDUM 2: COMPLEX EXPOSURE

A.2.1. QUANTITATIVE EVALUATION

In Chapter 6 a brief account was given of some methods for the quantitative assessment of the toxic effects resulting from concomitant exposure to two or more substances entering the body from some one ("isolated") source or medium, such as the air of work areas.* In real life man may of course be exposed to a toxic chemical or a combination of toxic chemicals that enter the body from different media (air, water, food) and consequently by different routes (by inhalation, by ingestion, through the skin). For example, it has been estimated that many of the pesticides (which are the most ubiquitous contaminants of the biosphere) are absorbed in food, air, and water in the proportions 92 to 95%, 5%, and 3%, respectively (Izmerov, 1975). The percentage

---

* It may be noted that, in this context, the air of work areas and the atmosphere of, for example, urban areas are considered to be two different media because the respective MACs are different for most toxic substances.

absorptions by different routes may of course vary for different pesticides, but the overall pattern will presumably be the same.

In the USSR, exposure to a given toxic substance entering the body from different media is described as complex exposure. Korbakova et al. (1971) and Izmerov (1975) have recommended assessing the resulting toxic effect in the same way as for combined exposure, that is, by using a formula of simple summation (see p. 285). Then

$$\frac{C_{ind}}{MAC_{ind}} + \frac{C_{atm}}{MAC_{atm}} + \frac{C_{water}}{MAC_{water}} + \frac{D_{food}}{PRA_{food}} \leq 1$$

where the subscripts "ind" and "atm" refer to the industrial environment and the atmosphere, respectively, and PRA_{food} is the permissible residual amount in food.

Although this formula has been recommended for the tentative evaluation of hazards from complex exposure to substances for which permissible values have been established for the different media (i.e., air of work areas, atmosphere, drinking water, and foods), one cannot but agree with Izmerov (1975) that this principle is of limited use, since different approaches are often employed to establish MACs for the same substance in different media. Thus, whereas the MACs in the air of work areas for many, though not all, toxic substances are set from absorption data (i.e., on a toxicological basis), the MACs of some of these substances for the air of residential areas are established from data on their unfavorable effects on vegetation, and the MACs of the same substances for water are based on the effects they produce on the sanitary state of water bodies or on the organoleptic properties of water, such as odor, taste, color, or turbidity (see the addendum to Chapter 8). This is a difficult problem that has been very little studied, especially as regards methodology.

Even more difficult is the quantitative assessment of human hazards from environmental pollution by two or more toxic substances entering the body from different sources, that is, the problem of concomitant combined *and* complex exposure. Such situations are typically encountered in large cities. In this case a formula of simple additivity may sometimes be employed as well:

$$\sum \frac{C_{i,j}}{MAC_{i,j}} \leq 1$$

where i refers to the different substances and j to the different sources. In using this formula one must of course remember the limitation referred to in the preceding paragraph.

Sidorenko and Pinigin (1976) have proposed determining the maximum permissible total-body burden on man from combined and complex exposure, as calculated from the following formula of simple additivity:

$$\text{MPB} = \frac{a_1}{x_1} + \frac{a_2}{x_2} + \cdots + \frac{a_n}{x_n} + \frac{b_1}{y_1} + \frac{b_2}{y_2} + \cdots + \frac{b_n}{y_n}$$

$$+ \frac{c_1}{z_1} + \frac{c_2}{z_2} + \cdots + \frac{c_n}{z_n} = 1$$

where MPB is the maximum permissible burden; a, b, and c are the levels of harmful substances as measured in the different media; and x, y, and z are the maximum permissible values of these substances in the respective media (e.g., in air, water, and food).

Reference was made above to the urban environment. The quantitative assessment of combined and complex exposure in an urban environment is particularly difficult. Various kinds of noise, vibration, and radiation, temperature fluctuations, and a number of other "components" of the human environment (e.g., socioeconomic and other stresses) combine to create an almost inevitable "background" which must be taken into account in any toxicity study designed to evaluate human hazards of toxic agents. But here, too, the problem of combined and complex exposure has not been clearly formulated, either quantitatively or methodologically. One would agree with Ulvedal (1976) that "we are just beginning on this track, and we have a long way to go".

Nevertheless, to the question of whether or not we assess correctly man's total exposure to pollutants and his total body burden from this exposure and the resulting health effects, Ulvedal has answered an unequivocal "yes." He has come to this conclusion from an analysis of studies where attempts were made to apply epidemiological approaches to assess the impact of environmental pollutants, unfavorable physical factors (noise, radiation), and certain psychosocial stresses such as overcrowding, unemployment, and malnutrition. Unfortunately the information presently available is obviously inadequate to permit any definite conclusions or generalizations. As regards the methodology of quantitative assessment of the factors mentioned above, this question has not yet been considered, as can be seen, for example, from the technical discussions held during the Twenty-Seventh World Health Assembly in 1974 (*Promoting Health in the Human Environment*, 1975).

A.2.2. EXAMPLES OF STUDIES ON COMPLEX EXPOSURE

As in the case of combined exposure, the effect of complex exposure may be additive, more than additive, or less than additive, depending on the physicochemical properties, sites and mechanism of action of the poison, its routes of entry, and other factors. So far no attempts appear to have been made to review the studies on complex exposure carried out so far and to arrive at more or less broad generalizations. Only results of individual studies can therefore be discussed.

Chernukha (1974) has carried out experiments with benzene administered simultaneously by inhalation and by mouth, using low and high doses and concentrations. The effect varied with exposure level, being more than additive at high levels and becoming just additive as the doses and concentrations were reduced.

Pavlenko et al. (1972, 1973, 1975) have studied the chronic toxicities of several alcohols (methyl, ethyl, heptyl, nonyl), formaldehyde, cyclohexanone, benzene, and gasoline concomitantly administered by inhalation and by mouth. It is noteworthy that these authors mainly used threshold and even maximum permissible levels (MPLs) rather than lethal ones. The results were found to depend on the index used to assess the complex effect. If the MPL was based on absorption (i.e., toxicological) data, the effect was just additive; but if, for example, the MPL for air was based on toxicological data while that for water was derived from organoleptic data, no summation occurred. The practical aspects of these studies have been summarized by Pavlenko (1974) in her recommendations for the study of complex exposure to industrial poisons entering the body simultaneously in water and in air.

ADDENDA REFERENCES

Bokov, A. N., V. I. Kiseleva, V. N. Kovalenko, N. P. Strogacheva, and L. I. Shpak, On the joint action of vibration and volatile components of expoxy resins in experiment, in E. P. Moskalenko, Ed., *Khimicheskiy Faktor—Vneshnaya Sreda— Zdoroviye Cheloveka* (*Sbornik Trudov Konferentsii*), pp. 45–48, Rostovskiy Meditsinskiy Institut, Rostov-on-Don, 1975.

Chernukha, T. M., Characterization of the complex action of benzene entering the body by ingestion and inhalation, *Gig. Sanit.*, **4**, 18–21 (1974).

Combined Action of Chemical and Physical Agents in the Industrial Environment. See *Kombinirovannoye Deistviye Khimicheskikh i Fizicheskikh Faktorov Proizvodstvennoi Sredy.*

Demidenko, N. M., and M. G. Mirgiyazova, Joint action of high ambient temperature and the pesticide Anthio, *Gig. Sanit.*, **7**, 18–21 (1974).

Dmitriyeva, O. V., Sequential exposure to a set of pesticides used in agriculture: a hygienic assessment, *Gig. Sanit.*, **9**, 107–109 (1974).

Fridliand, I. G., *Znacheniye Neblagopriatnykh Proizvodstvennykh Faktorov v Vozniknovenii i Techenii Nekotorykh Zabolevanii* [*Relevance of Unfavorable Occupational Factors to the Natural History of Some Diseases*], Meditsina, Leningrad, 1966.

Gabovich, R. D., I. A. Mikhaliuk, I. N. Motuzkov, and I. I. Shvaiko, Effect of various levels of exposure to ultraviolet radiation on the deposition of lead in the body, *Gig. Tr. Prof. Zabol.*, **3**, 9–11 (1973).

Gabovich, R. D., V. A. Murashko, and Ya. G. Timoshenko, Bodily resistance to hexachlorobenzene as studied using various combinations of altered environmental temperature and UV radiation, *Gig. Sanit.*, **8**, 17–21 (1975).

Genin, V. A., A. G. Medvedovsky, and V. M. Voronin, Enhancement of carcinogenic activity on combined exposure to hydrazobenzene and benzidine sulfate, *Gig. Tr. Prof. Zabol.*, **6**, 28–31 (1975).

Gusev, M. I., A practical approach to the study of combined action of low concentrations of toxic substances in the ambient air, *Gig. Sanit.*, **8**, 99–101 (1970).

Guseva, V. A., Effect of formaldehyde administered concurrently by inhalation and *per os*, *Gig. Sanit.*, **6**, 7–11 (1973).

Izmerov, N. F., Estimation of the maximum permissible level of complex exposure to chemical agents in the industrial, community, and domestic environments, in *Vsestoronniy Analiz Okruzhaiushchei Prirodnoi Sredy. Trudy Sovetsko-Amerikanskogo Simpoziuma, Tbilisi, 25–29 Marta 1974 g. [Comprehensive Analysis of the Environment. Proceedings, Soviet-American Symposium, Tbilisi, March 25–29, 1974]*, pp. 138–144, Gidrometeoizdat, Leningrad, 1975.

Kagan, Yu. S., E. I. Liublina, I. V. Sanotsky, N. A. Tolokontsev, I. M. Trakhtenberg, and I. P. Ulanova, Principles for the study of combined action of chemicals and methods for establishing their hygienic standards, in F. G. Krotkov, Ed., *Materialy XV Vsesoiuznogo Siezda Gigiyenistov i Sanitarnykh Vrachei, Kiev 22–27 Maya 1967 g.*, 113–135, Moscow, 1967.

Katsnelson, B. A., Some mechanisms of combined action relevant to the etiology and pathogenesis of silicosis, in *Kombinirovannoye Deistviye Khimicheskikh i Fizicheskikh Faktorov Proizvodstennoi Sredy*, pp. 10–19, Sverdlovskiy Institut Gigiyeny Truda i Profzabolevaniy, Sverdlovsk, 1972.

Katsnelson, B. A., L. G. Babushkina, and L. N. Yelnichnykh, Effect of high ambient temperature on the development of silicosis in experiment, *Gig. Tr. Prof. Zabol.*, **3**, 14–19 (1967).

Kombinirovannoye Deistviye Khimicheskikh i Fizicheskikh Faktorov Proizvodstvennoi Sredy [Combined Action of Chemical and Physical Agents in the Industrial Environment], Sverdlovskiy Institut Gigiyeny Truda i Profzabolevaniy, Sverdlovsk, 1972.

Korbakova, A. I., N. I. Shumskaya, G. N. Zayeva, and T. K. Nikitenko, Some considerations relating to the comprehensive evaluation of exposure to chemical environmental agents, in I. V. Sanotsky, Ed., *Nauchniye Osnovy Sovremennykh Metodov Gigiyenicheskogo Normirovaniya Khimicheskikh Veshchestv v Okruzhaiushchei Srede*, pp. 35–40, Institut Gigiyeny Truda i Profzabolevaniy Akad. Med. Nauk SSSR, Moscow, 1971.

Kustov, V. V., L. A. Tiunov, and G. A. Vasiliev, *Kombinirovannoye Deistviye Promyshlennykh Yadov [Combined Action of Industrial Poisons]*, Meditsina, Moscow, 1975.

Lazarev, N. V., *Obshchiye Osnovy Promyshlennoi Toksikologii* [*General Principles of Industrial Toxicology*], Medgiz, Moscow and Leningrad, 1938.

Lazarev, N. V., *Biologicheskoye Deistviye Gazov pod Davleniyem* [*The Biological Action of Gases under Pressure*], Voenno-Morskaya Meditsinskaya Akademiya, Leningrad, 1941.

Lazarev, N. V., Two types of action of organic solvents, in *Trudy Yubileinoi Nauchnoi Sessii, Posviashchennoi Nauchnoi Deyatelnosti Gosudarstvennykh Nauchno-Issledovatelshkih Instititov Gigiyeny Truda Ministerstva Zdravookhraneniya RSFSR*, pp. 331–343, Institut Gigiyeny Truda i Profzabolevaniy, Leningrad, 1967.

Litau, V. G., and V. I. Soloviyev, Contribution of the oil aerosol to the toxic effect from a mixture of volatile breakdown products resulting from heat oxidation of a lubricating oil synthesized on the basis of adenylic acid esters, *Gig. Tr. Prof. Zabol.*, **9**, 58–60 (1973).

Pavlenko, S. M., Patterns of action of industrial poisons (nonelectrolytes) entering the body concurrently in water and in air, *Gig. Sanit.*, **1**, 40–45 (1972).

Pavlenko, S. M., *Izucheniye Kompleksnogo Deistviya Promyshlennykh Yadov v Usloviyakh ikh Odnovremennogo Postupleniya v Organizm s Vodoi i Vozdukhom. Metodichesliye Rekomendatsii* [*Recommendations on Methods for the Study of Complex Exposure to Industrial Poisons Entering the Body Concomitantly in Water and in Air*], Meditsina, Moscow, 1974.

Pavlenko, S. M., and V. A. Guseva, Development of adaptation during complex exposure to toxic nonelectrolytes, *Gig. Sanit.*, **1**, 15–20 (1973).

Pavlenko, S. M., T. V. Yudina, and V. A. Guseva, Possible approaches to evaluating the latent reactions of some regulatory systems in response to toxic substances entering the body by different routes, *Gig. Sanit.*, **10**, 55–60 (1975).

Promoting Health in the Human Environment, World Health Organization, Geneva, 1975.

Sanotsky, I. V., Current status of studies into combined actions of gases, vapors, and aerosols, *Toksikologiya Novykh Promyshlennykh Khimicheskikh Veshchestv*, No. 11, pp. 6–13, Meditsina, Moscow, 1969.

Shchipacheva, A. D., Combined action of industrial ultrasound and ethanol on the nervous system of rats, *Gig. Sanit.*, **10**, 27–30 (1970).

Sidorenko, G. I., and M. A. Pinigin, Hygienic criteria of the maximum permissible stress, in *Vsestoronniy Analiz Okruzhaiushchei Prirodnoi Sredy. Trudy II Sovetsko-Amerikanskogo Simpoziuma, Gonolulu, Gavayi, 20–26 Oktiabria 1975 g.* [*Comprehensive Analysis of the Environment. Proceedings, Second Soviet-American Symposium, Honolulu, Hawaii, October 20–26, 1975*], pp. 119–128, Gidrometeoizdat, Leningrad, 1976.

Tiunov, L. A., and N. V. Savateyev, Some aspects of ship toxicology, *Voyenno-Med. Zh.*, **6**, 64–66 (1962).

Ulvedal, F., Are we on track in assessing environmental stress on man? in *Vsestoronniy Analiz Okruzhaiushchei Prirodnoi Sredy. Trudy II Sovetsko-Amerikanskogo Simpoziuma, Gonolulu, Gavayi, 20–26 Oktiabria 1975 g.* [*Comprehensive Analysis of the Environment. Proceedings, Second Soviet-American Symposium, Honolulu, Hawaii, October 20–26, 1975*], pp. 49–56, Gidrometeoizdat, Leningrad, 1976.

Volkova, Z. A., and Yu. M. Bagdinov, Occupational hygiene for workers engaged in rubber production, *Gig. Sanit.*, **9**, 33–40 (1969).

Vozovaya, M. A., Effect of low concentrations of benzine dichloroethane and their combinations on the reproductive function of animals and on their offspring, *Gig. Tr. Prof. Zabol.*, **7**, 20–23 (1975).

Yusupov, A. M., Toxicity of some pesticides for warm-blooded animals at high altitudes, *Gig. Sanit.*, **8**, 96–97 (1975).

7

THE RELATIONSHIP
BETWEEN STRUCTURE
AND TOXICITY

1. GENERAL CONSIDERATIONS

The scientific study of the relationships between the structures of chemical
compounds and their toxic actions was begun more than a century ago.
Since then, it has given rise to a theory which continues to develop and is one
of the cornerstones of several biological disciplines, primarily pharmacology
and toxicology. Yet the very fact that the interaction of substances and the
living organism has a chemical nature was not recognized until after a long-
continued clash of opinions, because the rapid reversal of many pharmacological and toxic effects led many investigators to deny their chemical basis.

Convincing evidence for the dependence of toxic effects on the chemical
compositions of poisons was presented by E. V. Pelikan (1854, 1855), one of
the first Russian toxicologists. It is an interesting historic fact that the prominent Russian chemist and composer, A. P. Borodin (1858), wrote in his dissertation, which had a direct bearing on toxicology, as follows:

> . . . By comparing poisonous substances with each other one came to
> realize that their toxicological properties and chemical makeup are
> closely interrelated. The first thing to be noted was the fact that many
> substances consisting of the same elements or taking part in similar re-
> actions also exert similar actions on the organism.

The development of a theory relating toxicity to structure was marked by
a number of outstanding works, some of which will be discussed in this and
the next chapter.

It is not our purpose here to dwell on the individual accomplishments of
pharmacology in establishing important relationships between the chemical
structures and medicinal effects of compounds. We will confine ourselves to a
consideration of the more general principles underlying the structure-action

312

relationships of poisons, with special reference to current and future problems of industrial toxicology. It must be emphasized that such relationships, if firmly established, are of great importance for industrial toxicology because they can serve as a basis for predicting, at least to a certain extent, the types of action and potencies of chemicals being newly applied in industry and elsewhere. One should not underestimate this opportunity today when new chemical products appear in numbers far too great for toxicologists to cope with their evaluation in good time.

That tangible practical benefits can be derived from structure-activity studies, which at first seemed to be of only academic interest, became evident, for example, when physicochemical constants came to be used to predict (by calculation) the approximate values of maximum allowable concentrations of harmful substances in the air of workplaces—a very important index in industrial toxicology and occupational hygiene.

Thus differences in the actions of various industrial poisons are due mainly to differences in the chemical structures of their molecules. Without taking this statement to the extreme, it is correct to say that it is the chemical structure of the molecules of a substance which determines most of its biological properties. The only exception appear to be the properties related to the degree of dispersion of the substance or, say, the structure of the crystal lattice of certain compounds.

It should be made clear that the biological actions of substances also depend, of course, on their physicochemical properties, but these in turn are determined by their chemical structures. This interrelationship is clearly illustrated by the following diagram (Lazarev, 1958):

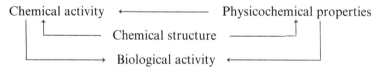

This diagram shows that the chemical structure of the molecules of a substance determines not only its physicochemical properties but also its capacity for chemical reactions. A biological effect may result from a chemical reaction between the substance and a certain chemical substrate in the body; at the same time the biological activity of the substance may be influenced by its physicochemical properties—either directly or indirectly through a change in chemical activity.

This does not mean that knowledge of the chemical structure is sufficient to predict unerringly the type of action and potency of any compound. Many instances are known of similar toxic actions by substances with quite dissimilar structures and of very different actions by substances with similar structures. This is not surprising, since the chemical structures of poisons are far more varied than the responses which they elicit in the body. Many of these responses are of a fairly standard, nonspecific type, although the substances concerned differ greatly in chemical structure. On the other hand, the specific actions of poisons are in most cases predetermined by their chemical structures.

This chapter will be chiefly concerned with the quantitative side of structure-toxicity relationships, especially those which can serve as a real basis for calculating approximate values of toxicity parameters for various biological objects. More promising in this respect are of course the relationships established in homologous series. However, consistent structure-related changes in toxicity are also traceable, and may be put to practical use, by properly considering other series of congeneric compounds.

Whereas initially structure-activity relationships were almost invariably established for organic compounds, since then, as will be shown later, a number of important relationships of practical use have been found among inorganic substances also.

In addition to more or less quantifiable relationships there are others that at least enable one to foresee the direction in which the toxicity of a compound will change as its chemical structure is altered. Clearly, it is the latter relationships which were first discovered and dealt with in the literature. The book by Lazarev (1938) was the first work to collect and present a critical review of data on changes in the narcotic potencies of compounds caused by an increase in the number of carbon atoms and by the branching or closure of the carbon chain. This book contains numerous examples showing how the potencies and, sometimes, even the nature of toxic action of substances are changed by the insertion into their molecules of multiple bonds or specific chemical groups such as polar OH groups. Serious alterations in toxicity were shown to result from the introduction of various halogens or amino, nitro, or nitroso groups into the molecules. It was already known four decades ago that the potency of a substance depends strongly on the spatial arrangement of substituting radicals in its molecule (position isomerism). Facts making it possible to relate toxicity to chemical structure for some inorganic substances were also known.

Subsequently, repeated attempts were undertaken to make generalizations as more evidence was accumulated on structure-toxicity relationships (e.g., Albert, 1957; Fairhall, 1957; Lohs, 1958; Golubev and Rusin, 1963; Sexton, 1963).

A reduction or an increase in the toxicity of a substance brought about by one of the above-mentioned changes in its chemical structure is related to the fact that the resulting changes in physicochemical properties may produce marked, even dramatic, changes in the absorption, distribution, and elimination of the substance, that is, in the relationship between its transport and distribution in the body. A change in the chemical structure may also strongly affect the way in which the poison is transformed in the body, and this may lead to toxic effects that are not only quantitatively but also qualitatively different. Such changes were thoroughly investigated as early as 1932 by Quick, who traced the metabolic transformations of benzene and its derivatives in relation to their chemical structures. The particular way in which substances are transformed in the body, depending on their chemical structures, explains the very high toxicity of certain methane derivatives (methanol, formaldehyde, formic acid, and methyl chloride, bromide, and iodide)—a fact of which toxicologists are well aware. The high toxicity of ethylene glycol compared with other saturated dihydroxy alcohols of the fatty series is accounted for by the formation of toxic oxalic acid and other intermediates during ethylene glycol oxidation in the body.

The comprehensive development of analytical toxicology entailed further studies on the metabolism of poisons in relation to their chemical structures (Filov and Gadaskina, 1970). Many interesting results obtained in these studies were presented by Williams in his monograph (1959) and, with reference to aliphatic organofluoric compounds, by Pattison (1959). A large number of important structure-action relationships were established within the vast class of organophosphorus compounds widely used in industry and agriculture. Kodama et al. (1955) made a special study of the structure-related toxicity for laboratory animals and for man of many phosphates, phosphites, phosphonates, and phosphinates. A detailed account of structure-activity relationships for organosphosphorus compounds, based on data from the literature and his own extensive studies, was presented by Kagan (1963a) in his comprehensive monograph.

Long-term studies on the toxicology of organosilicon compounds enabled Kulagina et al. (1961) and Kulagina and Kochetkova (1968) to reveal a number of consistent relationships between the chemical structures of these compounds and their toxic actions. Of the many other investigations where clear-cut structure-toxicity relationships were established in various series or groups of compounds, mention may be made of studies on propylamines (Guseinov, 1967), organoboron compounds (Zalesov et al., 1967), cyclic imino compounds (Zayeva et al., 1968), oxygen-containing heterocyclic compounds (Stasenkova and Kochetkova, 1968; Sochava, 1969), and toluene derivatives following the introduction of various substituents into the toluene molecule (Khalepo, 1969).

Structure-activity studies are of considerable interest not only to industrial toxicologists, but also to synthetic chemists, because their results may be of help in undertaking purposive syntheses of new nontoxic or slightly toxic compounds to replace highly toxic industrial poisons. In this connection the importance of cooperation between synthetic chemists and industrial toxicologists must be specially emphasized.

One example of successful collaboration of this kind can be seen in the work of Broitman (1964) and Broitman et al. (1966). In their studies clear-cut structure-toxicity relationships were established for various substituted phenols used as antioxidants, and it was suggested that the least toxic would be the phenols substituted in positions 4 and 6 by alkyl or aryl and condensed in position 2 with alkylene or, preferably, sulfur. Indeed, the antioxidants so synthesized—2,6-di(2'-oxy-3'-*tert*-butyl-5',4'-methylphenol), 2,2'-thiobis(4'-methyl-6-α-phenylethylphenol), and 2,2'-thiobis(4'-methyl-6-α-isobornylphenol)—proved to be practically nontoxic.

Another example is the project undertaken jointly by synthetic chemists and toxicologists for the purpose of developing and evaluating fireproof liquids for high-power turbines to replace petroleum oils, which present increased fire hazard. The main component in the first specimen of the newly developed liquid was tricresyl phosphate containing 37% of ortho isomers. This product, however, produced neuroparalytic effects, as was shown in experiments and in the course of its industrial application (Ryzhik, 1967). On the basis of animal experiments in which the neurotoxic properties of tricresyl phosphate with various isomeric compositions were studied, a specimen with a limited level of ortho isomers (which were mainly responsible for toxicity) and five to six times less toxicity was developed and applied industrially (Zilber, 1963). Further structure-activity studies of organophosphorus compounds made it possible to replace tricresyl phosphate first by trixylenyl phosphate, which reduced toxicity 12- to 15-fold (Zilber and Lykhina, 1964), and then by 3,5-trixylenyl phosphate, which was practically free from neurotoxic effects (Dvorkin, 1970).

So far, sustained structure-action relationships have been established, for the most part, among organic compounds, especially nonelectrolytes.* As far as their nature and mechanisms are concerned, the narcotic effects exerted by nonelectrolytes are manifestations of the simplest way in which a poison interacts with bodily receptors. The absence of any specific chemical reaction between a narcotic and its biological substrate creates the picture of nonspecificity of the biological effects produced by different narcotics.

Although it has long been recognized that the narcotic potencies of nonelectrolytes are determined by their physicochemical properties, it was comparatively recently that the qualitative characteristics of narcotic action were also shown to change as a consequence of quantitative changes in those

---

* The terms "physical toxicity," "nonspecific activity," and "structural nonspecificity" used by various authors are usually synonymous with "nonelectrolytic activity."

properties. By considering the physicochemical constants of a large number of nonelectrolytes in relation to their effects on the organism, Liublina divided all narcotics into two types. Narcotics of type I are more hydrophilic (ethanol, ethyl ether, acetone, etc.), and those of type II are strongly hydrophobic (gasoline, benzene, toluene, trichloroethylene, etc.). The former are readily soluble in water and have low oil/water partition coefficients, while the latter, on the contrary, are sparingly soluble and have high partition coefficients. The wide differences between the narcotic states induced by type I and by type II narcotics are well documented (e.g., Liublina, 1954, 1956, 1957) and need not be described here.

The validity of this classification was later confirmed in several investigations, in particular, by an experimental study of Abasov (1967), where the toxicities of automobile gasolines from Baku oil were considered in relation to environmental temperature, and by the electroencephalographic studies of Razumeyev (personal communication), where the effects of type I and type II narcotics on the lability of various brain structures were measured directly.

More recently, however, studies by Shekhtman (e.g., 1966, 1969) have indicated that the division of narcotics into these two types is rather arbitrary because, given suitable concentrations and exposure durations and frequencies, responses to narcotics of types I and II are identical. It may be argued, however, that the very fact that substances of types I and II are narcotics implies that they must show not only differences but also similarities in their actions. At certain concentrations and under certain exposure conditions the actions of the different types of narcotics may be so similar as to conceal the distinctions due to differences in their physicochemical properties. As shown by Liublina (1970), the actual differences in action between type I and type II narcotics are too great to be ignored in predicting, for example, the likelihood of acute poisoning or other adverse effects from exposure to a new chemical being applied industrially. Hence it seems quite logical that the validity of the division of narcotics into these two types is one of the conclusions reached in many toxicological studies.

Consistent structure-action relationships are also evident if we turn from narcotic to other relatively simple actions of poisons in homologous series. Thus it has long been known that the hemolytic and bactericidal effects of nonelectrolytes increase as a homologous series is ascended. The nonspecific irritant action of nonelectrolytes likewise changes as their chemical structures are altered. Augmentation of the irritant effect of the vapors of acetic esters with a growing number of carbon atoms was noted long ago by Flury and Wirth (1933). A special experimental study by Levina (1952) revealed a similar relationship for aliphatic hydrocarbons, alcohols, and ketones. The reverse relationship was observed, however, in certain series of unsaturated compounds. Thus Wang Weng-Yang (1957) found that the irritant effect in the aldehyde series decreased in going from formaldehyde to butylaldehyde, while Golubev (1957) demonstrated a similar reduction in the esters of vinyl alcohol from vinyl acetate to vinyl butyrate. Special studies can reveal the reasons for such deviations from the typical pattern of toxicity rise in homologous series. For example, Filov (1959b) has shown that vinyl esters are rapidly broken down in the body with the formation of acetaldehyde in a quantity that is smaller the larger the number of carbon atoms in the molecules of these esters.

That the irritant effect tends to increase in homologous series was further confirmed by Larson et al. (1956), who studied the capacity of alcohols, aldehydes, ketones, and acids to produce edema of the conjunctiva in experimental animals. Using their own simple quantitative method for registering edema, the authors found that the edema-producing potencies of monobasic organic acids tend to increase with rising molecular weight (formic acid as a methane derivative is an exception). A similar relationship was found to hold in the homologous series of saturated aldehydes (with the exception of formaldehyde) and primary unsaturated fatty alcohols. This study shows that, while unsaturated compounds are generally more liable to induce edema than saturated ones, this effect may decrease rather than increase with molecular weight. Thus acrolein and crotonaldehyde have greater edema-producing powers than propionaldehyde and butyraldehyde, respectively.

In general it seems that many other aspects of the toxicity of industrial poisons can be related to their chemical structures if structure-action relationships are specifically sought. One example is the study of Klinskaya (1956), in which the chemical structures of a number of substances were considered in relation to their capacities to be concentrated by the kidneys. It was found that foreign organic compounds containing an amino or imino group (amino compounds, amides of acids, some antibiotics), compounds with several alcohol groups (trihydric and hexahydric alcohols), and some glycol ethers (diglycolic and polyglycolic) are all concentrated by the kidneys in the urine, while hydrocarbons, chlorinated hydrocarbons, ketones, monohydric fatty alcohols, paraldehyde, and diethyl ether are not.

For more complex interactions of chemical agents with the living organism, which result, for example, in carcinogenic, mutagenic, or teratogenic effects, structure-action relationships are much more difficult to trace. Nevertheless, within certain limits and for some groups of poisons, they are evident enough to be of practical value to physicians or chemists.

The most sustained efforts in this area appear to have been directed at the study of carcinogenic effects. The results were summarized by Badger (1962) in his monograph *The Chemical Basis of Carcinogenic Activity*.

Of the several hundred carcinogenic agents known today, most are polycyclic aromatic hydrocarbons, but carcinogenic activity is also displayed by aromatic amines, azo compounds, urethanes, yperites, ethylenimines, some inorganic compounds, and a large number of miscellaneous substances from quite different chemical classes. Given such a great variety of chemical structures, it is of course very difficult to predict the carcinogenic activity of newly synthesized compounds. The problem is further complicated by the lack of structure-activity relationships expressible in quantitative terms. Nevertheless, the mere fact that a new chemical belongs to a particular class or group should place hygienists and toxicologists on guard and prompt them to test the chemical for possible carcinogenic activity.

An addendum to the Russian edition of Badger's book, prepared by N. I. Wolfson and M. A. Zabezhinsky, surveys studies on the electronic structure of carcinogenic hydrocarbons and their derivatives—a line of research that has gained much popularity in recent years. Encouraging results have been reported by the Pullmans and by Szent-Györgi and his school in establishing correlations between some electronic structure parameters of chemical compounds and their carcinogenic activity. Such studies are all the more important because they shed more light on the mechanism of carcinogenesis.

Very useful information of predictive value was collected by Shugayev et al. (1969) in their review of the carcinogenic activity of polycyclic aromatic hydrocarbons and products containing them, as well as of amines, azo compounds, hydroxy compounds, alkylating agents, some metals and metalloids, and a number of other carcinogens.

Increasing attention of hygienists and toxicologists is focused on the mutagenic activity of chemicals, and several hundred chemical mutagens from various classes have been identified. Much attention to searches for relationships between mutagenic activity and chemical structure has been given by I. A. Rapoport, founder of the Soviet theory of chemical mutagenesis. In his review of the progress made in the field of chemical mutagenesis Rapoport (1966) points out many interesting relationships; for example, high mutagenic activity is frequently shown by only one member of a homologous series, in many cases by the first. A number of structural features of compounds exhibiting mutagenic activity are indicated by Fomenko (1969) in his comprehensive review. This review also contains a useful list of about 120 chemical mutagens and presents an interesting attempt to classify them according to their chemical structures. Work along this line is continuing, and it may be hoped that this first classification, which can already be used for practical purposes, will be elaborated and improved.

Since the so-called thalidomide disaster in 1961, workers in many biomedical fields have concentrated their efforts on the study of teratogenic (i.e., causing fetal malformation and monstrosity) effects of drugs and other chemical agents. Chernukh and Aleksandrov (1969) point out in their monograph that by 1963 some 400 compounds that produced teratogenic effects in experimental animals were known. That this subject is receiving close attention is attested by the fact that it took several decades to discover a similar number of carcinogenic compounds. Of the various factors responsible for teratogenic effects, a prominent role must be played by chemical structure. So far, however, very few attempts have been made to relate chemical structure to teratogenic activity although, as the Chernukh–Aleksandrov monograph indicates, such relationships do exist. The problem is compounded by the fact that the progress made in this area has not yet reached the stage where animal data can be extrapolated to man to safeguard him against the teratogenic effects of new chemicals—hence the added importance of structure-activity studies in this field.

2. THE QUANTITATIVE ASPECTS OF STRUCTURE-RELATED CHANGES IN THE TOXICITY OF ORGANIC SUBSTANCES

2.1. Homologous Series

The groundwork for quantitative structure-toxicity studies was laid by Richardson. In 1869 he demonstrated that the narcotic efficiencies of fatty alcohols increased with a growing number of carbon atoms, that is, with molecular weight. This observation contained a quantitative concept which underlay all more or less consistent changes in toxicity established later in homologous series.

Richardson's observation remained unheeded for a long time, and it was not until after the turn of the century, when interest in anesthesia had been spurred by its successful application in surgery, that studies were made into the narcotic effects of compounds in various homologous series. It was soon discovered that the relationship observed by Richardson also held good in series of saturated and unsaturated hydrocarbons, chlorinated hydrocarbons, cycloparaffins, ketones, esters, and so on (see Lazarev, 1940a, for a review). It also applied to toxic effects other than narcotic (hemolytic, bactericidal, nonspecific irritant, etc.). The next important advance was made by Fühner (1904, 1905), who showed that the toxic concentrations declined, and the toxicities correspondingly increased, from one member of a homologous series to the next in an approximate ratio of 3:1. This meant that the toxic potency in a series could be described by the proportion $3^0:3^1:3^2:3^3:\ldots$

It is now known that Fühner's proportion is far from being generally true. The value of the multiplying factor may vary from one homologous series to another. This, however, does not preclude a simple mathematical description of the relationships between the toxic properties of homologues and the size of their carbon skeletons. Moreover, similar relationships were found to exist between the toxicities of compounds and a number of their physicochemical characteristics, including, among others, solubility, coefficient of partition between immiscible liquids, surface activity, and adsorptive capacity. A major contribution to the study of such relationships was made by N. V. Lazarev (1940a, 1944), and it is primarily due to him that they are well known to toxicologists in the USSR. These relationships can be and are used to advantage for various purposes, in particular, for predicting the unknown toxicity of one member of a homologous series from the known toxicities of other members. Theoretical interpretation of toxicity augmentation in homologous series and of the phenomenon of cutoff in toxicity, which is invariably seen to occur as a series is ascended to reach the member having a sufficiently large molecular size, became definitely possible because of Ferguson's idea of expressing toxicity in terms of thermodynamic activity (see Chapter 3).

The possibility of estimating the toxicities of individual homologues is of considerable importance. It is possible to calculate any of the commonly used indices of toxicity, such as the threshold, narcotic, and lethal doses or concentrations, and also the maximum allowable concentration (MAC), which is a particularly important index from the practical point of view. In calculating a given index for the homologue under study, the equitoxic values of that index for the studied members of the series should be used, and, to permit inter- or extrapolation, these values must of course be known for at least two members. It is essential that none of these homologues be the methyl one because the first member of a series often deviates from the general trend in the series. The calculation can be conveniently done on a graph, where the ordinal numbers of the homologues, the sums of carbon atoms, the molecular weights, or the values for some other property correlating with the toxicities of the homologues are plotted on the horizontal axis, and the logarithms of the concentrations or doses corresponding to the index to be calculated are plotted on the vertical axis. The known values of the toxicity index are then plotted as points, and a straight line is drawn through these points. The logarithm of the index for the homologue in question is found at the intersection of this line with the perpendicular erected from the point on the horizontal axis which corresponds to the homologue.

The regular pattern of toxicity variation within a homologous series and the differences in these patterns between series led Zayeva (1964) to suggest another method of calculation. In this method the overall numerical value of a given toxicity index (however expressed) of an organic compound is formally distributed among the individual chemical bonds of the compound. To observe the principle of additivity, parent bonds in homologues are assigned the same toxicity values. At the same time, parent bonds in different series may have different values, because of the different effects on these bonds of various atoms and their groups. With this approach the toxicity of a compound can be calculated from its structural formula. Clearly, it is necessary first to establish the toxicity values to be assigned to the different bonds by considering the homologues that have been studied toxicologically. Although this method was proposed by Zayeva for calculating MACs in the air of work areas, it can also be used to calculate other toxicity indices, provided that the appropriate additive values for the toxicity index concerned have been established. The principle just discussed has been successfully employed in various physicochemical calculations, and it is worthwhile to develop the approach further with a view to its wider application in toxicology and pharmacology.

2.2. Various Groups of Congeneric Compounds

A prominent role in the study of the relationships between the structures of substances and their biological, including toxic, properties is played by correlation analysis. After its successful use in organic chemistry, correlation analysis has been applied also in biochemistry, biochemical toxicology, and other disciplines, where it has put structure-activity studies on a quantitative basis, though of course within certain limits.

A most important correlational equation in organic chemistry is the Hammett equation (Hammett, 1940):

$$\log\left(\frac{K_X}{K_H}\right) = \rho\sigma \tag{1}$$

where K_H is the equilibrium constant or the rate of any reaction in which the compound takes part; K_X is the same, but for a similar compound in which hydrogen has been substituted for by X; ρ is a constant whose value depends only on the nature of substituent X; and σ is a constant which depends only on the type of reaction shown by the group of compounds concerned, and not on the substituent.

The Hammett equation describes a process in a system of related chemical compounds having a common nucleus and differing only in the nature and position of X. This equation was first used to determine dissociation constants for benzoic acid derivatives differing only in substituent X:

The constant ρ for benzoic acid dissociation in aqueous solution at 25°C was taken as unity, making it possible to estimate the values of σ for various substituents. The Hammett equation was widely used also to determine other constants for various benzene derivatives. Later it was applied to derivatives of aliphatic compounds in the form of the Taft equation:

$$\log\left(\frac{K_X}{K_H}\right) = \rho^*\sigma^* \tag{2}$$

the constants σ and σ^* being different for the same substituents. To determine the numerical value of σ^*, the value of ρ^* for the hydrolysis of ethyl acetate at 25°C was taken as unity.

Physically, Hammett's and Taft's equations are based on the capacity of any substituent X to interact with the electron system of the nucleus of the molecule. This interaction is approximately the same in different reactions of benzene derivatives having the same substituent. This also applies to aliphatic compounds. The constants σ and σ^* thus allow for the effect of the substituent on the reactivity of the molecule.

It is worth stressing that (1) and (2) are not strict, only correlational. Nevertheless they allow one to calculate equilibrium constants and rates of various reactions, as well as to arrive at certain conclusions regarding their mechanisms, the latter possibility being largely due to digressions from the equations. Other equations have also been proposed in organic chemistry which allow for various steric or other effects and give better correlations. Their applicability is, however, more limited than that of (1) and (2).

The use of the principles embodied in Hammett's equation in biochemistry is discussed by Zhdanov (1966). Here we will consider at some length how these principles can be applied to establish correlations between the structure of a chemical compound and its biological activity, primarily the magnitude of its toxic action.

Proceeding from the assumption that the biological activity of an organic compound is determined by only one reaction, Zahradnik (1962a, 1962b) proposed an equation identical in form to those of Hammett and Taft:

$$\log\left(\frac{\tau_i}{\tau_{et}}\right) = \alpha\beta \tag{3}$$

in which τ_i is the biological activity of the ith homologue; τ_{et} is the same, but for the ethyl derivative; β is a constant characterizing the biological activity of the substituent, β for ethyl being equal to 0; and α is a constant characterizing the main interacting system, that is, the biological object and the ethyl derivative. The constant β is independent of the biological object used, and of the basic structure of the compound; in this sense it is analogous to constants σ and σ^* in (1) and (2). The analogy, however, may prove to be only apparent if future studies on the mechanism of bioactivity show that β, unlike σ and σ^*, is not a measure of the polar properties of the substituents, but is associated with some other properties.

Equation 3 holds good for many organic compounds, both aliphatic and aromatic, particularly in homologous series (Zahradnik et al., 1962; Trčka and Dlabač, 1962; Zahradnik, 1962a). It is valid for different biological test objects and for different criteria of toxicity. For example, it has been successfully applied to sets of congeners using the following criteria: inhibition of barley germination; inhibition of catalase, amylase, and oxidase activities; hemolysis of erythrocytes; inhibition of development of sea-urchin eggs; inhibition of movement of worms; narcosis of goldfish, gudgeons, and tadpoles; inhibition of action of tortoise heart; intravenous and intraperitoneal LD_{50} for white mice; and lethal doses for rabbits.

If the toxicities of the members of a series of congeners obey (3), two conclusions can be reached. First, it can be concluded that the toxicities of the members are indeed determined by only one reaction or process, since such was the assumption on which the equation was derived. The mechanism of the process remains undisclosed. It may be a chemical reaction (in the case of chemically very active compounds exhibiting so-called chemical toxicity), or it may be a process by which the compound moves accross a biological membrane and accumulates in a sensitive biophase (in the case of substances with so-called physical toxicity). Second, it can be concluded that all members of the series have the same type of action. Whenever a member of a homologous series fails to obey (3), it is most likely that this member acts by a different mechanism. This is often the case with methyl derivatives (methanol, formic acid, etc.), a fact which led Zahradnik to use the ethyl derivative (τ_{et}) in (3) as the reference substance in comparing the biological potencies of homologues.

For some series of congeners Zahradnik's equation is not applicable at all. The main reason is that the biological effect in the series is not determined by one reaction. Thus it is easy to consider that the biological effect under study is determined by two processes to an equal or commensurate degree: by the physical transport of the agent to the site of its action, and by its chemical interaction with the receptor. This leads to a more complex equation (Zahradnik, 1968):

$$\log\left(\frac{\tau_i}{\tau}\right) = \varepsilon\chi_i + \gamma\delta_i \tag{4}$$

where δ_i and χ_i are constants allowing for the structural difference of the ith substituent from the reference substance as far as the effects on the physical (χ) and chemical (δ) properties involved in biological activity are concerned.

If the contribution of one effect to the biological activity greatly exceeds that of the other, (4) will be converted to (3).

As indicated by Zahradnik et al. (1968), the constant δ in (4) can be used for the constant σ in Hammett's equation (1), while the constant χ can be replaced by the partition coefficient.

Zahradnik's equation is likewise inapplicable to disubstituted compounds such as those of benzene:

$$X-\!\!\left\langle\bigcirc\right\rangle\!\!-Y$$

where the substituents X and Y may be in the meta and para positions* and may be quite varied.

Boček et al. (1964, 1967), Kopecký et al. (1965), and Zahradnik et al. (1968) attempted to establish structure-toxicity correlations for such compounds. They determined the LD_{50} of 45 disubstituted benzene derivatives for white mice, using NO_2, CL, H, CH_3, OH, and NH_2 as the X and Y substituents.

Boček et al. (1964) tested these equations:

(1) $\quad \log\!\left(\dfrac{[LD_{50}]_{HH}}{[LD_{50}]_{XY}}\right) = a_X + a_Y$

(2) $\quad \log\!\left(\dfrac{[LD_{50}]_{HH}}{[LD_{50}]_{XY}}\right) = d_X \cdot d_Y$

(3) $\quad \log\!\left(\dfrac{[LD_{50}]_{HH}}{[LD_{50}]_{XY}}\right) = b_X + b_Y + e_X \cdot e_Y$

Only the third combined model proved satisfactory. The structure-toxicity relationships for 1,4-disubstituted butane derivatives, however, best fitted the first, additive model. The authors have pointed out the difficulties involved in the physicochemical interpretation of the constants a, b, and e (personal communication) and have not proposed any working hypotheses. What is clear is that these constants reflect the effect of the substituents on toxicity and that the term $e_X \cdot e_Y$ is related to the interaction of the substituents.

Equations 1 to 4 satisfactorily fit into a complex parabolic equation proposed by Hansch:

$$\log\!\left(\frac{1}{C}\right) = k_1\pi^2 + k_2\pi + k_3\sigma + k_4 \tag{5}$$

---

* Because of steric effects, the ortho position is not covered by Hammett's equation or by any of those derived from it.

Hansch, alone and with other authors, has published in recent years many papers giving a large number of correlational equations describing structure-activity relationships for various series of congeneric compounds. A historic and logical presentation of his ideas is given in the review by Zhdanov (1966); for a more detailed account, reference should be made to the original papers (Hansch, 1968, 1969; Hansch et al., 1968). One of them (Hansch, 1969) presents an equation more complex than (5), taking account of the steric effects of substituents on biological activity.

In (5), C is the molar concentration producing a standard response in a standard time interval, σ is Hammett's constant, π is a certain function of the partition of the compound between immiscible solvents, and k_1, k_2, k_3, and k_4 are constants obtained for each set of congeners by statistical methods such as the method of least squares. The π, which may be called Hansch's constant, is a measure of the contribution of the substituent to the partition coefficient. This constant can be computed from the equation $\pi = \log P_X - \log P_H$, where P_X is the octanol/water partition coefficient of the derivative and P_H is that of the parent compound. It has been pointed out that the parameter π can also be calculated from the parachor of a compound (McGowan, 1963).

The main concept behind (5) is that it is very difficult for highly hydrophilic molecules to penetrate lipid barriers, so the probability of their reaching the sites of action within a given time interval is small. On the other hand, substances which have high partition coefficients are firmly retained by the first lipids with which they come into contact, so that they likewise find it difficult to reach their sites of action.*

If k_1 and k_2 in (5) are set to zero, we get Hammett's equation (1). Setting to zero k_1 and k_3 will give an equation which linearly relates the potencies of substances to their partition coefficients and which may be called the Overton-Mayer equation after the investigators who were the first to establish this relationship in a qualitative form for the narcotic activities of organic compounds. For sets of congeners whose biological activity is determined by physical factors only, an excellent correlation of the π constants of Hansch with the β constants of Zahradnik has been demonstrated (Kopecký and Bŏcek, 1967). Equation 4 is equivalent to (5) on condition that $k_1 = 0$.

Specific examples of (5) are equations correlating structure with activity

---

* This concept of the passage of molecules across lipid barriers is highly schematic and can represent only the most general model of permeability. The movement of nonelectrolytes across lipid barriers, primarily biological membranes, is now the subject of intensive study. The main ideas proposed in this field are discussed, for example, by Albert (1973) and by Krolenko and Nikolsky (1970).

for thyroxine analogues in rodents:

$$\log\left(\frac{1}{C}\right) = -1.13\pi^2 + 7.44\pi - 16.32\sigma + 0.29$$

and for chloramphenicol analogues on *Staphylococcus aureus*:

$$\log\left(\frac{1}{C}\right) = 0.54\pi^2 + 0.48\pi + 2.14\sigma + 0.22$$

An idea of the applicability of (5) is given by Table 25.

A good correlation can be sometimes described by a shortened form of (5). Thus the linear correlation for the narcotic activity of 28 alcohols, ketones, and esters on tadpoles is given by the equation $\log(1/C) = 0.869\pi + 1.242$, and for the toxicity of mono- and polysubstituted benzoic acids to mosquito larvae, by the equation $\log(1/C) = 0.519\pi + 1.540$. Another example is the equation describing the effect of phenols on *Salmonella typhosa*:

$$\log\left(\frac{1}{C}\right) = -0.288\pi^2 + 1.312\pi + 0.139$$

It is of interest that correlational equations can relate physicochemical

Table 25. Calculation of Growth-Stimulating Properties of Substituted Phenoxyacetic Acids for Barley Seedlings

$$\text{Log}\left(\frac{1}{C}\right) = -2.14\pi^2 + 4.08\pi + 2.78\sigma + 3.36$$

Substituent and Site of Its Attachment to Nucleus	σ	π	Log(1/C) Calculated	Log(1/C) Found Experimentally
CF$_3$, 3	0.55	1.09	6.8	6.5
Cl, 4	0.37	0.80	6.3	6.4
I, 3	0.28	1.08	6.1	6.3
F, 4	0.34	0.20	5.0	6.3
Br, 3	0.23	0.97	5.9	6.0
Cl, 3	0.23	0.82	5.9	5.7
NO$_2$, 3	0.78	0.04	5.7	5.3
SCH$_3$, 3	-0.05	0.59	4.9	5.3
OCH$_3$, 3	-0.27	0.13	3.1	4.7
CH$_3$, 3	-0.17	0.44	4.3	4.3
OH, 3	-0.36	-0.73	-1.8	3.7
n-C$_4$H$_9$, 3	-0.15	2.03	2.4	0

properties not only to toxic and other biological effects but also to purely bio-chemical changes in organic compounds. Without discussing this question in detail, we will merely note that Hansch et al. (1968) have presented many equations similar to (5) and its derivatives which relate the constants π and σ to a number of metabolic reactions for sets of congeners. Examples are the formation of glucuronides from derivatives of benzoic acid or aliphatic alcohols in rabbits and the oxidative deamination of primary amines by cat and cattle liver extracts.

Ideally, the mathematical expression of a structure-biological activity relationship should not merely be a statement of the actually existing correlation, but also be explanatory. It should explain, to some extent, the mechanism by which the substance interacts with the biological substrate, for it is this interaction which determines the ensuing biological effect. The assumption that a greater interaction results in a higher biological activity led Ostrenga (1969) to formulate a so-called molar attraction constant as an indicator of biological activity. This constant, which takes into account the electrostatic forces of attraction and the molar volume of the compound, has been shown to correlate rather well with the magnitude of biological action in series of structurally related compounds.

In the preceding section we discussed a method for the additive description of the toxicities of homologues in terms of the sum of the toxicities of the chemical bonds in their molecules. A similar principle was used by Free and Wilson (1964) to describe biological activity in various series of chemical analogues. Their method is predicated on the assumption that each substituent can be assigned a certain positive or negative contribution to the biological activity, these contributions being additive. A comparison of Free and Wilson's method with that of Hansch, made in a study where these two methods were used to evaluate the inhibitory potencies of 1-decyl-3-carbamoylpiperidines against butyrylcholinesterase, has shown that the Hansch method gives better results (Clayton and Purcell, 1969). However, Craig (1974) has reported that these two methods give similar results when applied independently to predict the antimalarial potencies of phenanthrene amino-carbinols and has advised using both techniques whenever possible. Cammarata (1972) has pointed to the interrelationship between these methods.

Much earlier, a similar approach was used by McGowan (1951a, 1952b) to calculate the toxicity of compounds not necessarily organic but having so-called physical toxicity, that is, showing no specific chemical interaction with the biological substrate. In particular, he proposed a method for calculating the toxicity of a substance from the parachor, a parameter which, as is known, can always be calculated from the structural formula of the compound. McGowan's principles have been employed for practical calculations in toxicology.

2.3. Relationships outside Series of Congeneric Compounds

It has been shown repeatedly that the toxicity parameters of organic substances tend to correlate with some of their physicochemical properties. The range of substances for which such correlations may be found is very large; in fact it extends to practically all organic substances. Clearly, the correlations established here are not as good as those described above for series of congeners.

Many broad correlations of this kind were described by Lazarev (1944). They include correlations between physicochemical properties and various biological responses to substances applied to test objects in air or in water. Lazarev was the first to call attention to the importance of such correlations for the classification of organic nonelectrolytes in terms of their biological activities. In his monograph *Nonelectrolytes* he succeeded in constructing a system of organic compounds which can give a general concept of their biological actions from data on only one property—lipophilicity.

In this system, nonelectrolytes are arranged in order of increasing oil/water partition coefficients. Each successive group includes compounds having partition coefficients 10 times higher than those of the preceding group. The first group includes substances with partition coefficients in the range 10^{-3} to 10^{-2}; the ninth and last group, those with coefficients of 10^5 upward.

Lazarev's system not only represents an important theoretical generalization of the relationship between physicochemical properties and biological activity, but can also be used to considerable practical advantage in a number of biomedical disciplines. In particular, if it is known to which group a substance belongs, it is possible to predict to some extent the magnitude of its harmful effect, even if no data on its biological activity are available.

This biological and physicochemical system was devised more than three decades ago. Since then, it has become apparent that a system similar to Lazarev's may have an important role to play in the field of toxicology, in particular, for the quantitative prediction of toxicity parameters. However, the oil/water partition coefficient, on which Lazarev's system relies, is not a readily available physicochemical constant, and it is usually unknown for newly synthesized chemicals. The use of this coefficient also has other disadvantages which, incidentally, were pointed out by Lazarev himself. Now that a wealth of data on relationships between the structures, properties, and activities of compounds has been accumulated, it is feasible to develop a biological system of substances based on a more precise and readily accessible or easily measurable physicochemical constant or, perhaps, on a combination of such constants.

A simple structure-activity relationship was presented in mathematical form by Kobozev (1955). His attention was drawn to the previously known relationship between the biological activities and molecular sizes of substances. That such a relationship exists is indicated, in particular, by what he called an "aggravation effect": the activities of substances belonging to various groups (vitamins, alkaloids, chemotherapeutic agents, etc.) generally tend to increase with increasing molecular weight, irrespective of the qualitative features of their action. Kobozev illustrated this correlation for 80 biologically active substances to which the following equation applies:

$$-\log(\text{dose}) = 1 \pm 1.1 + \tfrac{1}{115} M \tag{6}$$

where the dose is expressed in moles, M is the molecular weight, and the constant ± 1.1 or, to be more exact, $\pm(0 - 1.1)$ is a quantitative measure of the closeness of the correlation.

More recently, a strictly quantitative study was made of the relationships between the most commonly used indices of toxicity for laboratory animals and the more readily accessible physicochemical constants (Filov and Liublina, 1965). This study was designed to reveal close correlations with a view to their subsequent use primarily for practical purposes, namely, for the calculation of toxicity indices. The following five indices were considered: the LD_{50} for white mice of substances administered by intragastric intubation in 0.2 ml of refined sunflower-seed oil; the inhalation LC_{50} for white mice after a 2-hr exposure and for an observation period of 7 days; the NC_{50} for white mice upon 2-hr exposure; the C_{min} (threshold concentration) causing changes in the unconditioned flexor reflex in rabbits after 40-min exposure; and the MAC. All concentrations were expressed in millimoles per liter and all doses in millimoles per kilogram. The logarithms to base 10 of the doses and concentrations were used. Data were collected on 38 chemical, physical, thermodynamical, and other properties of 218 organic compounds from different classes for which all or some of the five toxicity indices specified above were known. These properties and the corresponding ranges of values are listed in Table 26.

Of course, not all the values of physicochemical properties and toxicity indices were available for each of the 218 compounds. Consequently the number of data points (n) was different for different pairs. For instance, when the LC_{50} was considered in relation to t_{melt} (no. 6 in Table 27), both these parameters were known for only 148 of the 218 substances, so that correlations for this pair were sought using those 148 substances; similarly, only 40 substances were used in correlating the MAC and parachor (no. 31 in Table 27); and so on. The correlation coefficients (r) were calculated on a computer and expressed in percentages (Table 27). Coefficients whose statistical significance is less than 99% ($p > .01$) are given in parentheses; those of higher

Table 26. Values of Physicochemical Properties

Number	Symbol	Name	Units	Conditions under Which Values Were Measured	Range of Values
1	M	Molecular weight			28–280
2	ρ	Density	g/cm^3	20°C, compared with water at 4°C	0.645–2.89
3	V_m	Molar volume	$cm^3/mole$	$V_m = M/\rho$	36.8–223.0
4	n_D	Refractive index		20°C	1.283–1.685
5	R_m	Molar refraction[a]	$cm^3/mole$		6.7–52.0
6	t_{melt}	Melting point	°C		−190 to +178
7	t_{boil}	Boiling point	°C	760 mm Hg	−103 to +258
8	P	Saturated vapor pressure	mm Hg	25°C	0.15–10^5
9	P_t	Saturated vapor pressure	mm Hg	At temperature t_e	429–1324
10	t_e	Equilibrium temperature	°C	1 mole of vapor of the substance in a volume of 22.414 liters, and vapor and liquid in equilibrium	−113 to +239
11	dt/dP_t	Rate of change of t_{boil} with pressure	°C/mm Hg	25°C	0.02–82
12	dt/dP_p	Rate of change of t_{boil} with pressure	°C/mm Hg	10 mm Hg	0.33–0.58
13	ρ_{crit}	Critical density	g/cm^3		0.230–0.776
14	t_{crit}	Critical temperature	°C		92–611
15	P_{crit}	Critical pressure	atm		22.4–74.2
16	L_f	Latent heat of fusion	kcal/mole		0.4–5.0
17	L_{vap}	Latent heat of vaporization	kcal/mole	At t_{boil}	3.2–12.0
18	L_{comb}	Heat of combustion	kcal/mole	Gas at constant pressure and 25°C	63–3963

331

Table 26. (*Continued*)

Number	Symbol	Name	Units	Conditions under Which Values Were Measured	Range of Values
19	L_{form}	Heat of formation of gas	kcal/mole	25°	−90 +44
20	ΔA_{form}	Free energy of formation of gas	kcal/mole		−84.0 to +88.4
21	$\log K$	Logarithm of olive oil/water partition coefficient			−1.5 to +5.5
22	$\log \lambda$	Logarithm of water/air partition coefficient			−1.72 to +4.77
23	σ	Surface tension	dynes/cm	20°C	12.5–51.0
24	ν	Kinematic viscosity	cSt	20°C	0.2–108
25	η	Dynamic viscosity	cP	20°C	0.2–143
26	S	Solubility	mM/liter	20°C	0–∞
27	c_p	Specific heat capcity	cal/(mole °K)	27°C and constant pressure	15.6–114.6
28	c_p^v	Specific heat of vapor	cal/(mol °K)	25°C and 1 atm	8.5–50.6
29	λ	Thermal conductivity	cal/(cm sec °C)	Liquid	$(0.24–0.65) \times 10^5$
30	P_a	Atomic polarization	cm³		0.4–6.7
31	$[P]$	Parachor	$g^{1/4} \cdot cm^3/(sec^{1/2}\ mole)$	Calculated	99–402
32	μ	Electric dipole moment	debye	25°C; solution in benzene	0–4.3
33	ε	Dielectric constant		25°C; liquid; measured at a frequency of 10^5	1.8–58.0
34	D'	Specific dispersion	cm³/g	25°C; $D' = D/\rho$	58–256
35	D	Absolute dispersion		25°C; $D = (n_f − n_c) \times 10^4$	55–254
36	V_i	Primary ionization potential	eV		7.7–12.4
37	S_l	Entropy of liquid	cal/(mole °C)	25°C	33.1–93.9
38	S_g	Entropy of gas	cal/(mole °C)	25°C	52–120

ᵃ Most of the values have been taken from tables where the refraction was calculated from the formula $R_m = [(n^2 − 1)/(n^2 + 2)](M/\rho)$, ... the method of Eisenlohr or Vogel.

Table 27. Correlation Coefficients (%) between Toxicity Indices and Physicochemical Properties

Number	Symbols	LC$_{50}$ r^a	n^b	NC$_{50}$ r	n	C$_{min}$ r	n	LD$_{50}$ r	n	MAC r	n
1	M	−39.5	201	−57.1	96	[−34.3]	66	(−2.2)	60	−39.2	124
2	ρ	−35.3	183	−45.3	94	[−34.2]	63	(−23.1)	55	−47.7	117
3	V_m	(−14.5)	182	(−26.2)	94	(−13.9)	63	(15.6)	55	(−1.0)	117
4	n_D	−31.2	177	−55.1	92	−45.1	62	(−19.7)	55	−36.2	113
5	R_m	[−23.0]	181	−44.6	95	(−21.9)	63	(−4.7)	55	(−13.8)	116
6	t_{melt}	−41.0	148	−52.5	84	[−40.6]	54	(−16.1)	52	−44.2	101
7	t_{boil}	−45.8	189	−56.9	94	[−30.3]	66	(−18.7)	60	[−29.9]	123
8	log P	40.9	185	48.7	95	(−29.0)	65	(20.8)	59	[23.5]	119
9	P_t	[−41.3]	54	−52.3	42	−73.6	17	(−19.3)	18	[−50.6]	34
10	t_c	−65.9	53	−68.5	41	[−72.1]	17	(−18.7)	18	(−40.7)	34
11	dt/dP_t	−46.5	52	[−44.5]	39	[−42.1]	17	(−36.2)	18	(−43.1)	32
12	dt/dP_p	(−21.6)	61	[−43.9]	45	−61.4	27	(−4.2)	28	[−43.4]	43
13	ρ_{crit}	−47.6	59	−49.5	50	[−52.4]	24	(−22.3)	25	−65.0	43
14	t_{crit}	−62.2	78	−58.7	61	[−47.0]	34	(−13.9)	32	(−30.9)	58
15	P_{crit}	(−11.7)	71	(16.3)	57	(−20.7)	32	(−32.9)	29	[−36.1]	53
16	L_f	[−37.4]	66	−54.5	52	[−42.1]	26	(−5.1)	27	(−16.2)	46
17	L_{vap}	−22.8	91	−73.0	62	−17.0	35	(−29.8)	30	(−12.7)	60
18	L_{comb}	(30.2)	51	(−21.4)	48	(−2.6)	24	(30.6)	23	(36.8)	38
19	L_{form}	(7.8)	51	(−3.1)	38	(−45.3)	21	(−3.4)	19	(−38.4)	36
20	ΔA_{form}	(27.5)	55	(−23.9)	46	(−40.0)	24	(13.6)	20	(−4.4)	38
21	log K	(20.1)	83	(−19.3)	70	(−8.8)	43	(15.6)	39	(21.9)	66
22	log λ	[−28.8]	89	(1.4)	74	(−7.2)	52	(−30.9)	47	(−19.9)	77
23	σ	−47.0	100	−55.0	66	−67.8	38	(−22.4)	36	−52.1	64

Table 27. *(Continued)*

Number	Symbol	LC$_{50}$ r^a	n^b	NC$_{50}$ r	n	C$_{min}$ r	n	LD$_{50}$ r	n	MAC r	n
24	ν	(−18.2)	96	(7.4)	65	(−21.1)	35	(−5.5)	35	(−20.2)	61
25	η	(−20.2)	96	(−3.4)	65	(−35.7)	35	(−6.2)	35	(−21.1)	61
26	log S	(4.1)	95	(16.2)	73	(9.5)	52	(−12.5)	49	(7.5)	76
27	c_p	(−11.6)	72	[−37.5]	52	(−13.8)	33	(7.1)	33	(20.5)	52
28	c_p^v	(19.5)	58	(−18.5)	48	(−12.3)	21	(−23.9)	19	[44.5]	35
29	λ	[−42.7]	40	34.3	36	(35.6)	20	(29.4)	24	(5.8)	35
30	P_a	(−41.3)	36	(−25.9)	30	(−0.6)	19	−78.5	14	(−25.3)	32
31	[P]	(−11.0)	58	−49.9	46	(−11.9)	18	(42.7)	20	(15.1)	40
32	μ	−34.9	137	(−20.2)	82	(−24.7)	52	(−21.6)	50	[−30.5]	93
33	ε	−45.0	99	(−2.4)	68	(3.8)	41	(−24.2)	40	(−19.5)	65
34	D'	(−0.1)	59	(−26.6)	40	(−46.9)	26	(−7.4)	24	(−25.4)	36
35	D	(−27.8)	59	−53.9	40	−66.2	26	(−27.4)	24	−59.4	36
36	V_i	(−2.0)	60	(23.2)	46	(2.5)	29	(6.0)	28	(3.6)	45
37	S_i	(28.0)	45	(−31.4)	38	(−12.7)	23	(16.7)	22	(37.2)	31
38	S_g	(13.6)	69	[−42.6]	55	(−1.1)	29	(16.9)	24	(26.4)	42

^{a} r = correlation coefficient.
^{b} n = number of pairs.

significance, with a probability ranging from 99 to 99.9%, are enclosed in brackets; the remaining coefficients have a probability greater than 99.9%.

Even a cursory inspection of Table 27 reveals that different toxicity indices show different correlations with physicochemical properties. The poorest correlation is found for the LD_{50}, where coefficients are low and relatively insignificant ($p > .01$). The only exception is the correlation with P_a, but more data are needed to test it, for it may have been due to chance. The low correlations for the LD_{50} can be readily explained by the fact that absorption from the gastrointestinal tract, which depends on a large number of factors, is superimposed on toxic activity as such; this complicates the poisoning picture and makes the correlations more difficult to detect.

As was to be expected, the highest correlation with physicochemical properties is shown by the narcotic concentration, which is the most unequivocal indicator of toxicity, for it is determined at the moment the animal falls on one side, that is, at the time of onset of narcosis, which appears to reflect some standard mechanism of action of substances. In the case of the LC_{50}, the correlation is somewhat poorer because of the diversity of mechanisms resulting in a lethal outcome. The same is true of the correlation with C_{min}.

Worthy of note are the fairly high correlations of the MAC with some physicochemical properties. The MAC is a highly integral toxicity index, reflecting, as it does, many aspects of toxic action, and has considerable practical importance. The established correlations may be used for the approximate calculation and tentative prediction of MACs (see Chapter 8).

As regards the physicochemical properties studied, some of them (V_m, P_{crit}, L_{comb}, L_{form}, ΔA_{form}, $\log K$, $\log \lambda$, v, η, S, c_p, c_p^v, $\log \lambda$, P_a, D', V_i, S_l, S_g) do not have satisfactory correlations with the toxicity indices; others (M, ρ, n_D, t_{melt}, ρ_{crit}, σ) show good correlations; still others correlate well with some of the indices.

We tried to classify the 38 physicochemical properties considered. (Although we are well aware that this classification has a number of shortcomings and may have to be modified, we consider the attempt worthwhile.) All the properties were divided into three classes (I, II, and III), class II being then divided into three categories (A, B, and C), and category C into two groups (1 and 2), as follows:

I. Properties determined by the supramolecular level of substance organization: ΔA_{form}, S_l, S_g, dt/dP_t, dt/dP_p.
II. Properties determined at the molecular level:
   A. Properties related to the molecular structure: M, ρ, ρ_{crit}, V_m, $[P]$.
   B. Properties related to the kinetic (or vibrational) energy of the molecule: P_{crit}, λ, c_p, c_p^v.

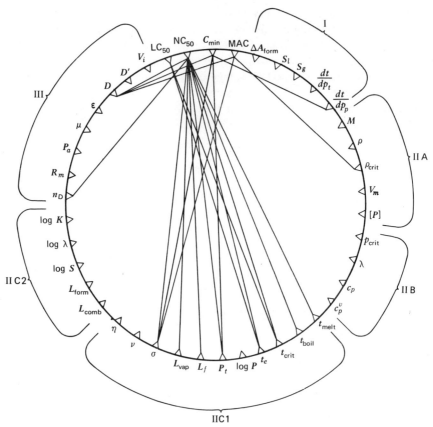

Figure 43. Correlations between toxicity indices (in mM/liter of air) and physicochemical properties of volatile organic compounds at the level of $r > 50\%$ ($p < .001$). See text for explanation. All concentrations are in logarithmic form.

    C. Properties related to the energy of molecular interaction:
       1. Between molecules: t_{melt}, t_{boil}, t_{crit}, t_e, $\log P$, P_t, L_f, L_{vap}, σ, v, η.
       2. With other molecules: L_{comb}, L_{form}, $\log S$, $\log \lambda$, $\log K$.
III. Properties determined at the nuclear-electronic level: n_D, R_m, P_a, μ, ε, D, D', V_i.

An interesting result emerged when the toxicity indices studied were considered in relation to the properties grouped in this way. Straight lines in Figure 43 connect toxicity indices (the LD_{50} was omitted because of the poor correlation) with physicochemical properties for correlations with $r > 50\%$ and $p < .001$. It will be seen that most (13 out of 20) of the correlations are with properties determined at the molecular level and related to the energy of interaction of molecules with one another (group C1). In this group only viscosities (v and η) and saturated vapor pressure (log P) fail to give high correlations, whereas in IIB and IIC2 such correlations are not found at all. Elsewhere high correlations are few, although D (absolute dispersion) from class III correlates with three toxicity indices (incidentally, D is related to n_D belonging to the same class and likewise correlating with the NC_{50}).

The overall pattern persists if we narrow or broaden the range of correlations, say by including all those with $r > 60\%$ or only those with $r > 40\%$.

At this stage, we are unable to explain these facts but deem them worthy of attention.

The above study appears to have covered all possible correlations between the considered toxicity indices and physicochemical properties for volatile organic compounds.

The following circumstance is of interest. It is now known, for some groups of organic compounds, that a reversal occurs in the direction of correlation between log LD_{50} and molecular weight, t_{boil}, t_{melt}, and molar refraction among nonvolatile or slightly volatile compounds. For example, in the case of aromatic amines the lethal dose decreases with the molecular weight only up to a molecular weight of about 150, while the reverse relationship holds for amines of higher molecular weight (Liublina, 1973b).

It may be added that the MACs of nonvolatile organic compounds were found to be less dependent on the four physicochemical constants mentioned above than those of volatile compounds when these two kinds of compound were considered separately.

There can be no doubt that correlations similar to those discussed in this section will be increasingly used for both practical and theoretical purposes as more understanding is gained of the chemical basis of life processes; at the same time a knowledge of these correlations should promote such understanding.

3. THE TOXICITIES, STRUCTURES, AND PHYSICOCHEMICAL PROPERTIES OF INORGANIC SUBSTANCES

This section will not present correlations at all comparable to the excellent ones established for organic compounds and described above. Such correlations have not yet been reported, nor are they likely to be ever found in view of the immense diversity of inorganic substances, particularly as regards their capacity for various physicochemical interactions.

The mechanisms of interaction of various chemical substances with living cells are now being gradually unraveled. A leading role in this is played by quantum-chemical concepts. It can be stated with certainty that, as more information is gained about the mechanism of action of inorganic substances, prospects will open for establishing correlations between their structures, properties, and biological activities. Such correlations, although not as good as those detected for organic substances, will be used to advantage for gaining further insights into the mechanism of biological activity of inorganic substances, as well as for a variety of calculations to serve practical purposes. Work along this line has been started, and some results have been reported, although they often leave much to be desired and cannot be quantified (see Liublina et al., 1967, for a review). Here we will discuss some of the more interesting and promising results. The correlations established between toxicity indices and some physicochemical constants of gases and vapors, which can already be used for calculations in toxicology, will be discussed in Chapter 8.

Inorganic substances, when introduced into the biological environment of the organism, are usually broken down into ions and interact as such with the constituents of cells and tissues. For this reason the toxic effect produced by an inorganic compound is determined by the toxicity of its ions, in most cases by some one ion which exerts the greatest biological effect. Therefore the biological activity should be expected to correlate best with the characteristics of such ions. In 1904 Matthews pointed out a relationship between the toxicity of metal ions and the standard potential of the corresponding metals (the ions formed in solutions of salts of the metals). More recently, the toxic concentrations of metal ions, as determined for various model systems such as enzyme solutions or for animals with a low level of organization, have been related to the molecular weight, valency, ionic radius, electric charge, and other characteristics of the metals. Thus Shaw (1961) found the toxicities of bivalent ions of transition metals to correlate closely with the stability of metal complexes (see Table 28, where toxicities are expressed as negative

Table 28.   Toxicities of Bivalent Ions of Transition Metals

Test Object	Ion					
	Mn	Fe	Co	Ni	Cu	Zn
Urease	2.5	4.1	4.2	4.5	6.5	5.7
Fundulus eggs	0.3	1.1	1.1	1.2	4.2	0.6
Daphnia magna	3.4	4.0	4.6	5.3	6.8	6.0

Source.   Shaw (1961).

Table 29.   Correlations between the Toxicities and Some Physicochemical Properties of Metals

Constants Correlating with Log LD_{50}	Standard Potential	Primary Ionization Potential	Atomic Radius	Solubility of Sulfides (log S)	Density of Oxygen Compounds
Correlation coefficient	-0.77	-0.54	0.59	0.66	-0.47
Number of pairs	35	42	41	34	41
Probability of absence of correlation	$p < .001$	$p < .01$	$p < .001$	$p < 001$	$p = .01$

logarithms of the metal ion concentrations needed to produce a particular level of biological response). The high correlation was attributed by the author to the formation of complexes of the metals with vitally important enzymes, and this determined the toxicities of the metals.

In another study (Liublina, 1965) correlations were established between the toxicities of metal ions (the criterion of effect was the intraperitoneal LD_{50} of soluble metal compounds for white mice) and the physicochemical properties of the metals or their compounds (Table 29). It can be seen from Table 29 that the correlations are significant and in three cases (with atomic radius, standard potential, and solubility) are rather high. The correlations made it possible to derive the following two equations:

$$\log LD_{50} = -0.63SP - 1.0$$

$$\log LD_{50} = -0.21 \log S + 0.75$$

where SP is the standard potential.

Rabotnikova (1965) determined the interperitoneal LD_{50} of metal oxides for mice in an attempt to correlate the toxicities with properties of both the oxides and the corresponding metals. The correlations obtained are of interest, especially the one between the LD_{50} and the normal body level of a metal, which has a correlation coefficient of $+0.55$ at $p < .01$. Consequently, the lower the toxicity of the metal oxide, the more metal is contained in the body.

Kist (1967), in a similar study, tried to correlate the relative lethal toxicity of an element with the normal content of that element in the human body. The term "relative lethal toxicity" (RLT) was used by the author to mean the ratio of the average normal body concentration (C) of the element to the additional concentration attained on condition that all the administered lethal dose is evenly distributed in the body. Seventeen elements (P, K, Fe, Cu, F, Cr, As, Ba, Hg, B, Co, Li, Mn, Ni, Sb, Ag, Ga) were studied. The RLTs of trace elements proved to be very small. Thus, to produce a lethal effect, the body concentration of cobalt or nickel had to be raised 1000-fold or more above the normal level. On the other hand, a lethal concentration of an element widely represented in the body, such as phosphorus or potassium, was reached when the normal concentration was increased only insignificantly.* It was concluded that the lower the normal body content of an element, the greater is the range of fluctuations of its level that may be harmless for man. The author proposed the equation

$$\log \text{RLT} = 1.2 \log C + 36$$

It appears that the periodic table, which classifies the elements with such extraordinary logic and enables us to foretell the properties of many chemical compounds, may also be used to advantage to evaluate the bioactivities of substances. At any rate, if a biological effect correlates with physicochemical properties, the periodic table must contain a key to the existing correlation. This key has not yet been found, although models of it, perhaps still far from the original, are being developed.

The first attempt to relate the toxicities of elements to their positions in the periodic table was undertaken by Saccardo (1955), who depicted the periodic system of elements in the form of a spiral with 12 coils crossed by 16 radii. In his system all the elements are found at the points of intersection of the radii and the coils, being arranged clockwise beginning with the outermost coil and proceeding toward the center. Saccardo proposed many rules for estimating the approximate values of physicochemical properties of elements. Unfortunately, it is not practicable to relate the toxicity of an element to its place on the spiral because of the large number of reservations and exceptions to the rules.

Interesting work has been done by Bienvenu et al. (1963), who reported LD_{50} values for soluble salts of 38 metals obtained in the course of their attempt to relate ion toxicity to the position of the element in the periodic table. These salts had chlorine or, in some cases, sulfate or nitrate as their anions. When the intraperitoneal LD_{50} values for white mice were expressed

---

* It may seem that these results are opposite to those of Rabotnikova (1965) mentioned above. The results of these two studies are, however, incomparable because Rabotnikova determined the toxicities of metal oxides and Kist those of elements; also, the toxicity indices were different: unlike the LD_{50}, the RLT characterizes the range of toxic concentrations.

in milliatoms per kilogram of body weight, a periodicity related to cation toxicity was observed, except at the level of transition elements.[†]

The next attempt (Nofre et al., 1963) concerned compounds differing in their anions but having the same cation, sodium. It was found that the toxicity of an anion may vary with its valency. Toxicity increased with increasing valency in the halogens and phosphorus and decreased in arsenic, selenium, tellurium, sulfur, and nitrogen. In view of this, the authors did not feel it practicable to relate the toxicities of anions to their positions in the periodic table. According to Levina (1972), some metals likewise become more toxic, and others less toxic, with rising valency. The same difficulty therefore holds for cations also.

The relationship between toxicity and valency is a rather complicated matter. Some correlations have been established, but all of them are too narrow in scope to be of real value. This question is discussed in detail by Levina (1972).

It would seem that the above difficulty can be circumvented if one considers only compounds of like type, say those with highest or lowest valencies or those with a certain medium valency chosen according to some rule common for all compounds (Liublina, 1967).

In Figure 44, LD_{50} data of Bienvenu et al. (1963) and Nofre et al. (1963), supplemented with those from other sources, are arranged in order of the atomic numbers of the toxic elements of the compounds concerned. In all cases the logarithms of doses for inert gases were taken to be > 1.75, since the intraperitoneal doses corresponding to that figure did not reach the LD_{50} level; higher doses could not be tested because the volume of administered gas would have been too great. Compounds of lanthanides and transuranic elements were omitted.

One cannot fail to notice a certain, though incomplete, periodicity in the diagram. Each period ends with an element from the zero group, that is, the most inert substance whose LD_{50} was not reached (in Figure 44 this is indicated by arrows pointing upward), so there is a peak at the end of each period. In addition there are at least two bulges in each of the long periods (4, 5, and 6). Thus, in period 4, the first bulge extends from vanadium (23) to copper (29), and the second from copper (29) to arsenic (33); in period 5 the first bulge is

[†] Here and in the following discussion of the toxicity of inorganic compounds, LD_{50} values are given in terms of milliatoms of the elements listed in Figure 44 according to their atomic numbers. An LD_{50} in milligrams per kilogram is converted to one in milliatoms per kilogram by dividing it by the molecular weight and multiplying the result by the number of atoms of the element concerned. Therefore, if there is one atom of the element in the molecule, the dose in milliatoms per kilogram will be equal to that in millimoles per kilogram; if there are two atoms, it will be twice that in millimoles per kilogram; if three atoms, thrice that in millimoles per kilogram; and so on.

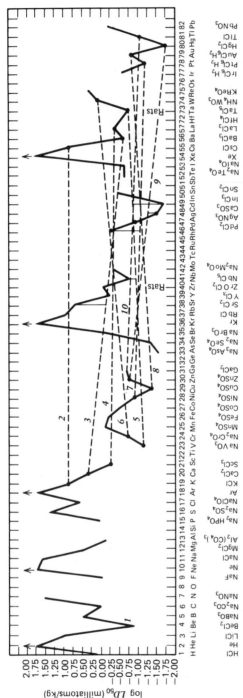

Figure 44. Toxicity (LD_{50}) as a function of the atomic number of the toxic element. *Abscissa*, the two upper lines indicate the numbers and symbols of the elements; the lower line shows the compounds whose log LD_{50} values (calculated in terms of the toxic element concerned) are given on the ordinate. *Ordinate*, log LD_{50} values for white mice with intraperitoneal injection in aqueous solution. *1*, Segments of the thick, broken lines connect log LD_{50} values of compounds containing toxic elements, listed according to their atomic number; the dotted lines connect log LD_{50} values of compounds of metals from the same subgroups in the fourth and sixth long periods, as follows: *2*, from the first principal subgroup (K and Cs); *3*, from the second principal subgroup (Ca and Ba); *4*, from the third principal subgroup (Sc and La); *5*, from the fifth principal subgroup (V and Ta); *6*, from the sixth principal subgroup (Cr and W); *7*, from the eighth subordinate subgroup (Ni and Pt); *8*, from the first subordinate subgroup (Cu and Au); *9*, from the second subordinate subgroup (Zn and Hg); *10*, from the third subordinate subgroup (Ga and Tl). The vertical lines in period 5 denote the distances between true LD_{50} values and those found by interpolation. Arrows above LD_{50} values for inert gases indicate that the LD_{50} was not attained. *Periods*: *2*: Li → Ne, *3*: Na → Ar, *4*: K → Kr (long), *5*: Rb → Xe (long), *6*: Cs → (long).

342

from niobium to indium (41 to 49) and the second from indium to antimony or tellurium (49 to 51 or 52); in period 6 the first is from tantalum to mercury (73 to 80), while the second is left incomplete because no data were available. Within the three long periods many log LD_{50} values for the second long period lie close to the straight lines drawn through the corresponding points in the first and third long periods (dotted lines in Figure 44). The unusual trend of toxicity variation for subordinate groups in periods 4, 5, and 6 (decreasing toxicity with increasing atomic number of elements in these subgroups: V > Nb > Ta; Cr > Mo > W; Cu > Ag > Au) does not abolish periodicity but only complicates it.*

An attempt to relate the log MAC to the position of the toxic ion in the periodic table led to a similar result. It is of interest that the periodicity of toxicities presented in Figure 44 resembles in form that of the ionization potentials of elements in the periodic table.

Using the same more or less homogeneous material, the atomic structures of the most and least toxic elements were then compared (Table 30). It can be seen that an atom can be very toxic when at least four electronic shells are present. The outer shells of all toxic atoms are far from being filled—not only p^6 but also p^5 is absent; moreover, there is no p^2, whereas the shell next to the outermost one is completely or nearly filled (d^{10}, d^9). It is only in uranium that the intermediate shell d is filled by four electrons.

The least toxic elements, belonging to the zero group of the periodic table, have their outer and inner shells completely filled. Each of the elements of low toxicity from the first principal subgroup has only one electron in its outermost shell.

The structural features mentioned above of the more toxic elements are shared also by Zn, Ga, Ag, Sb, Au, Tl, Bi, and Po. Comparable LD_{50} values are available only for Zn, Ga, Ag, Au, and Tl. These five elements are all similar in their LD_{50}s to particularly toxic elements.

The above relationships between toxicity and electronic structure have been discussed in greater detail elsewhere (e.g., Brakhnova and Samsonov, 1966; Suvorov, 1968). So far, however, the only unequivocal conclusion that has emerged from these discussions is that the toxicity of an element increases as its electronic stability decreases. In other words, the more active the element chemically, the more toxic it is. (This statement is valid only in the most general sense.) It is of interest in this context that the chemical activity of metals has been reported to decline with increasing electronic stability of their d configurations (Samsonov, 1966). This explains why toxicity declines in

---

* The unusual pattern of toxicity change in the subordinate subgroups may be associated with some other anomalies observed in these subgroups.

Table 30.   Structures of the Most and Least Toxic Elements

Element Number in the Periodic Table	Symbol	Structure[a]
		Most Toxic
29	Cu	$1s^2\, 2s^2\, 2p^6\, 3s^2\, 3p^6\, 3d^{10}\, 4s$
33	As	$1s^2\, 2s^2\, 2p^6\, 3s^2\, 3p^6\, 3d^{10}\, 4s^2\, 4p^3$
34	Se	$1s^2\, 2s^2\, 2p^6\, 3s^2\, 3p^6\, 3d^{10}\, 4s^2\, 4p^4$
48	Cd	$1s^2\, 2s^2\, 2p_6\, 3s^2\, 3p^6\, 3d^{10}\, 4s^2\, 4p^6\, 4d^{10}\, 5s^2$
49	In	$1s^2\, 2s^2\, 2p^6\, 3s^2\, 3p^6\, 3d^{10}\, 4s^2\, 4p^6\, 4d^{10}\, 5s^2\quad 5p$
52	Te	$1s^2\, 2s^2\, 2p^6\, 3s^2\, 3p^1\, 3d^{10}\, 4s^2\, 4p^6\, 4d^{10}\, 5s^2\quad 5p^4$
78	Pt	$1s^2\, 2s^2\, 2p^6\, 3s^2\, 3p^6\, 3d^{10}\, 4s^2\, 4p^6\, 4d^{10}\, 4f^{14}\, 5s^2\; 5p^6\quad 5d^9\;\; 6s$
80	Hg	$1s^2\, 2s^2\, 2p^6\, 3s^2\, 3p^6\, 3d^{10}\, 4s^2\, 4p^6\, 4d^{10}\, 4f^{14}\, 5s^2\; 5p^6\quad dd^{10}\; 6s$
92	U	$1s^2\, 2s^2\, 2p^6\, 3s^2\, 3p^6\, 3d^{10}\, 4s^2\, 4p^6\, 4d^{10}\, 5s^2\quad 5p^6\; 5d^{10}\; 6s^2\quad 6p^6\; 6d^4\; 7s^2$
		Least Toxic
2	He	$1s^2$
10	Ne	$1s^2\, 2s^2\, 2p^6$
18	Ar	$1s^2\, 2s^2\, 2p^6\, 3s^2\, 3p^6$
36	Kr	$1s^2\, 2s^2\, 2p^6\, 3s^2\, 3p^6\, 3d^{10}\, 4s^2\, 4p^6$
54	Xe	$1s^2\, 2s^2\, 2p^6\, 3s^2\, 3p^6\, 3d^{10}\, 4s^2\, 4p^6\, 4d^{10}\, 5s^2\quad 5p^6$
3	Li	$1s^2\, 2s$
11	Na	$1s^2\, 2s^2\, 2p^6\, 3s$
19	K	$1s^2\, 2s^2\, 2p^6\, 3s^2\, 3p^6\, 4s$
37	Rb	$1s^2\, 2s^2\, 2p^6\, 3s^2\, 3p^6\, 3d^{10}\, 4s^2\, 4p^6\, 5s$
55	Cs	$1s^2\, 2s^2\, 2p^6\, 3s^2\, 3p^6\, 3d^{10}\, 4s^2\, 4p^6\, 4d^{10}\, 5s^2\quad 5p^6\; 6s$

[a] Figures before letters denote the principal quantum number, showing the ordinal number of the electronic shell. Letters characterize the orbit, and superscripts to these letters indicate the number of electrons on the orbit. Each line as a whole characterizes the number of electronic shells and the degree to which they are filled.

subordinate groups in going from vanadium to tantalum and from chromium to tungsten (see p. 343 and Figure 44).

The relationships, and especially the correlations, existing between the chemical structures and toxic activities of industrial poisons described in this chapter have been used for practical purposes. The next (and last) chapter describes methods for calculating the approximate values of various toxicity indices and maximum allowable concentrations in the air of workplaces.

ADDENDUM: QUANTITATIVE RELATIONSHIPS BETWEEN STRUCTURE AND BIOLOGICAL ACTIVITY

In Chapter 7 the progress made by industrial toxicology in the study of quantitative structure-activity relationships (now commonly abbreviated as QSAR) was surveyed up to the year 1970. The research conducted in the USSR was summarized also in our later English-language publications (Filov, 1976; Liublina and Filov, 1975). This section discusses the work that, in our view, is the most interesting or promising carried out in the QSAR area in the past few years.

A1. CORRELATIONS BETWEEN TOXIC PROPERTIES AND PHYSICOCHEMICAL PARAMETERS

Of the studies where attempts were made to relate biological effects to the more generally known properties such as density, molecular weight, and boiling point, of special interest appears to be the work of Andreeshcheva (1975), in that the olfactory threshold was used as criterion. The relationships found are presented in Table A1. Differences between the experimentally determined and the calculated threshold values ranged from 1.2- to 2-fold.

Table A1. Correlation Coefficients between Physical Properties of Benzene Derivatives and Olfactory Thresholds for Man as Assessed from Electroencephalographic Data

Property	r
Saturated vapor pressure	0.87
Density	0.56
Heat of formation	0.66
Molecular weight	-0.45
Boiling point	-0.72
Refractive index	-0.61
Molar refraction	-0.68
Surface tension	-0.63
Dipole moment	-0.50
Viscosity coefficient	-0.45
Heat capacity	-0.55
Melting point	-0.41

Source. Andreeshcheva (1975).

Vrbovsky (1974) studied the acute toxicity of piperidine derivatives for mice of both sexes in relation to molecular weight, using the intravenous, intraperitoneal, and oral routes of administration. The rectilinear relationships obtained for log LD_{50} values in narrow groups of compounds permitted assessment of the relative mechanisms of their toxic actions. The properties of four newly synthesized compounds proved to be similar to those predicted from the correlations discovered.

Encouraging results have been reported from a study of the relationships between the biological properties of stable nonelectrolytes and their polarizabilities (Dmitriyeva, 1972). A relationship close to a functional one was established for narcotic concentrations (NC):

$$NC \text{ (mg/liter)} = kP_m^{-2.5} \qquad (n = 56; \text{error} = +8 \text{ to} -10\%)$$

where P_m is the molar polarization and $k = 2.7 \times 10^5$. It is also possible to calculate the maximum allowable concentration, though, of course, less accurately:

$$MAC \text{ (mg/m}^3) = 6.5 \times 10^7 \times P_m^{-4} \qquad (\text{error} = +12 \text{ to} -17\%)$$

The relationship between MAC (mg/m^3) and NC (mg/liter) is

$$MAC = 0.185(NC)^{1.5}$$

In another study the toxicity for rats of aliphatic and aromatic halo derivatives was considered in relation to their reactivity (Eitingen and Ulanova, 1975). The measure of reactivity was the relative death rates of free radicals in solution as estimated by electron paramagnetic resonance. The correlation coefficients were found to be 0.68 for LD_{50} (mM/kg) and 0.86 for LC_{50} (mM/liter).

The last two studies are representative of the current interest in searching for correlations between biological parameters and the electronic characteristics on which molecular reactivity depends to varying degrees. Another example is the study of Hetnarski and O'Brien (1975), in which the inhibitory actions of various methyl carbamate derivatives on acetylcholinesterase were found to correlate with their ability to donate π electrons to form a charge-transfer complex. The charge-transferring capacity was measured from methyl carbamate interaction with a model electron acceptor, tetracyanoethylene, and was characterized by a charge-transfer constant found from the equation

$$C_t = \log K_X + \log K_H$$

where K_X and K_H are association constants for the interaction with tetracyanoethylene to form charge-transfer complexes for substituted and nonsubstituted compounds, respectively.

Another constant not previously used in correlation analyses is the magnitude of σ charges on atoms of a molecule (Amatuni and Krylov, 1974). These charges are considered by the authors to be a highly specific property of each theoretically possible molecule and to reflect adequately any changes in the chemical structure of the compound; moreover, their values can be readily calculated on a computer in a standard manner.

The criterion selected was the percent inhibition of a given biochemical reaction by 24 compounds having the general formula

$$R_3-\underset{\underset{R_2\quad R_1}{\diagup}}{\diagup}-NH-CO-NH-CO-CH_2-R$$

Use was made of a multiple linear correlation equation of the type $Y = a + b_1 x_1 + \cdots + b_i x_i$, where Y is the activity of the compound; $a, b_1, \ldots, b_i$ are constant factors; and $x_1, \ldots, x_i$ are the atomic charges. The correlation coefficient was found to be 0.97. Similar calculations for compounds with the general formula $(C_6H_5)_2-COH-CO-CH_2-C(R_1,R_2)-N(R_3,R_4)$ yielded a correlation coefficient of 0.999 ($n = 12$). Calculations by this method made for 13 compounds gave higher correlation coefficients than did Hansch's method.

Clearly, such virtually linear functional relationships are obtainable only in the case of a fairly standard biological response similar to the one used in the above study (inhibition of a biochemical reaction *in vitro*). Lower correlations should be expected for far more complex toxic effects in mammals (LD_{50}, carcinogenic acitivity, etc.).

Kagan et al. (1976) have employed quantum-chemical parameters to calculate MACs and other indices for several new organophosphorus pesticides.

A2. FURTHER DEVELOPMENT OF EXTRATHERMODYNAMIC APPROACHES TO QSAR PROBLEMS

A.2.1. Hammett-Taft's Approach

This approach has been applied to correlate acute toxicities of xylenol isomers for mice, rats, and rabbits (Kirso and Maazik, 1970). The results are shown in Table A2, where $\Sigma\sigma_i = \Sigma(\sigma_m + \sigma_p + \sigma_o)$. As might have been expected, the less toxic ortho-substituted dimethyl phenols somewhat deviated from the overall trend. Similar correlations have been obtained for other substituted phenols. Log LD_{50} values for mice of 49 organophosphorus compounds of the type

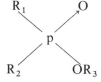

Table A2. Relationship of LD_{50} Values of Xylenols to Hammett–
Taft's Constants for Three Species

Species	Equation	n	r	$\bar{S}$
Mouse	$\log LD_{50} = 0.755\Sigma\sigma_i + 2.744$	4	0.968	0.018
Rat	$\log LD_{50} = 1.001\Sigma\sigma_i + 2.898$	5	0.799	0.081
Rabbit	$\log LD_{50} = 0.844\Sigma\sigma_i + 3.145$	4	0.918	0.039

Source. Kirso and Maazik (1970).

have been satisfactorily correlated to Hammett's constants (Vilceanu et al., 1972). The quadratic regression equation obtained was processed using a FORTRAN program to yield an r of 0.85—a good result considering the large differences among the compounds used.

A.2.2. Free and Wilson's Method

Hudson et al. (1970) have discussed the conditions for the application of the correlational approach of Free and Wilson and have presented its statistical interpretation. Free and Wilson's method is further discussed in Section A2.4.

A.2.3. The Extrathermodynamic Approach of Hansch

Hansch's equations have been applied much more extensively than any others to various problems in the QSAR area. In our view, there are at least three reasons for this. First, Hansch's parabolic equation can describe with reasonable accuracy many more experimental results than can any other approach. Second, Hansch's lipophilic constants are readily available. Octanol/water partition coefficients are not difficult to determine in experiment or by calculation. Last, but not least, Hansch himself has been extremely active in this field.

The principles underlying Hansch's method and his basic equations were described in sufficient detail in Chapter 7. Here only some of the more recent and, in our judgment, most interesting publications will be discussed.

Hansch's approach was the subject of a symposium held in 1970 (*Biological Correlations—The Hansch Approach*), as well as of many papers presented to several conferences, including those held in Prague, Czechoslovakia, in 1973 and in Suhl, German Democratic Republic, in 1976, both under the title "Chemical Structure-Biological Activity Relationships: Quantitative Approaches."

Hansch's concepts have been detailed by the author himself in several theoretical reviews (e.g., Hansch, 1971, 1973). The possible reasons for the parabolic relationship between biological effect and lipophilic character are discussed in a review paper by Hansch and Clayton (1973). Among a variety of explanations these authors adduce nine regarded by them as the most important. These include, among others, the kinetic features of substance transport across a lipid membrane (considered with reference to a three-compartment catenary model simulating substance passage from the aqueous to the lipid and back to the aqueous phase), conformational changes in the receptors caused by members of a congeneric series, and metabolic transformations.

Mention should be made of papers by Tute (1971, 1975), where Hansch's approach is expounded in a popular manner; the first of these papers offers a kind of guideline for the practical application of the method and may be used for teaching purposes. An outline of the history and current status of the method can be found in Hansch (1976). In another paper Hansch (1972) analyzes the quantitative relationships between the lipophilic character and the metabolism of organic xenobiotics both at the microsomal level and *in vivo*. Mention may also be made of the work of Ordukhanian et al. (1976), who used Hansch's approach to establish correlations for the LD_{100} (mice) of a group of phosphoryl derivatives of pyrimidine.

The complete quadratic correlation equation of Hansch has the form

$$\log\left(\frac{1}{C}\right) = k_1\pi^2 + k_2\pi + k_3\sigma + k_4E_s + k_5 \qquad (A1)$$

The meaning of all parameters in (A1), except E_s, is explained on p. 326; E takes account of the steric effects of substituents. In certain cases a dummy variable is introduced into the equation to account for various changes, such as the effect of the ortho position of substitution or the contribution of a *de novo* group. As mentioned in Chapter 7, some values of k may be equal to zero and the equation then simplifies.

In considering experimental results for a group of compounds, the form of the correlation equation is not known beforehand and it is not clear which parameters determine the selected biological effect. With the aid of a computer, a large number of equations with different parameters and their superpositions can be screened to discard statistically insignificant equations and to select those with high correlation coefficients and small standard errors. A search for the most satisfactory equation may be fairly time-consuming. Thus Silipo and Hansch (1974) tested 1920 equations to select only one of them. It is important that an equation thus selected is particularly valuable because it enables one not only to reach conclusions from inter- and extrapolations but also to form a judgment about the mechanism of action of the set of compounds under study.

In recent years the chromatographic parameters R_f have come to be used to characterize the lipophilicities of substances in view of the correlation of this quantity with log P and π. Tomlinson (1975) has discussed, in all possible aspects, the use in QSAR studies of the parameter $R_m = \log(1/R_f - 1)$ and has suggested that it could find wider applications in this field. This quantity is related to Hansch's constant π in a simple manner: $\pi_X = R_{mX} - R_{mH} = \Delta R_{mX}$, that is, π is analogous to ΔR_m. Examples were given of correlations described by linear

$$\log\left(\frac{1}{C}\right) = aR_m + b$$

and nonlinear

$$\log\left(\frac{1}{C}\right) - a(R_m)^2 + b(R_m) + c$$

relationships. Henry et al. (1976) have proposed using high-pressure liquid chromatography for this purpose.

A.2.4.   Comparison of Free and Wilson's and Hansch's Methods; New Models

Cammarata (1972) and Craig (1972) have discussed the assumptions underlying Free and Wilson's and Hansch's analyses and have shown these two methods to be fundamentally interrelated, as well as pointing out their differences. It has been emphasized that the Free–Wilson approach is to be preferred when considering a group of very closely related compounds and that it cannot be applied to a group of widely differing substances, for which Hansch's approach gives better results.

Mathematically, Free and Wilson's approach can be expressed as follows:

$$\log\left(\frac{1}{C}\right) = \sum_i a_i + \mu \tag{A2}$$

where a_1 is the group contribution of substituent X_i, provided that $a_H = 0$, and $\mu = \log(1/C)$ of the unsubstituted compound. The parameter a_i can be interpreted as a weighted sum of the physical properties ϕ_j of the substituent:

$$a_i = \sum_j b_j \phi_j \tag{A3}$$

where b_j are coefficients of physical properties, for example such substituent parameters as π, σ, and E_s. Substitution of the value for a_i into the Free–Wilson equation (A2) gives

$$\log\left(\frac{1}{C}\right) = \sum_i \sum_j b_j \phi_j + \mu = b_1 \sum_i \phi_1 + b_2 \sum_i \phi_2 + \cdots + b_n \sum_i \phi_n + \mu$$

(A4)

or, in the more common form,

$$\log\left(\frac{1}{C}\right) = b_1 \phi_1 + b_2 \phi_2 + \cdots b_n \phi_n + \mu \tag{A5}$$

This equation can be interpreted by Hansch's linear model:

$$\log\left(\frac{1}{C}\right) = k_1 \pi + k_2 \sigma + k_3 E_s + k_4 \tag{A6}$$

On this basis Kubinyi and Kehrhahn (1976) made a precise practical comparison of these methods, using concrete numerical examples. Free and Wilson's and Hansch's approaches were then combined into a mixed approach (Kubinyi, 1976a).

Indeed, in view of the equivalence of (A2) and (A6), Hansch's approach can be modified in three ways.

1. Equation A2 can be substituted for the nonparabolic part of the complete Hansch equation (A1) to give the equation

$$\log\left(\frac{1}{C}\right) = k_1 \pi^2 + \sum_i a_i + \mu \tag{A7}$$

which may be called the Free–Wilson equation with an additional term $k_1 \pi^2$ that imparts to it a parabolic character.

2. A linear combination of $\sum_i a_i$ (Free and Wilson's part for substituents X_i) and $\sum_j k_j \phi_j$ (Hansch's part for substituents Y_i) gives a mixed equation:

$$\log\left(\frac{1}{C}\right) = \sum_i a_i + \sum_j k_j \phi_j + k \tag{A8}$$

3. Equations A2 and A1 (or A7 and A8) can be combined to give

$$\log\left(\frac{1}{C}\right) = k_1 \pi^2 + \sum_i a_i + \sum_j k_j \phi_j + k \tag{A9}$$

in which the second term on the right is Free and Wilson's part for substituents X_i, the third is Hansch's part for substituents Y_i, and the first term accounts for the parabolic relationship (π must be equal to $\pi_X + \pi_Y$).

Equations A7 to A9 widen the applicability of correlation analysis, since the limitations that are inherent in either one of the two approaches discussed and that could be overcome by the use of the other simply do not exist in the mixed approach. Mention has been made above of the dummy variables introduced into a Hansch equation in order to "correct' it and thus make it applicable to describing some specific set of data. This fairly uncertain parameter becomes quite unequivocal in the mixed model, for its part is now played by the Free–Wilson additive parameter $\sum_i a_i$.

Hansch's parabolic model fits the experimental results better the closer these approach optimal lipophilicity P_0 (P being the octanol/water partition coefficient). The farther the P values are from the P_0 value, the less suitable is the parabola, and closer approximations are obtainable with a linear approach. For this reason Kubinyi (1976b) has proposed what he calls a bilinear model:

$$\log\left(\frac{1}{C}\right) = a \log P - b(\log \beta \cdot P + 1) + c \qquad (A10)$$

where C is the molar concentration. The nonlinear term β has to be derived by an iterative method of nonlinear regression analysis. The author presents two examples to demonstrate that this model compares favorably with Hansch's model in the case of groups of compounds with a wide range of $\log P$ values. If this range is small, however, Hansch's model is to be preferred as being simpler.

A.2.5.   Application of Pattern Recognition Methodology

In recent years there has been mounting interest in the use of pattern recognition approaches in QSAR studies. It has been claimed that these approaches can yield better results than regression analysis. One of their advantages is that only a relatively small sample of substances whose biological activities have been studied is needed to find the characteristics shared by a whole class of compounds with a given type of biological activity; or, speaking in the language of cybernetics, the sample acts as a teaching sequence. These characteristics can then be used to judge whether or not compounds with unknown activities belong to the class under consideration.

The application of pattern recognition methods to predict the toxicities of chemical compounds is based on the following premises. First, there exists an objective structure-activity relationship: activity is a function of structure. Second, once this function has been established for a group of compounds, it can be extrapolated to new compounds. And, third, the structure of a chemical compound can be represented as a certain set of structural parameters. These may include chemical functional groups, as well as quantities characterizing spatial or electronic structure. For instance, in screening potential anticancer drugs for their chemotherapeutic activities, Kowalski and Bender (1974) used a dictionary of structural parameters comprising 20 input features, namely, (1) number of oxygen atoms, normalized to the total number of atoms in the molecule (number of oxygens/number of atoms); (2) number of phosphorus atoms/number of atoms; (3) number of sulfurs/number of atoms; (4) number of halogens/number of atoms; (5) number of carbons/number of atoms; (6) number of C-S bonds/number of carbons; (7) number of C-C double bonds/number of carbons; (8) number of C-N bonds/number of carbons; (9) number of C-O bonds/number of carbons; (10) number of C-O double bonds/number of carbons; (11) number of N-H bonds/number of nitrogens; (12) number of O-H bonds/number of oxygens; (13) number of PO_4 groups; (14) number of S-H bonds; (15) purine derivative; (16) pyrimidine derivative; (17) number of oxygen atoms in rings; (18) number of nitrogen atoms in rings; (19) number of phenyl groups; and (20) substitution at the primary nitrogen in purine or pyrimidine.

Generally speaking, the problem of constructing an appropriate dictionary to describe the structures of compounds is central to the cybernetic prediction of their biological properties. If such a dictionary is available, pattern recognition techniques can be used to train the computer to discriminate active from inactive or toxic from nontoxic compounds. Giller et al. (1972) have considered three approaches to the problem of finding the function activity $= f$ (structure) that differ in the methods of representing the information on the structure of compounds and in the pattern recognition algorithms. These are a combined perceptronic, a logical-structural (the one used in the above-mentioned 20-feature dictionary), and a topological approach.

A3. STRUCTURE-ACTIVITY RELATIONSHIPS AMONG INORGANIC COMPOUNDS

First, a word on the negative side is in order. Levina (1972a) has checked out the hypothesis that the toxicities of various compounds of a given metal correlate with their solubilities and has concluded that solubility does not provide any clue to differences in toxicity, nor can it account for variations in the rates of clearance of tissues (in particular, pulmonary tissue) from different compounds of the same metal or, for that matter, in the levels of their accumulation in the body and the rates of their elimination from it as a whole. Explanations for differences in potency among compounds of the same metal should evidently be sought in the biotransformations undergone by the compounds. Important considerations here are binding of the compound to the receptors, rate of release of the metal from the compound, binding of the metal to biological complexones and firmness of the resulting bonds, physical properties of the compound, and its transport across biomembranes.

As stated on p. 343, the toxicities of elements tend to rise as their electronic stability diminishes. It may be noted that the greatest influence on the properties (including biological ones) of an element is exerted by the electronic structure of the outermost shell. The next shell is less influential, while the third has only a slight effect (this effect is appreciable, though, in the lanthanide and actinide series). The differences in electronic configuration among the inner shells occurring with electrons of identical valency determine the differences among group analogues; the nuclear charge is screened to different degrees, the least effective shielding being shown by the s^2 shell, a more effective one by d^{10}, and the most effective by s^2p^6.

The stability of electronic configurations is a measure of the chemical activity of an element. The bonding energy of the outer electrons responsible for this stability depends on the magnitude of the atomic charge and varies in a periodic manner. The capacity of an atom for chemical reactions and its toxic properties both decrease with increasing statistical weight of stable electronic configurations, with increasing energy stability, and with decreasing proportion of unlocalized electrons (Brakhnova et al., 1973). The latter authors have demonstrated that the toxic properties of metal ions display a periodicity related to increases in their charge and have indicated some features of this periodicity associated with the filling pattern of atomic orbitals and the stability of electronic configurations. Thus the toxic properties of elements diminish in groups of the periodic table with rising energy stability (with an increase in the principal quantum number) in going from titanium to zirconium and hafnium, from vanadium to niobium and tantalum, from chromium to molybdenum and tungsten, from manganese to rhenium, and from metals of the iron triad (iron, cobalt, nickel) to those of the ruthenium triad (ruthenium, rhodium, palladium) and the osmium triad (osmium, iridium, platinum). One should probably agree with the above authors that the potential for gaining an understanding of changes in the ion toxicities of inorganic substances from a knowledge of the periodicity in the formation of electron shells is very great.

As is known, several types of crystal lattices of the elements can be distinguished in the periodic table. The crystal lattice structure is determined by the electronic structure of atoms within the lattice; the lattice is in fact a derivative of the energy state of the electronic structure. The type of crystal lattice has been shown to correlate with the MAC, which is an integral index of the toxicity of inorganic compounds (Brakhova and Bazhenova, 1971). The type of crystal lattice reflects the electronic state of the substance: a decrease in lattice symmetry tends to result in greater toxicity. Substances having a body-centered cubic lattice are least toxic. Their biological activity is characterized predominantly by a slight pneumoconionic effect. For these substances MACs between 6 and 10 mg/m^3 may be recommended (such MACs have been adopted for titanium, niobium, and tungsten). In the case of a face-centered cubic lattice (copper, silver, gold) a MAC of 3 to 5 mg/m^3 may be advised. Substances of this group tend to produce chronic systemic effects with involvement of parenchymatous organs. An extremely dense hexagonal packing of the magnesium type is typical of substances causing severe toxic effects, both acute and chronic. In this case MACs of about 1 to 2 mg/m^3 are acceptable. Substances with lattices of low symmetry (rhombic, rhombohedral, monoclinic, etc.) are even more toxic, and their tentative MACs should not exceed 0.5 mg/m^3.

The above relationships between type of crystal lattice structure and toxicity have been confirmed in a study with hydrides of transition metals (Brakhnova and Shkurko, 1972).

Mention should be made of two relatively recent monographs where, among other things, evidence is presented for structure-toxicity relationships among inorganic compounds (Levina, 1972b; Izraelson et al., 1973). The first of these contains a well-compiled review, while the second presents many new facts, in particular, a number of correlations between the physicochemical properties of metal salts and their toxicities (Table A3).

The considerable negative correlation seen between log LD_{50} and the stabilities of metal complexes with cthylenediaminetetraacetic acid (EDTA)

Table A3. Correlations of Toxicities (log LD_{50} in milliatoms/kg for mice with intraperitoneal injection) with Physicochemical Properties of Metal Salts

Property	r	n	P
Electronegativity (according to Pauling)	−0.66	45	.999
Electron affinity (kcal/g atom)	−0.67	25	.999
Electron work function (eV)	−0.35	42	.988
Ionic radii (Å)	0.30	50	.972
Atomic radii (Å)	0.51	43	.999
Atomic diameters (Å)	0.85	33	.999
Atomic volumes (cm^3/g atom)	−0.40	20	.964
Stability of complexes with EDTA	−0.65	29	.999
Stability of hydrocomplexes	−0.44	24	.979
Stability of citrate and oxalate complexes	−0.56	17	.981

Source.   Levina (1972b).

is indicative to a degree of cation behavior in biological media. Metal complexes with EDTA are invariably more stable than those of the same metal with such bodily complexones as proteins, amino acids, and carboxylic acids. However, the stability constants (i.e., reciprocals of dissociation constants) of the same metals having different ligands in biological substrates correlate with the stability constants of complexes of these metals with EDTA.

The negative correlation between log LD_{50} values and the stabilities of metal complexes with EDTA means that the toxicities of the corresponding metal ions show positive correlation with the stabilities of these complexes.

The stabilities of metal complexes correlate also with ionization potentials, the correlation coefficient being 0.424 ($n = 24$, $p = .02$) according to Levina (1972b), as well as, in a similar manner, with electronegativities. The toxicities of metals correlate with both these characteristics.

To sum up, there exist certain correlations between several physicochemical properties of atoms and ions that characterize the structure, electronic shell, and chemical reactivity of the atom, on the one hand, and the toxicity of the metal (in the form of a salt), on the other. In this context one may recall the study of Rabotnikova (1965), who determined the intraperitoneal LD_{50} of metal oxides for mice (see p. 339). More recently Rabotnikova (1971) has also estimated threshold doses, using various indices. The threshold dose (D_{min}) was taken to be the minimal dose of a given oxide that caused significant changes in at least one of the indices measured, during the course of 1 week.

This study revealed coefficients of 0.50 or more for correlations of the log LD_{50} (in milliatoms/kg body weight) with the melting point and molecular mass of a given oxide and the standard potential of the element. Similar correlation coefficients have been obtained between the log LD_{50} and log MAC values of the same oxides. Therefore not only the toxicities of metal salts but also those of their oxides show correlations with the standard potentials of the corresponding elemental metals, while the toxicities of oxides at the lethal level correlate with the concentrations at levels considered safe for persons in the working environment.

Our calculations of correlation coefficients between threshold doses of metal oxides and lethal doses of the same oxides as determined by Rabotnikova have shown a high degree of correlation and even a possibility of estimating D_{min} from the LD_{50} when both these indices are stated in milliatoms per kilogram ($r = 0.87$, $n = 24$). Given such a close correlation, threshold doses may be expected to correlate also with constants found to correlate significantly with the LD_{50}. To test this assumption, we have considered log threshold doses of 24 metal oxides in relation to electronegativities (according to Pauling), atomic radii, standard ionization potentials, atomic weights, and boiling and melting points of the elemental metals (Table A4).

Table A4.   Correlations of Log D_{min} and Log MAC Values of Metal Oxides with Some Constants of Metal Atoms (log D_{min} in milliatoms/kg body weight of mice with single intraperitoneal injection)

Const.	Electro-negativity (according to Pauling)	Atomic Radii (Å)	Standard Ionization Potential	Atomic Weight of Metal	Boiling Point of Metal at 10^{-6} mm Hg	Melting Point of Metal
	Correlations with log D_{min}					
	0.071	−0.226	−0.427	−0.438	0.446	0.451
	21	21	20	20	20	20
	≪ .90	< .90	> .90 < .95	> .95 < .98	> .95 < .98	> .95 < .98
	Correlations with log MAC					
	0.492	−0.359	−0.597	−0.465	0.444	0.415
	15	15	15	16	14	16
	> .90 < .90	< .90	> .98	> .90 < .95	< .90	< .90

Comparison of the data contained in Table 29 and in Table A3, as well as of Rabotnikova's (1965) LD_{50} data for oxides (see p. 339), with our results summarized in Table A4, indicates that the correlation of standard ionization potentials is lower with log D_{min} values than with log LD_{50} and log MAC values. In the case of electronegativity, too, the correlation of this constant has proved to be closer and more significant with log MAC than with D_{min}. Thus correlations between toxicity and constants of elemental metals are traceable at different toxicity levels.

ADDENDUM REFERENCES

Amatuni, V. N., and S. S. Krylov, On the relationship between structure and biological activity, *Dokl. Akad. Nauk SSSR*, **217**, 949–952 (1974).

Andreeshcheva, N. G., Predicting the biological efficiency of organic compounds depending on their chemical structure and basic physicochemical properties, in G. I. Sidorenko, Ed., *Materialy Pervogo Itogovogo Sovetsko-Amerikanskogo Simpoziuma po Probleme "Gigiyena Okruzhaiushchei Sredy"*, *Riga, 1974*, pp. 31–35, Institut Obshchei i Kommunalnoi Gigigeny im. A. N. Sysina, Moscow, 1975.

Biological Correlations—The Hansch Approach. Symposium, Los Angeles, Calif., 1970, American Chemical Society, Washington, D.C., 1972.

Brakhnova, I. T., and L. N. Bazhenova, Crystal lattice structure of elements and compounds as an index of their toxic action, *Gig. Sanit.*, **10**, 95–100 (1971).

Brakhnova, I. T., and G. I. Shkurko, Hygienic evaluation of the biological action of hydrides of transition metals taking into account their electron and crystal structure, *Gig. Sanit.*, **7**, 36–39 (1972).

Brakhnova, I. T., A. V. Roshchin, and S. V. Suvorov, On the relationship of toxicity of metal ions to the filling patterns of electronc shells, *Gig. Tr. Prof. Zabol.*, **10**, 33–38 (1973).

Cammarata, A., Interrelationship of the regression models used for structure-activity analyses, *J. Med. Chem.*, **15**, 573–577 (1972).

Craig, P. N., Comparison of the Hansch and Free–Wilson approaches to structure-activity correlation. Biological correlation—the Hansch approach, *Adv. Chem. Ser.*, No. 114, 115–129 (1972).

Dmitriyeva, N. V., Calculation of narcotic and maximum allowable concentrations of nonelectrolytes, in *Aktualniye Voprosy Gigiyenicheskoi Toksikologii*, pp. 35–36, Ministerstvo Zdravookhraneniya RSFSR, Sanitarno-epidemiologicheskaya Stantsiya g. Moskvy, Moscow, 1972.

Eitingen, A. I., and I. P. Ulanova, The relationship of biological action of halo derivatives of organic compounds to their reactivity, *Gig. Tr. Prof. Zabol.*, **9**, 36–39 (1975).

Filov, V. A., Correlation between physico-chemical properties of chemical compounds and indices of their toxic action: use for prediction, *Experientia*, Suppl. No. 23, 99–113 (1976).

Giller, S. A., A. B. Glaz, V. E. Golender, L. A. Rastrigin, and A. B. Rozenblit, Use of pattern recognition for predicting the pharmacologic activity of chemical substances, *Khim.-Farm. Zh.*, **6**(12), 18–24 (1972).

Hansch, C., Quantitative structure-activity relationships in drug design, in E. J. Ariëns, Ed., *Drug Design*, Vol. 1, pp. 271–342, Academic Press, New York, 1971.

Hansch, C., Quantitative relationships between lipophilic character and drug metabolism, *Drug. Metab. Rev.*, **1**, 1–13 (1972).

Hansch, C., Quantitative approaches to pharmacological structure-activity relationships, in *International Encyclopedia of Pharmacology and Therapeutics*, Vol. 1: C. J. Cavallito, Ed., *Structure-Activity Relationships*, pp. 75–166, Pergamon Press, Oxford, 1973.

Hansch, C., On the structure of medicinal chemistry, *J. Med. Chem.*, **19**, 1–6 (1976).

Hansch, C., and J. Clayton, Lipophilic character and biological activity of drugs. II. The parabolic case, *J. Pharm. Sci.*, **62**, 1–21 (1973).

Henry, D., J. H. Block, J. L. Anderson, and G. R. Carlson, Use of high-pressure chromatography for quantitative structure-activity relationship studies of sulfonamides and barbiturates, *J. Med. Chem.*, **19**, 619–626 (1976).

Hetnarski, B., and R. D. O'Brien, The charge-transfer constant for structure-activity relationships, *J. Med. Chem.*, **18**, 29–33 (1975).

Hudson, D. R., G. E. Bass, and W. P. Purcell, Quantitative structure-activity models; some conditions for application and statistical interpretation, *J. Med. Chem.*, **13**, 1184–1189 (1970).

Izraelson, Z. I., O. Ya. Mogilevskaya, and S. V. Suvorov, *Voprosy Gigiyeny Truda i Professionalnoi Patologii pri Rabote s Redkimi Metallami* [*Occupational Health for Workers Handling Rare-Earth Metals*], Meditsina, Moscow, 1973.

Kagan, Yu. S., E. A. Yershova, O. P. Mintser, and E. P. Larionova, Predicting toxic properties of and hygienic standards for organophosphorus pesticides, in *Primeneniye Matematicheskikh Metodov dlya Otsenki i Prognozirovaniya Realnoi Opasnosti Nakopleniya Pestitsidov vo Vneshnei Srede i Organizme. Materialy Vtorogo Simpoziuma*, pp. 86–87, Institut Gigiyeny i Toksikologii Pestitsidov, Polimernykh i Plasticheskikh Mass, Kiev, 1976.

Kirso, U. E., and I. Kh. Maazik, On toxicity-structure relationships in phenols, *Trudy Inst. Eksp. Klin. Med. Minist. Zdravookhr. Est. SSR*, 3(2). 177–183 (1970).

Kowalski, B. R., and C. F. Bender, The application of pattern recognition to screening prospective anticancer drugs, *J. Am. Chem. Soc.*, 96, 916–918 (1974).

Kubinyi, H., Quantitative structure-activity relationships. 2. A mixed approach, based on Hansch and Free–Wilson analysis, *J. Med. Chem.*, 19, 586–600 (1976a).

Kubinyi, H., Quantitative structure-activity relationships. 4. Nonlinear dependence of biological activity on hydrophobic character: a new model, *Arzneimittelforsch.*, 26, 1991–1997 (1976b).

Kubinyi, H., and O.-H. Kehrhahn, Quantitative structure-activity relationships. 1. The modified Free–Wilson approach, *J. Med. Chem.*, 19, 578–586 (1976).

Levina, E. N., On relationships between solubility of metal compounds and their toxicity, distribution, and elimination from the body, *Gig. Tr. Prof. Zabol.*, 1, 40–43 (1972a).

Levina, E. N., *Obshchaya Toksikologiya Metallov* [*General Toxicology of Metals*], Meditsina, Leningrad, 1972b.

Liublina, E. I., and V. A. Filov, Chemical structure, physical and chemical properties and biological activity, in *Methods Used in the USSR for Establishing Biologically Safe Levels of Toxic Substances*, World Health Organization, Geneva, 1975.

Ordukhanian, A. A., A. S. Kabankin, M. A. Landau, and B. T. Garibdzhanian, Correlations between toxicity and structural parameters of some phosphoryl derivatives of pyrimidine, *Khim.-Farm. Zh.*, 10(12), 42–46 (1976).

Rabotnikova, L. V., The toxicity of metal oxides in relation to the physicochemical properties and normal body levels of the metal, in I. D. Gadaskina, A. A. Golubev, and E. T. Lykhina, Eds., *Voprosy Obshchei i Chastnoi Promyshlennoi Toksikologii*, pp. 52–55, Institut Gigiyeny Truda i Profzabolevaniy, Leningrad, 1965.

Rabotnikova, L. V., A comparative single-dose study of biological activities of metal oxides at the threshold level, *Gig. Tr. Prof. Zabol.*, 8, 33–36 (1971).

Silipo, C., and C. Hansch, The quantitative structure-activity relationship of 9-(X-phenyl)guanines reversibly inhibiting guanine deaminase: quantitative comparison of enzyme from two sources, *Mol. Pharmacol.*, 10, 954–962 (1974).

Tomlinson, E., Chromatographic hydorphobic parameters in correlation analysis of structure-activity relationships, *J. Chromatogr.*, 113, 1–45 (1975).

Tute, M. S., Principles and practice of Hansch analysis: a guide to structure-activity correlation for the medicinal chemist, *Adv. Drug. Res.*, **6**, 1–77 (1971).

Tute, M. S., Lipophilicity, *Chem. Ind.*, No. 3, 100–105 (1975).

Vilceanu, R., Z. Szabadai, A. Chiriac, and Z. Simon, Multiple structure-toxicity correlation of organic phosphorus compounds, *Stud. Biophys.*, **34**, 1–6 (1972).

Vrbovsky, L., The study of relationships between chemical structure and toxicity, in *Proceedings, European Society for the Study of Drug Toxicity, 1974*, Vol. 15, pp. 331–336, Excerpta Medica, Amsterdam, 1974.

8

METHODS FOR THE CALCULATION OF TOXICITY PARAMETERS AND MAXIMUM ALLOWABLE CONCENTRATIONS, AS WELL AS OF LESS ACCESSIBLE CONSTANTS FROM THOSE MORE READILY ACCESSIBLE

In the USSR the groundwork for the estimation of toxicities of substances by calculation was laid more than three decades ago by N. V. Lazarev, one of the founders of Soviet prophylactic toxicology. In his book *Nonelectrolytes* (1944) he demonstrated correlations, in particular, between narcotic and lethal concentrations of nonelectrolytes in the blood, on the one hand, and their oil/water partition coefficients and solubilities in water, on the other. The equations proposed by Lazarev made it possible to calculate approximate values of these concentrations in aqueous solution in the blood of white mice from data on the oil/water partition coefficient or water solubility. His equations could also be used to estimate lethal and narcotic concentrations in ambient air if the blood/air partition coefficient and the degree of saturation of the organism with the substance concerned were known.

More recently, work on methods for the approximate calculation of toxicity parameters based on correlations with physicochemical constants has been pursued mainly by Lazarev's former pupils, among whom the present authors belong. First, correlations were established between some physical constants of volatile organic compounds and their toxicity indices, expressed as fractions of the saturation concentrations or in millimoles per liter of air

(Liublina, 1959, 1960; Liublida and Golubev, 1963). Later, a large number of various constants of miscellaneous organic compounds (mainly volatile) were considered in relation to several indices of biological potency, and a number of general equations based on the correlations discovered were derived. Still later, correlations were established and equations proposed for particular groups of organic compounds for which sufficient toxicological data were available.

The values of maximum allowable concentration (MAC), calculated on the basis of correlations with such physicochemical constants as the oil/water partition coefficient and aqueous solubility (i.e., with distributive properties), could give only an indication of the magnitude of the nonelectrolytic (nonspecific) actions of the toxic substances concerned. Any specific action exhibited by a poison, in addition to nonspecific action, increases its toxicity so that calculations from the above constants can show only the upper limit of MACs in such cases. The establishment of correlations with physical constants has made it possible to obtain closer approximations to true MAC values.

In these studies the effective doses and concentrations as well as the MACs were most often expressed in logarithmic form, in view of the linear relationship between log doses of toxic substances and their potencies. Effective doses and concentrations were usually stated in millimoles per liter (mM/liter) and MACs in millimoles per cubic meter (mM/m^3). The statistical methods used by the authors for the establishment and analysis of correlations can be found in many books on the application of statistics in biology and in various manuals of mathematical statistics (e.g., Pomorsky, 1935; Lukomsky, 1958; Baily, 1959; Ezekiel and Fox, 1959; Terentiev, 1960; Kaminsky, 1962; Plokhinsky, 1967; Snedecor and Cochran, 1968).

1. METHODS USED FOR THE CALCULATION OF INDICES OF BIOLOGICAL POTENCY IN HOMOLOGOUS AND OTHER SERIES

In Chapter 7 mention was made of Zahradnik's constants β, which make it possible to calculate indices of the biological potencies of aliphatic homologues from data on two members of the series, excluding the methyl derivative (see Equation 3 on p. 323). It is convenient to make calculations in graphic form. In the diagram proposed by Zahradnik, β values are plotted on the horizontal axis and logarithms of the molar concentration (dose) producing the selected effect or of the MAC are plotted on the vertical axis. The points corresponding to the two known members of the series are first plotted, and a line is then drawn through the two points thus obtained. The value of the biological index for the member in question is found at the point of inter-

Table 31.   Values of Constant β for Aliphatic Homologues

Alkyl	R	Number in Figure 45	Value of β
Methyl	CH_3	1	0.38
Ethyl	CH_2CH_3	2	0.00
Isopropyl	$CH(CH_3)_2$	3	-0.24
tert-Butyl	$C(CH_3)_3$	4	-0.41
n-Propyl	$CH_2CH_2CH_3$	5	-0.47
Isobutyl	$CH_2CH(CH_3)_2$	7	-0.82
tert-Neopentyl	$CH_2C(CH_3)_3$	9	-0.95
sec-Butyl	$CH(CH_3)CH_2CH_3$	6	-0.72
tert-Amyl	$C(CH_3)_2CH_2CH_3$	8	-0.89
n-Butyl	$CH_2(CH_2)_2CH_3$	10	-1.02
sec-Amyl	$CH(CH_3)CH_2CH_2CH_3$	11	-1.20
Isoamyl	$CH_2CH_2CH(CH_3)_2$	12	-1.31
n-Amyl	$CH_2(CH_2)_3CH_3$	14	-1.41
n-Hexyl	$CH_2(CH_2)_4CH_3$	17	-1.95
Isohexyl	$CH_2(CH_2)_2(CH_3)_2$	16	-1.66
tert-Hexyl	$C(CH_3)_2(CH_2)_2CH_3$	13	-1.35
n-Heptyl	$CH_2(CH_2)_5CH_3$	19	-2.43
tert-Heptyl	$C(CH_3)_2(CH_2)_3CH_3$	15	-1.60
n-Octyl	$CH_2(CH_2)_6CH_3$	20	-2.92
sec-Octyl	$CH(CH_3)(CH_2)_5CH_3$	18	-2.22
n-Nonyl	$CH_2(CH_2)_7CH_3$	—	-3.46
n-Decyl	$CH_2(CH_2)_8CH_3$	—	-3.80

Source.   Zahradnik (1962a).

section of this line with the perpendicular erected from the point on the horizontal axis corresponding to that member. Values of the constant β are given in Table 31. Clearly, the volatility must be taken into consideration when calculating the LC_{50} and the solubility when determining the LD_{50}, that is, the constant on which the upper limit of LC_{50} or LD_{50}, respectively, depend.

According to Zahradnik, the log dose or concentration of the ethyl derivative is taken as zero, so it is necessary to have data on the ethyl derivative and at least one other derivative (but excluding the methyl derivative). It is possible, however, to calculate toxicity indices when data are available on any two homologues other than the ethyl and methyl derivatives. To do this, two points are plotted on the diagram (Figure 45) corresponding to the two known

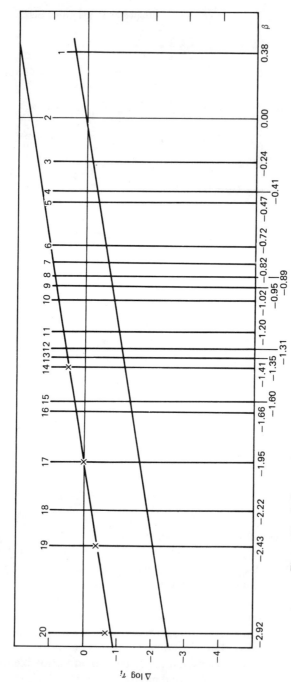

Figure 45. A diagram for calculating effective doses and concentrations (according to Zahradnik) for compounds of the RX type. Crosses denote experimentally found NC_{50} values, the ordinates giving their logarithms. Numbers above vertical lines correspond to homologues shown in Table 31. The τ_i refers to the biological activity of the ith homologue.

members of the series, and a line is then drawn through these points until it cuts all vertical lines (numbers above vertical lines in Figure 45 refer to homologues listed in Table 31). The distance between the point of intersection of this line with vertical line 2 (for the ethyl derivative, whose $\beta = 0.00$) and the $\Delta \log \tau_i = 0$ is then subtracted from the two initial points. A straight line is again drawn through the two points thus obtained. The new line, parallel to the first one, corresponds to the position of the points on Zahradnik's diagram, where all the lines intersect at the origin and which gives values of the toxicity index in question for all aliphatic homologues. The ordinate gives the log value, to which the true or calculated value of the log dose or concentration of the ethyl derivative should be added. Of course, a different logarithmic scale of doses or concentrations can be used each time, as appropriate to the case under consideration. The values required will be found on the vertical axis, at the points where it is cut by the line joining the known points.

The constants β were derived by Zahradnik from experimental data, mostly LD_{50} values for white mice with intravenous or intraperitoneal administration of the substances. Such data allow one to obtain reproducible results with little variation. Unfortunately, toxicity data reported by various authors using other routes of administration are highly variable. Thus, according to Rabotnikova (1970), the oral LD_{50} values reported by different authors for the same substances ($n = 20$) vary by as much as a factor of 5 on the average, the largest difference being 13-fold. These differences may be due not only to different degrees of purity of the chemical compound assayed, but also to such factors as type and amount of diluent used, state of gastrointestinal mucosa, and diet. With regard to inhalational toxicities of organic vapors and gases ($n = 25$), Rabotnikova found interlaboratory variations up to 11-fold, the average difference being 3.8-fold. Much smaller interlaboratory variations were noted with the subcutaneous and intraperitoneal routes of administration. Thus subcutaneous LD_{50} values ($n = 30$) varied 1.87-fold on the average, the largest difference being 4.8-fold; the corresponding figures for the intraperitoneal LD_{50} ($n = 25$) were 1.25 and 1.8. Such relatively small variations are accounted for by more accurate dosages and the fact that the substance is introduced into a closed space or cavity, from which it can escape only through blood or lymph vessels. The smaller differences for intraperitoneal LD_{50} values may be explained by the rapid absorption of substances from the peritoneal cavity. With slower absorption from the subcutaneous fat, many foreign substances bring into play defense mechanisms, which may delay absorption to varying degrees and thus contribute to the variability of the data.

According to Zayeva (1964, 1970), the MAC can be calculated by adding up the biological activity values corresponding to the chemical bonds of the compound (see Chapter 7, p. 321). The sum of the biological activities thus obtained $(\sum A)$ is placed in the denominator, and the molecular weight (M) multiplied by 1000 in the numerator, to give the formula

$$\text{MAC (mg/m}^3\text{)} = \frac{M \times 1000}{\sum A} \tag{1}$$

It seems interesting to compare MAC values calculated by Zayeva's and Zahradnik's methods. However, since the MAC depends not only on the physical and chemical properties of the compound but also on the long-term effects of intoxication, it is only in rare cases that the MAC can be related to the molecular structure. For this reason a MAC calculated by any method based on molecular structure will be a cruder approximation to the true value than a LC_{50} or LD_{50} calculated by the same method. For this reason comparisons of different methods for the calculation of the MAC are often inconclusive: a more accurate method may give results very similar to those obtained by a less accurate method. This was demonstrated by Liublina (1962) by comparing MACs calculated (1) by interpolation (from regular changes in the MACs of normal alkyls seen to occur with each increase of their chain by one carbon atom), (2) according to Zahradnik, and (3) according to Zayeva.

Comparison of calculated LC_{50} values for normal compounds showed roughly the same applicability of Zahradnik's method and of interpolation from the number of carbon atoms. As regards iso compounds, the difference between β values for such compounds is in some cases greater than that for successive normal members of a homologous series; there is in fact no alternative to the use of β constants for the calculation of toxicity indices for aliphatic iso compounds.

For aromatic compounds Boček et al. (1964, 1967) have developed an equation for the calculation of intravenous LD_{50} values for disubstituted benzene derivatives in the meta and para positions for white mice (see Chapter 7, p. 325). Since their equation, like that of Zahradnik, involves relative magnitudes of toxicity, it seemed worthwhile to try to apply it to the calculation of other indices. Accordingly, Liublina made an attempt to calculate the LC_{50} $(n = 8)$ and the MAC $(n = 15)$ values for disubstituted and monosubstituted benzene derivatives, but the results were unsatisfactory. Although, in some cases, the disagreement with experimentally found values was fairly small (e.g., less than ± 0.01 for the log LC_{50} in two cases), in others it amounted to more than 1 for both the log LC_{50} and the log MAC (i.e., to a factor of more than 10 for the antilogarithms). In calculating a rather more closely related index, namely, the oral LD_{50} for disubstituted benzene derivatives $(n = 6)$, the deviations were much smaller and did not exceed -0.78 and $+0.42$. In view of interlaboratory differences in oral LD_{50} values by a factor of 5 on the average (see above), such deviations cannot be regarded as very great. More satisfactory results may be expected for the intraperitoneal LD_{50}.

2. CALCULATION METHODS BASED ON CORRELATIONS BETWEEN PHYSICAL PROPERTIES AND BIOLOGICAL INDICES OF VOLATILE ORGANIC COMPOUNDS

It is clear that any equation based on correlations is subject to modification as more data become available. All the equations given below are those that have not yet lost their importance; where calculations were later made on more extensive material, the original equation is omitted.

The logarithm of the MAC expressed as a fraction of the saturation concentration in air was found to be inversely correlated with the logarithm of the saturated vapor pressure P (expressed in mm Hg), and the following equation was derived:

$$\log \text{MAC (as a fraction of the saturation value)} = -0.71 \log P - 2.92 \quad (2)$$

$$(n = 252, r = -0.75, \bar{S}_{YX} = 0.96)$$

When the log MAC was expressed in millimoles per cubic meter of air rather than as a fraction of the saturation value, it showed a direct correlation with the log P to give the equation:

$$\log \text{MAC (mM/m}^3) = 0.28 \log P - 1.51 \quad (3)$$

$$(n = 252, r = 0.44, \bar{S}_{YX} = 0.92)$$

Consequently, the higher the saturated vapor pressure of the substance, the smaller is the fraction of this saturation value represented by the MAC, but the greater is the value of the MAC (expressed in mM/m^3 or mg/m^3). To convert the log MAC from millimoles per cubic meter to milligrams per cubic meter, it is sufficient to add the logarithm of the molecular weight (log M) to the right-hand side of (3):

$$\log \text{MAC (mg/m}^3) = 0.28 \log P - 1.51 + \log M \quad (4)$$

For various volatile organic compounds, approximate MAC values can be found not only from saturated vapor pressures but also from a number of other constants (Liublina and Golubev, 1967). Thus:

$$\log \text{MAC} = 1.12 - 0.058\sigma + \log M \quad (5)$$

$$\log \text{MAC} = 14.2 - 10n_D + \log M \quad (6)$$

$$\log \text{MAC} = -1.2 - 0.012t_{\text{melt}} + \log M \quad (7)$$

$$\log \text{MAC} = 0.40 - 0.01M + \log M \quad (8)$$

$$\log \text{MAC} = -0.4 - 0.006t_{\text{boil}} + \log M \quad (9)$$

$$\log \text{MAC} = 1.6 - 2.2\rho + \log M \quad (10)$$

where the MAC is in milligrams per cubic meter, and σ is the surface tension (dynes/cm at 20°C), n_D is the refractive index, t_{melt} is the melting point (°C), M is the molecular weight, t_{boil} is the boiling point (°C), and ρ is the density (g/cm³).

Equations 2 through 10 are usable only if the values of the constants lie within certain limits, namely, $M = 30$ to 300, $\rho = 0.6$ to 2.0, $t_{boil} = -100$ to $+300$, $t_{melt} = -190$ to $+180$, and $n_D = 1.3$ to 1.6. Those are the ranges of values of these constants for substances whose log MACs were used in deriving the above equations.

In calculating the MAC, all the available constants—at any rate, at least two—should be used. The mean value of the log MAC is first calculated, and only then is the antilogarithm taken. For (4) through (10) correction factors for the effect of the chemical structure (and making some allowance for substance reactivity) have been proposed. These equations represent average correlations between the quantities considered, so the correction factors are positive ($+$) for substances having predominantly nonelectrolytic (nonspecific) action and negative ($-$) for those producing pronounced specific effects (Table 32).

Table 33 presents equations for calculating the log LC_{50}, log C_{min}, and log NC_{50} (the median narcotic concentration for mice) from various physical constants, the concentration being expressed in millimoles per liter of air (Liublina and Filov, 1965).

Table 32. Corrections to Log MAC for the Chemical Structure of Compounds

Compounds	Correction
Saturated aliphatic hydrocarbons	+0.5
Saturated aliphatic ketones, alcohols, ethers, and esters	+0.5
Saturated cyclic hydrocarbons containing a benzene ring (excluding benzene and the first member of a homologous series	+0.5
Straight-chain compounds containing a triple bond	−0.5
Aliphatic amines	−1.0
Aniline and its derivatives	−1.0
Acid anhydrides	−1.0
Cyclic compounds containing an NO_2 group in a side chain	−1.0
Compounds containing the ONO_2 group in the straight chain	−1.0
Compounds having a double or triple bond together with an active element or group (Cl, Br, F, NO_2, OH) in the straight chain	−1.0
Substances containing an epoxy group	−1.5
Organophosphorus compounds	−1.5
Aldehydes	−1.5
Substances splitting off the CN group	−2.0

Table 33.   Equations Relating Toxicity Indices
(in mM/liter) of Volatile Organic Compounds
to Some of Their Constants

Equation	Equation Number
$\log \mathrm{LC}_{50} = 0.98 - 0.063\sigma$	(11)
$\log \mathrm{LC}_{50} = -0.02 - 0.009t_{\mathrm{boil}}{}^{a}$	(12)
$\log \mathrm{LC}_{50} = 0.08 - 0.011M^{a}$	(13)
$\log \mathrm{LC}_{50} = 0.11 - 1.20\rho^{a}$	(14)
$\log \mathrm{LC}_{50} = -1.6 - 0.010t_{\mathrm{melt}}$	(15)
$\log \mathrm{LC}_{50} = 9.2 - 6.8n_{\mathrm{D}}$	(16)
$\log C_{\mathrm{min}} = -0.5 - 0.88\sigma$	(17)
$\log C_{\mathrm{min}} = 12.5 - 10n_{\mathrm{D}}$	(18)
$\log \mathrm{NC}_{50} = 0.75 - 0.013M$	(19)
$\log \mathrm{NC}_{50} = 0.68 - 1.232\rho$	(20)
$\log \mathrm{NC}_{50} = 0.49 - 0.039R_{m}{}^{a}$	(21)
$\log \mathrm{NC}_{50} = 0.345 - 0.0094t_{\mathrm{boil}}$	(22)

[a] This equation was derived later than the
others and is based on a larger body of data.

To see what advantages, if any, might be gained by calculating a toxicity
index from several constants at a time, the $\log \mathrm{NC}_{50}$ was considered in rela-
tion to M, ρ, R_m (molar refraction), n_{D}, t_{melt}, and t_{boil} and was found to correlate closely with each of these properties. Multiple regression coefficients
showed, however, that the $\log \mathrm{NC}_{50}$ was strongly dependent on only four of
the constants, namely, M, ρ, R_m, and t_{boil}. All the regression coefficients computed after the elimination of n_{D} and t_{melt} were significant, and the following
regression equation was obtained:

$$\log \mathrm{NC}_{50} \,(\mathrm{mg/liter}) = 1.55 + 0.00916M - 1.537\rho - 0.03R_m$$

$$- 0.00732t_{\mathrm{boil}} + \log M \quad (23)$$

The mean deviations and the mean square deviations of the logarithms of
experimentally found NC_{50} values from the calculated values were then
compared on two random samples of 22 substances each. For each sample
the NC_{50} was computed (1) from each of the four constants separately, (2) as
the mean of the values thus obtained, and (3) from the multiple regression
equation. The deviations from experimentally determined values were smaller
in cases 2 and 3, which gave similar results. Accordingly, calculation of the

mean NC_{50} value from the results obtained for each of the available constants was recommended as being a simpler procedure than the use of multiple regression equations.

The above equations for the calculation of toxicity indices are of practical use only in respect to compounds for which no other, more satisfactory equations, specially derived for the particular classes to which the compounds belong, are available. Such equations are presented in the next section.

A correlation analysis was carried out for a number of readily accessible constants (M, ρ, n_D, t_{boil}, t_{melt}, and log P) in order to identify the properties most closely associated with biological indices expressed in millimoles per liter of air (Liublina, 1963a). The correlation coefficients were compared with the partial correlation coefficients calculated by eliminating, in turn, one of the constants concerned. It was found that the correlation between the LC_{50} and M or n_D remained significant in all cases. Therefore elimination of the effect of any one of the properties can only decrease the closeness of the correlation between the LC_{50} and M or n_D but cannot make it insignificant. The same is true for the correlations between the log MAC and M, ρ, or t_{melt} and between log C_{min} and n_D.

Thus it can be seen that M, ρ, t_{melt}, and n_D are the properties most closely correlated with indices of biological potency. Of these four properties, two (M and ρ) are determined at the molecular level and are related to the molecular structure, one (t_{melt}) is related to the molecular interaction energy, and one (n_D) is determined at the nuclear-electronic level (see Chapter 7, p. 335).

The degree of correlation between constants and the log MAC, log LC_{50}, log NC_{50}, and log C_{min} depends on the units in which the concentration is expressed (whether in mM/liter of air, in mM/liter of blood, or as a fraction of the saturation value). This can be seen from Figure 43 (p. 336), in which the logarithm of the oil/water partition coefficient (log K) and the logarithm of the water solubility (log S) are nowhere seen to correlate with the toxicity indices at the level of $r > 0.50$. High correlations between lethal or narcotic concentrations, on the one hand, and log K or log S, on the other, are observed only when the concentrations are expressed in millimoles per liter of blood. In Figure 43 the concentrations are in millimoles per liter of air, and so no close correlations are to be seen. Therefore it was thought necessary to calculate correlation coefficients and derive regression equations (when the correlations were high enough) for concentrations expressed in millimoles per liter of blood, in millimoles per liter of air, and as a fraction of the saturation value. Such calculations were made by Liublina (1963a). A comparison was made of the correlation coefficients between 12 constants and toxicity indices for volatile organic compounds whose concentrations were stated (1) in millimoles per liter of air, (2) in millimoles per liter in aqueous solution in blood,

In fractions of
saturation value

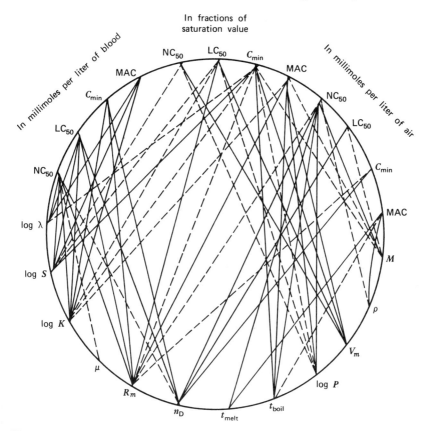

Figure 46. Graphic representation of values of the correlation coefficients between various constants of volatile organic compounds and their toxicity indices, expressed in millimoles per liter of blood (left), millimoles per liter of air (right), and as a fraction of the saturation concentration (top center). Solid lines correspond to correlation coefficients > 0.60; dotted lines, to those between 0.50 and 0.60. All concentrations are in logarithmic form.

and (3) as a fraction of the saturation value. The third statement of the effective concentration corresponds to the thermodynamic activity (see Chapter 3). It can be seen from Figure 46 that biological indices of different levels show reliable correlations with n_D, M, t_{melt}, t_{boil}, ρ, log P, and R_m when the concentrations are in millimoles per liter of air; with log K, log S, log λ, n_D, R_m, and μ when they are in millimoles per liter of blood; and with V_m, R_m, t_{boil}, log S, log P, log K, M, and log λ when they are stated as fractions of the saturation values (the physicochemical constants are listed in decreasing order of reliability of correlations). While each of the 12 properties shows reliable correlations, such correlations are seen in most cases for concentrations expressed in one or two ways. Correlations with the molecular weight are significant for all indices; but since the concentrations in air are given in millimoles per liter, a negative correlation between the molecular weight and a concentration thus expressed may represent the correlation between the logarithm of the fraction and its denominator. This possibility is ruled out only when the concentration is expressed as a fraction of the saturation value. Most of the properties showing high correlations with concentrations in millimoles per liter of air are again those characterizing the energy of molecular interaction (see p. 336). The three constants correlating most closely with the concentrations in millimoles per liter of blood are those related to aqueous solubility. Finally, both those kinds of constants plus the molar volume correlate well with the concentrations expressed thermodynamically, that is, as fractions of the saturation values.

Useful correlations were found to be the ones established between the molar volume (V_m) and the above biological indices expressed as fractions of the saturation concentrations. The indices thus expressed are easy to calculate, but it is difficult to go from them to concentrations in millimoles per liter of air, except for organic substances having low water/air partition coefficients ($\lambda < 300$, < 150, and < 14 for the calculation of the LC_{50}, MAC, and C_{min}, respectively), that is, for substances whose concentrations in the blood are more or less rapidly equilibrated with those in the air (Liublina, 1969). For such substances the following equations may be used:

$$\log \text{MAC} = 0.035 V_m - 7.23 + \log C_{20^\circ} \qquad (24)$$

$$\log LC_{50} = 0.034 V_m - 4.4 + \log C_{20^\circ} \qquad (25)$$

$$\log C_{min} = 0.037 V_m - 6.61 + \log C_{20^\circ} \qquad (26)$$

where C_{20° is the saturation concentration for air at 20°C, and the MAC, LC_{50}, and C_{min} are in milligrams per liter or millimoles per liter of air, depending on the units used for the saturation concentration. For substances with low λ values, (24) to (26) give better approximations to the true values than calculations from other constants.

3. CALCULATION OF TOXICITY INDICES FOR PARTICULAR CLASSES OF VOLATILE ORGANIC COMPOUNDS FROM READILY ACCESSIBLE CONSTANTS

As shown above, a number of general equations are available for the approximate calculation of the LC_{50}, C_{min}, and MAC from the values of various properties; on the other hand, there exist methods for more accurate calculations of these indices for particular homologous series when data on at least two members of the series are available. Some sort of intermediate approach seems to be desirable that, while not all-embracing, is also not confined to particular homologous series. Accordingly, an attempt has been made to derive equations enabling one to calculate toxicity indices for individual classes of organic compounds from the more readily available constants; for this purpose, toxicity indices of volatile organic compounds were considered in relation to their constants, with separate mathematical treatment of data for each class of compounds investigated (Liublina, 1969; Liublina and Rabotnikova, 1971).

Although these studies were concerned with volatile organic compounds, to avoid excessive fragmentation of material LC_{50} and C_{min} data were considered for all substances under investigation up to a boiling point of 250°C (except for aerosol concentrations), while MAC data were considered for all substances, regardless of their boiling points. The requirement that the constants be readily accessible and that the correlation be high was satisfied by the correlations with t_{boil} and M. Of the indices calculated, the highest correlation coefficients (and the lowest residuals) were obtained for the LC_{50}.

Equations for the calculation of the LC_{50} are presented in Table 34. It is evident from this table that satisfactory results ($\bar{S}_{YX} \leq 0.42$) in calculating the LC_{50} from both these constants (t_{boil} and M) are obtainable only for hydrocarbons, ethers, and amines. Since the equations for hydrocarbons were derived using a fairly large body of data, it seemed desirable to construct a diagram convenient for the estimation of the LC_{50} from these constants without resorting to calculation.

It was first determined what molecular weights corresponded to what boiling points for hydrocarbons, and the diagram was constructed for the range of the corresponding values. In the diagram (Figure 47), boiling point values are plotted along the horizontal axis and molecular weight values along the vertical axis. Each point of intersection of these two constants directly indicates the log LC_{50} in millimoles per liter, the corresponding figures being given in the scale of discontinuous lines just under the broad, slanting band. As a guide there are also shown solid lines connecting the points corresponding to equal LC_{50} values stated in more customary units (mg/liter). The scale for these lines, which are straight in the right-hand part of the diagram and curved in the left-hand part, is given just above the broad band.

The diagram makes it possible not only to find rapidly an approximate value of the LC_{50} for a new hydrocarbon but also to predict certain toxicological and hygienic characteristics of the hydrocarbon, as is illustrated by the example given below.

The molecular weight scale made it possible to give a scale of vapor density with respect to air, which indicates whether vapors of the hydrocarbon will

Table 34. Reliability of Correlations and Equations for the Calculation of LC_{50} from Molecular Weight (M) and Boiling Point (t_{boil}) for Individual Classes of Organic Compounds
(Correlation coefficients at $p < .001$ unless otherwise stated.)

Class of Compounds	n	r	$\bar{S}_{YX}$	Equation: $\log LC_{50}$ (mM/liter) =
Hydrocarbons	42	-0.90	0.34	$2.17 - 0.026M$
	42	-0.94	0.26	$0.79 - 0.011t_{boil}$
Alcohols	14	-0.90	0.44	$1.25 - 0.016t_{boil}$
Ethers	7	-0.96	0.19	$1.74 - 0.020M$
	7	-0.98	0.14	$0.74 - 0.011t_{boil}$
Ketones	14	-0.82	0.51	$1.16 - 0.015t_{boil}$
Amines (various)	23	-0.80	0.41	$-0.60 - 0.010M$
	22	-0.79	0.42	$-1.00 - 0.005t_{boil}$
Nitriles and cyanide compounds	10	-0.91	0.33	$-1.30 - 0.014M$
Nitro compounds	13	-0.71^{a}	0.77	$0.71 - 0.020M$
Heterocyclic compounds	17	-0.79	0.87	$2.80 - 0.041M$
Chlorohydrocarbons	40	-0.60	0.73	$0.20 - 0.012M$
	38	-0.71	0.63	$-0.10 - 0.011t_{boil}$
Bromohydrocarbons	16	-0.74^{a}	0.96	$-2.06 - 0.020M$
Miscellaneous organic compounds,	277	-0.52	0.96	$0.08 - 0.011M$
including those listed above	249	-0.62	0.84	$-0.02 - 0.009t_{boil}$

$^{a} .001 < p < .01$

tend to be concentrated near the ceiling (vapor density < 1) or near the floor (vapor density > 1).

The boiling point scale made it possible to indicate approximate values of the saturated vapor pressure calculated from the following formula (Levina, 1952): $\log P$ (mg Hg) $= 3.5 - 0.0202(t_{boil} + 3)$. The two lower rows of figures give saturation concentrations (mM/liter of air) under normal conditions and their logarithms, respectively. Knowledge of these concentrations is important for judging the rate of evaporation of the substance and for deciding whether or not the substance can reach a given concentration in the air.

The long, thick line sloping across the right-hand part of the broad band marks the boundary to the right of which are found hydrocarbons unlikely to develop concentrations equal to the LC_{50} at ordinary ambient temperatures.

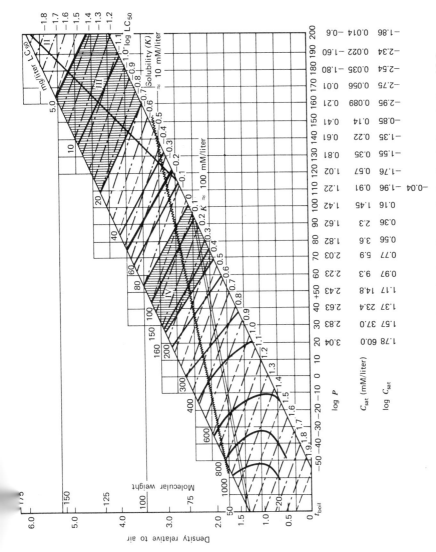

Figure 47. A diagram for the approximate determination of some physicochemical constants and LC_{50} values of hydrocarbons from their molecular weight and boiling point (see text for details).

375

Since the oil/water partition coefficient (K) and water solubility (S) of hydrocarbons most often correlate with their molecular weights and boiling points, two more lines were drawn. The double line across the band divides hydrocarbons according to their partition coefficients K; below this line, this coefficient is usually smaller than 100, and above it, greater than 100. Consequently, a hydrocarbon placed below this double line will probably belong to one of the lower groups (up to and including Group V) of Lazarev's system of nonelectrolytes (see Chapter 7, p. 329), while a hydrocarbon placed above the line will belong to a higher group. Type II narcotics may be expected to be found above the line, and type I narcotics below it (see Chapter 7, p. 317).

The zigzag line nearly parallel to the double line divides hydrocarbons on the basis of their water solubilities: above the line the solubility is usually less than 10 mM/liter, and toward the top and to the right-hand side of the diagram it becomes increasingly probable that the hydrocarbon will be insoluble. Below this line, hydrocarbons whose solubility exceeds 10 mM/liter are generally located.

Furthermore, the diagram shows toxicity ratings given in accordance with the classification adopted by the Section on the Establishment of Maximum Allowable Concentrations for Substances in the Air of Work Areas, Ministry of Health of the USSR. In this classification extremely toxic substances (Class I) are those whose LC_{50}s are less than 0.5 mg/liter; highly toxic (Class II), those whose LC_{50}s are between 0.5 and 4.9 mg/liter; moderately toxic (Class III), those with LC_{50}s between 5.0 and 49.9 mg/liter; and slightly toxic (Class IV), those whose LC_{50}s are 50 mg/liter and upward. In the diagram the boundaries between Classes II and III and between Classes III and IV are marked by short, thick lines.

The values of LC_{50} obtained from the diagram give a mean residual $(\bar{S}_{YX})$ of 0.34. This means that two thirds of the calculated values will not deviate from experimental data by a factor of more than 2.2; this is quite a satisfactory result for preliminary calculations. As a rule the deviations will be within the range of lethal concentrations from the LC_{min} to the LC_{100} and should help to obtain the LC_{50} in experiments more rapidly and on a smaller number of animals.

Here is an example to illustrate how the diagram can be used in practice. It was necessary to make a toxicological and hygienic evaluation of ethylidene norbornane and vinyl norbornane. The molecules of both these compounds consist of carbon and hydrogen atoms and have a CH_2 group inside their six-member ring. Hydrocarbons of such structure were not used in constructing the diagram, so it was all the more interesting to compare the prediction made from the diagram with the actual characteristics found experimentally.

The molecular weight (M) of ethylidene norbornane (ENB) is 120, and its boiling point (t_{boil}) is 150°C; therefore its log LC_{50} (in mM/liter), given on the diagram by the point of intersection of M and t_{boil}, is roughly equal to -0.96. (If this point lay on the line made up of equal dashes, the log LC_{50} would have been about -1.0—all such lines lead to log LC_{50} figures whose last digit is 0 or 5.) To convert millimoles per liter to milligrams per liter, we take the antilog of -0.96 (or $\bar{1}.04$), get 0.11 mM/liter, and multiply it by M to obtain 13.2 mg/liter. We could obtain a rougher estimate of the LC_{50} directly in milligrams per liter on the upper scale. We can now state that ENB belongs to Class III of toxicity, that is, it is moderately toxic. Next, we can see that ENB should be sparingly soluble or almost insoluble in water, since the point of intersection in our case lies well above the zigzag line corresponding to a solubility of about 10 mM/liter. Actually, ENB is virtually insoluble in water. Furthermore, since the point of intersection lies only slightly above the long, thick line dividing the hydrocarbons for which the LC_{50} is reached at normal temperatures (between 20° and 25°C) from those for which it is not, we can tell that the saturation concentration for ENB should be close to its LC_{50}, if these two concentrations are expressed in the same units. The saturation concentration for air is to be found in the second row of figures from the bottom; it is equal to 0.14 mM/liter, that is, is indeed close to the LC_{50} (0.11 mM/liter). The experimentally found average value for the LC_{50} of ENB is 16.9 $\pm$ 6.0 mg/liter, or 0.141 mM/liter. We thus see that the LC_{50} value found from the diagram lies within the confidence limits of the true LC_{50} value.

Now, from the distance between the point of intersection and the double line (this distance is greater than that between the point of intersection and the solubility line), we can conclude that ENB is likely to belong to one of the higher groups of Lazarev's system of nonelectrolytes and to be a narcotic of type II; this means that exposure to ENB should result in rapid acute poisoning.

Finally, we can readily find out from the left vertical scale that the vapor density of ENB in air is greater than 4; therefore it will tend to accumulate near the floor.

We will not make a prediction for vinyl norbornane from the diagram, leaving it to those who might be interested (the experimentally found LC_{50} of vinyl norbornane is 17.7 $\pm$ 2.6 mg/liter, $M = 120$, $t_{boil} = 140.4$°C, and it is virtually insoluble in water).

A similar diagram could be prepared for chlorinated hydrocarbons, for which nearly the same quantity of data on acute inhalational toxicity is available as for hydrocarbons. The CL_{50} values calculated from such a diagram, however, would be much less accurate because the residuals ($\bar{S}_{YX}$) are much higher (see Table 34).

The toxicity of halogen-containing hydrocarbons depends largely on the number of halogen atoms in the molecule. Figure 48 compares log LC_{50}

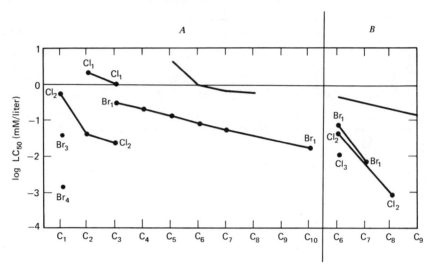

Figure 48. Plots of log LC_{50} as a function of the number of carbon atoms for hydrocarbons (lines without designations) and halogen-containing hydrocarbons (provided with indices Cl or Br with subscript figures denoting the number of halogen atoms in the molecule). A, Saturated aliphatic hydrocarbons; B, aromatic hydrocarbons.

values for saturated aliphatic hydrocarbons and aromatic hydrocarbons with those for their chlorine- and bromine-substituted derivatives. It can be seen that, as the number of carbon atoms increases, the augmentation of acute inhalational toxicity for aliphatic hydrocarbons differs only slightly from that for their chlorine and bromine derivatives; in contrast, the acute toxicity of aromatic hydrocarbons increases much less steeply than that of their halo derivatives. The acute toxicity of brominated aliphatic hydrocarbons is greater by one order or magnitude or more than that of the corresponding hydrocarbons. Monochlorinated hydrocarbons are less toxic than brominated ones, whereas dichlorinated hydrocarbons are more toxic than monobrominated ones by as much as one order of magnitude. Monochlorinated and monobrominated aromatic hydrocarbons become progressively more toxic, compared with the corresponding nonsubstituted hydrocarbons, as the number of carbon atoms increases.

Much less information was available about the acute inhalational toxicity of amines. As can be seen from Table 34, amines have the lowest regression coefficients, which means that their toxicities increase less with rising M and t_{boil} than do those of other compounds. At the same time the calculated log LC_{50} values for amines prove to be smaller than those for most other compounds listed in the table.

In addition to the groups of compounds shown in Table 34, data were considered for oxides and peroxides, aldehydes, and esters, but the correlations obtained were either insignificant or significant at the level of .05 > p > .02. Nevertheless it was found possible to calculate LC_{50} values for aldehydes, provided that corrections were made for the toxicity of the first member of a homologous series, the correction factors being -2.5 for the calculation from M and -2.1 for the calculation from t_{boil}. The equations for aldehydes are as follows:

$$\log LC_{50} = 1.3 - 0.027M \qquad (27)$$

$$\log LC_{50} = -0.008 t_{boil} \qquad (28)$$

These two equations, as well as those shown in Table 34, may serve as guides in the experimental determination of LC_{50}.

In graphic form, changes in acute toxicity with increasing t_{boil} and M are shown in Figures 49 and 50, respectively; these figures may be used as nomograms to estimate the $\log LC_{50}$ values of groups of compounds for which $\bar{S}_{YX} < 0.80$.

The equations presented in Table 35 give an indication of threshold concentrations (C_{min}); this table shows all significant correlations, beginning with $p < .05$.

There are far fewer data on C_{min} than on LC_{50} for organic compounds. Most of the C_{min} values used in the correlation analysis were obtained from measurements of the characteristics of the unconditioned flexor reflex in rabbits (Liublina, 1948), but some came from measurements of motor activity or the neuromuscular excitation threshold in rats. Since, as can be seen from

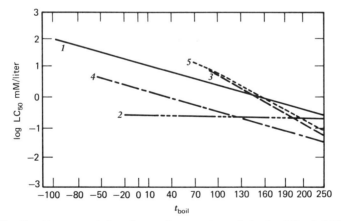

Figure 49.   Graphic representation of regression equations relating $\log LC_{50}$ (mM/liter) and boiling point for individual groups of volatile organic compounds. _1_, Hydrocarbons and ethers; _2_, amines; _3_, alcohols; _4_, chlorohydrocarbons; _5_, ketones.

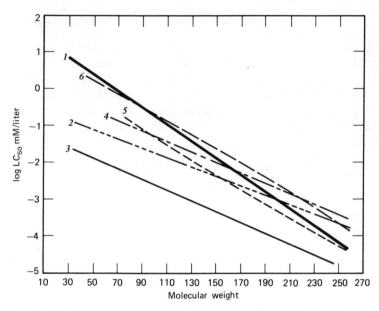

Figure 50. Graphic representation of regression equations relating log LC_{50} (mM/liter) and molecular weight for individual groups of volatile organic compounds. *1*, Hydrocarbons; *2*, amines; *3*, nitriles and cyanide compounds; *4*, chlorohydrocarbons; *5*, nitro compounds; *6*, ethers.

Table 35.   Reliability of Correlations and Equations for Calculating the Threshold Concentration (C_{min}) **from molecular weight** (M) **and boiling point** (t_{boil}) **for Particular Classes of Organic Compounds**

Class of Compounds	n	r	p	$\bar{S}_{YX}$	Equation: $\log C_{min}$ (mM/liter) =
Hydrocarbons	13	−0.89	<.001	0.47	$-0.95 - 0.010t_b$
	13	−0.82	<.001	0.60	$-0.51 - 0.015M$
Ketones	4	−0.97	<.05	0.20	$-0.72 - 0.011t_b$
Fatty amines and anilines	8	−0.71	<.05	0.60	$-2.33 - 0.005t_b$
Various amines	13	−0.63	<.02	0.65	$-2.29 - 0.008M$
Miscellaneous organic compounds,	92	−0.41	<.001	0.96	$-1.88 - 0.006t_b$
including those listed above	100	−0.55	<.001	0.92	$-1.31 - 0.011M$

Tables 34 and 35, the residuals ($\bar{S}_{YX}$) and the equations for miscellaneous compounds are rather different from those derived for particular groups of compounds, the latter equations are of course preferable. Unfortunately, for many groups of organic compounds, too few C_{min} data are available to permit the establishment of the reliable correlations necessary for deriving regression equations of practical use.

As more data are gathered in regard to different levels of toxicity for particular classes of organic compounds, it may be possible to prepare more diagrams similar to the one shown in Figure 47 for hydrocarbons.

4. CALCULATION OF BIOLOGICAL INDICES FOR NONVOLATILE ORGANIC COMPOUNDS

Experimental data on LC_{50} values for aerosols are very scanty because of the difficulty of setting up a stable concentration of an aerosol. Lethal doses rather than lethal concentrations are usually obtained in experiment. The oral route of administration is most common, but intraperitoneal lethal doses have also been determined for some substances.

When the first attempt was made to establish correlations between physicochemical constants and LC_{50}s for various pesticides that cannot present serious hazards in the form of gas or vapor because of their slight volatilities, the correlations obtained proved unreliable (Liublina, 1963b).

Later, a significant positive correlation was discovered for organophosphorus compounds between molecular weight and oral LD_{50} for rats, over a molecular weight range of 250 to 480. This correlation may be employed for the preliminary calculation of the LD_{50} despite a high value of the mean square deviation ($\bar{S}_{YX} = 1.23$, $n = 75$, $p < .001$, $r = 0.5$). In this case the experiment should be started on two groups of animals. The initial dose for one group is given by the equation

$$\log LD_{50} \ (\text{mM/kg } per \ os) = 0.014M - 4.83 \tag{29}$$

minus approximately one half of the $\bar{S}_{YX}$ value (i.e., $\log LD_{50} = 0.014M - 4.83 - 0.6$). For the other group the starting dose is given by the same equation, but 0.6 should be added to rather than subtracted from the value obtained.

Positive correlations were also found between molecular weight and oral LD_{50} for nonvolatile aromatic amines (beginning with $M = 150$) and for nonvolatile phenols (beginning with $M = 200$). The LD_{50} for an aromatic amine can be calculated from the equation

$$\log LD_{50} \ (\text{mM/kg}) = 0.010M - 1.25 \tag{30}$$

$$(n = 23, r = 0.75, p < .001, \bar{S}_{YX} = 0.40)$$

Table 36.   Reliability of Correlations and Equations for Calculating the MAC from the Molecular Weight (M) Separately for Volatile (V) and Nonvolatile (NV) Compounds (For comparison, data are also given for volatile and nonvolatile compounds together.)

Class of Compounds		n	$\bar{S}_{YX}$	Equation: log MAC (mM/m³) =
Saturated alcohols	V	10	0.25	$3.0 - 0.040M$
	NV	8	0.25	$-0.5 - 0.005M$
	All	18	0.85	$1.0 - 0.015M$
Nitro compounds without	V	10	0.25	$1.40 - 0.023M$
unsaturated bonds in open	NV[a]	20	0.35	$-1.35 - 0.0039M$
chains	All	30	0.71	$0.15 - 0.013M$
Amines and their nonchlorinated	V	14	0.55	$-0.30 - 0.013M$
derivatives	NV	26	0.35	$-1.2 - 0.0046M$
	All	40	0.56	$-1.04 - 0.006M$

[a] Including five nitrochlorobenzenes.

The equation for phenols is

$$\log LD_{50}\ (mM/kg) = 0.0036M + 0.18 \tag{31}$$

$$(n = 25, r = 0.55, p < .01, \bar{S}_{YX} = 0.30)$$

It is also possible to calculate the MAC for a nonvolatile organic compound from its molecular weight. At present, such calculations may be recommended for saturated alcohols, nitro compounds, and amines. The corresponding equations are shown in Table 36.

It should be noted that, as the separate calculation of correlations for nonvolatile organic compounds has shown, the log MACs of these substances show a smaller decrease with increasing molecular weight than in the case of volatile compounds.

5.   CALCULATION OF TOXICITY INDICES AND MAXIMUM ALLOWABLE CONCENTRATIONS FOR GASES AND VAPORS OF INORGANIC COMPOUNDS

Searches for correlations between various constants and toxicity indices of inorganic vapors and gases have shown that, although such correlations exist, their number is much smaller than that for organic compounds (Liublina, 1965). The values of the MAC calculated from the boiling point and molecular weight show roughly the same degree of agreement with the MACs in force for organic as for inorganic compounds, but in view of the scarcity of relevant information the equations presented in Table 37 for inorganic compounds should be regarded as highly tentative and far less accurate than those derived for organic vapors and gases. (For comparison, equations for organic vapors and gases are also given in the table.)

It follows from the table that the acute toxicities of inorganic substances are much higher (i.e., their LC_{50} values are much lower) than those of organic substances having the same molecular weights—by about one and a half orders of magnitude at $M = 100$ and by more than two orders at $M = 200$. The calculated values of MACs for inorganic compounds are lower by one and a half orders of magnitude than those for organic compounds having the same positive t_{boil}.

6. CALCULATION OF APPROXIMATE VALUES OF UNKNOWN TOXICITY INDICES FROM THOSE WHICH ARE KNOWN

In toxicological practice it is often necessary to estimate the MAC of an industrial poison from its lethal or threshold concentration as measured in a single-exposure experiment. A number of general (and simple) quantitative relationships between some parameters of inhalation toxicity of organic vapors and gases have been described by Zayeva (1970). By comparing the speeds of development of intoxication and the magnitudes of the corresponding concentrations, Zayeva has derived the following approximate relationship:

$$C_1 \sim C_2 \frac{\log V_1}{\log V_2} \tag{38}$$

where V_1 is the greater speed of intoxication development corresponding to the higher concentration C_1, and V_2 and C_2 are the smaller speed and the lower concentration, respectively. Zayeva showed this relationship to hold at lethal and threshold concentration levels for a number of substances. By inserting into (38) the logarithms of experimentally found average values of V for different toxicity levels (LC_{100}, LC_{50}, C_{min}, and MAC), she derived the following general quantitative relationships for gases and vapors of organic substances:

$$LC_{50} \sim 0.5 \, LC_{100} \tag{39}$$

$$LC_0 \sim 0.08 \, LC_{100} \tag{40}$$

$$C_{min} \sim 0.007 \, LC_{100} \tag{41}$$

Table 37. Equations for Calculating MAC and LC_{50} Values of Inorganic and Organic Gases and Vapors

Gases and Vapors	Equation	n	r	p	Equation Number
Inorganic	$\log$ MAC (mg/m^3) $= \log M - 2.0 - 0.0075 t_{boil}$	40	-0.45	$<.01 > .001$	(32)
Organic	$\log$ MAC (mg/m^3) $= \log M + 0.6 - 0.010 t_{boil}$	123	-0.30	$<.001$	(33)
Inorganic	$\log$ MAC (mg/m^3) $= \log M - 1.4 - 0.0077 M$	45	-0.42	$<.01 > .001$	(34)
Organic	$\log$ MAC (mg/m^3) $= \log M + 0.4 - 0.010 M$	124	-0.39	$<.001$	(35)
Inorganic	$\log LC_{50}$ (mg/liter) $= \log M - 0.90 - 0.017 M$	31	0.87	$<.001$	(36)
Organic	$\log LC_{50}$ (mg/liter) $= \log M + 0.08 - 0.011 M$	111	0.75	$<.001$	(37)

$$MAC \sim 0.0005 \, LC_{100} \tag{42}$$

$$MAC \, (mg/m^3) \sim 0.5 \, LC_{100} \, (mg/liter) \tag{43}$$

$$LC_{100} \sim 2 \, LC_{50} \tag{44}$$

$$LC_0 \sim 0.15 \, LC_{50} \tag{45}$$

$$C_{min} \sim 0.014 \, LC_{50} \tag{46}$$

$$MAC \sim 0.0013 \, LC_{50} \tag{47}$$

$$MAC \, (mg/m^3) \sim 1.3 \, LC_{50} \, (mg/liter) \tag{48}$$

$$MAC \sim 0.066 C_{min} \tag{49}$$

$$MAC \, (mg/m^3) \sim 66 C_{min} \, (mg/liter) \tag{50}$$

According to Zayeva, calculations from $LC_{50} \sim 0.5 \, LC_{100}$ (39) for 60 substances gave deviations not more than twofold from observed values, most of the calculated values being between 0.75 and 1.5 of the actual LC_{50}.

As for the MAC, calculations from LC_{50} values (48) for 48 substances gave deviations less than twofold from the MACs in force for half of the substances and not more than fivefold for most substances. Deviations greater than fivefold involved seven substances with marked specific activities. Similar results were obtained when the MAC was calculated from the LC_{100} (42). Calculations of the MAC from C_{min} showed greater disagreement, which was attributed by Zayeva to different sensitivities of the methods used for the experimental determination of C_{min}.

Rather different relationships were established by Liublina in a regression analysis of data for a much larger number of organic substances (including those having specific activity, but excluding pesticides). The equations obtained are shown in Table 38, which also gives equations for the calculation of concentrations from oral LD_{50} data for small laboratory animals. It can be seen from this table that the MAC can be estimated from the LD_{50} with greater approximation to reality than from the LC_{50} or the C_{min}, as the corresponding $\bar{S}_{YX}$ values indicate.

Zayeva's and Liublina's formulas cannot be compared directly because they use different units for concentration. It would have been possible to assess their relative values if Zayeva had determined the residuals.

According to Golubev (1970), the MACs of volatile substances correlate most closely with their irritant threshold concentrations. Golubev derived several equations for the calculation of MACs from threshold concentrations producing irritant effects on the upper air passages in animals and in man (Table 39). The closest approximation to the true values was attained when

Table 38. Reliability of Correlations between Toxicity Indices of Volatile Organic Compounds and Equations for the Preliminary Calculation of Unknown Indices from Those Which Are Known (MAC in mM/m^3, LC_{50} in $mM/liter$, C_{min} in $mm/liter$, LD_{50} in mM/kg)

n	r	p	$\bar{S}_{YX}$	Equation
178	0.72	$<.001$	0.65	$\log MAC = 0.72 \log LC_{50} - 0.31$
84	0.82	$<.001$	0.53	$\log C_{min} = 0.76 \log LC_{50} - 1.62$
94	0.73	$<.001$	0.55	$\log MAC = 0.77 \log C_{min} + 0.91$
112	0.66	$<.001$	0.60	$\log MAC = 0.88 \log LD_{50} - 2.29$
92	0.59	$<.001$	0.80	$\log LC_{50} = 0.84 \log LD_{50} - 2.33$
36	0.68	$<.001$	0.90	$\log C_{min} = 0.68 \log LD_{50} - 3.4$

the MAC was calculated from both the C_{min} of irritant action for man and the LC_{50} for mice.

At present, the use of general equations such as those shown in Tables 38 and 39 (with the possible exception of the last equation in Table 39) is justified only in cases where no equations specifically derived for particular classes of compounds are available. Indeed, an attempt to derive regression equations for correlations between the LC_{50} and MAC and between the LD_{50} and MAC for individual classes of organic compounds has revealed that such equations are different for different classes. The correlations and equations obtained are presented in Table 40; in graphic form the corresponding equations for the calculation of log MAC from the LC_{50} and LD_{50} are shown in Figures 51 and 52, respectively.

It is evident from Table 40 that one and the same increase in LC_{50} should lead to a greater increase in the MAC for hydrocarbons than for heterocyclic compounds and to a smaller increase in the MAC for hydrocarbons than for

Table 39. Reliability of Correlations and Equations for Calculating the MAC from the C_{min} Producing an Irritant Effect (C_{irrit}) in Animals and Human Beings (MAC in mg/m^3, C_{irrit} and LC_{50} in $mg/liter$)

n	p	$\bar{S}_{YX}$	Equation
21	$<.001$	0.65	$\log MAC = 0.88 + 0.61 \log C_{irrit}$ for cats
31	$<.001$	0.53	$\log MAC = 1.25 + 0.57 \log C_{irrit}$ for rabbits
70	$<.001$	0.41	$\log MAC = 1.94 + 0.76 \log C_{irrit}$ for human beings
30	$<.001$	0.31	$\log MAC = 1.16 + 0.37 \log LC_{50} + 0.47 \log C_{irrit}$ for human beings

Table 40. Reliability of Significant Correlations between Log LC_{50} and Log MAC and between Log LD_{50} and Log MAC and Equations for Calculating MACs from LC_{50} and LD_{50} for Some Classes of Organic Compounds

Class of Compounds	n	r	p	$\bar{S}_{YX}$	Equation: log MAC =
Hydrocarbons	26	0.72	$<.001$	0.64	$0.80 \log LC_{50} - 0.04$
Alcohols	11	0.86	$<.001$	0.64	$0.94 \log LC_{50} + 0.11$
Aldehydes	5	0.98	$<.01$	0.10	$0.43 \log LC_{50} - 0.86$
Nitro compounds	8	0.85	$<.01$	0.55	$0.64 \log LC_{50} - 0.14$
Amines	15	0.53	$<.05$	0.61	$0.86 \log LC_{50} - 0.27$
Heterocyclic compounds	11	0.85	$<.001$	0.29	$0.42 \log LC_{50} - 0.94$
Chlorohydrocarbons	30	0.86	$<.001$	0.60	$0.87 \log LC_{50} - 0.36$
Alcohols	5	0.91	$<.05$	0.40	$0.98 \log LD_{50} - 1.96$
Nitro compounds	6	0.98	$<.001$	0.19	$0.89 \log LD_{50} - 2.70$
Amines	24	0.40	$=.05$	0.40	$0.37 \log LD_{50} - 2.12$

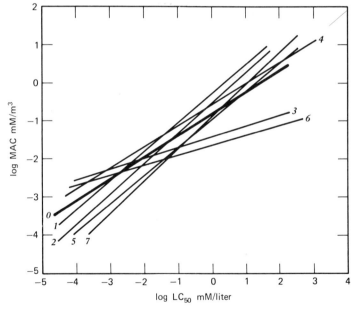

Figure 51. Graphic representation of regression equations relating log MAC and log LC_{50} for particular groups of organic compounds. *1*, Hydrocarbons; *2*, alcohols; *3*, aldehydes; *4*, nitro compounds; *5*, amines; *6*, heterocyclic compounds; *7*, chlorohydrocarbons; *0*, the general equation.

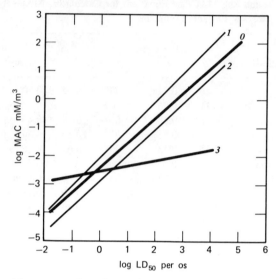

Figure 52. Graphic representation of regression equations relating log MAC and log LD_{50} for particular groups of organic compounds. *1*, Alcohols; *2*, nitro compounds; *3*, amines; *0*, the general equation.

alcohols. Differences between regression coefficients are particularly large for correlations between the MAC and LD_{50} (see Figures 51 and 52). The general equations of Table 38 are average equations which, when applied to a particular class of compounds, may greatly increase the deviation of calculated values from true ones, as can be seen from Figures 51 and 52. At the same time the total area taken up by the straight lines on the graphs is small, especially in Figure 51. Within the range of medium log LC_{50} values, calculation of the MAC from any of the equations in Table 40 gives a deviation from the general equation of less than ± 0.3, or less than by a factor of 2.

The differences between the equations in Table 40 are due, in the final analysis, to features of toxic action peculiar to low concentrations (functional cumulation, reversibility of chronic intoxication, etc.) that cannot be taken into account in calculating the MAC from a lethal concentration or dose, but that are allowed for in the safety factor, by which the threshold concentration determined in a chronic test is divided to obtain the MAC (see Chapter 5).

To ascertain the degree to which the correlations of the LC_{50}, C_{min}, and MAC with each other are affected by the physicochemical properties of volatile organic compounds, Liublina (1963b) computed partial correlation coefficients for the correlations between each of the above biological indices and 11 constants (molecular weight, specific weight, molar volume, boiling point, melting point, logarithm of saturated vapor pressure, refractive index, molar refraction, logarithms of oil/water and water/air partition coefficients, and logarithm of water solubility). It was found that the partial correlation coefficients of log MAC, log C_{min}, and log LC_{50} with each other remain high (no lower than 0.61) when some one constant (any of those listed above) is eliminated. The correlations between the indices remain reliable even after elimination of the effects of the two properties most closely associated with the indices concerned. Consequently the correlations between the different toxicity indices are much stronger than those between these indices and the physical and physicochemical constants considered. This implies that the MAC can be calculated for volatile organic compounds not only from their constants but also from such toxic indices as the C_{min} or LC_{50} when these have been determined experimentally (the constants then become of subsidiary importance).

It should be emphasized that the relationships described so far in this section concern volatile compounds only. For high-boiling (slightly volatile or nonvolatile) organic compounds used as pesticides, regression analysis made it possible to derive the following equation (Liublina and Golubev, 1967):

$$MAC \ (mg/m^3) = 0.0008 \ LD_{50} \ (mg/kg) \tag{51}$$

When data on organophosphorus and on organochlorine high-boiling pesticides were treated separately, two substantially different equations were obtained:

$$\log MAC = 0.6 \log LD_{50} - 3.0 \tag{52}$$

for organophosphorus compounds, and

$$\log MAC = 1.2 \log LD_{50} - 3.4 \tag{53}$$

for organochlorine compounds.

Of considerable interest appears to be the paper by Kagan et al. (1972) concerned with the prediction of toxicity indices and MACs for pesticides. The authors derived a regression equation for calculating the safety factor (F_s) on the basis of the cumulation coefficient (K_{cum}). This coefficient is a very important consideration in the selection of F_s: the lower the K_{cum}, the greater is the cumulative effect from low concentrations of the harmful substance and, consequently, the higher is the hazard of chronic poisoning (see Chapter 5). Kagan et al. proposed equations for the calculation of the MAC from one or two toxicity indices. Here are most of their equations:

$$MAC = 0.0008 \ LD_{50} + 0.146* \qquad (r = 0.56) \tag{54}$$

$$MAC = 0.1C_{chr} + 0.04 \qquad (r = 0.98) \tag{55}$$

* Compare with (51).

$$F_s = 2.26K_{cum}^2 - 39.2K_{cum} + 177.32 \qquad (\eta = 0.65) \tag{56}$$

$$MAC = 0.1 \times 10^{-3}\left(\frac{C_{min}}{C_{chr}}\right)^2 - 0.01\left(\frac{C_{min}}{C_{chr}}\right) + 0.265 \qquad (\eta = 0.47) \tag{57}$$

$$MAC = 0.07 - 0.5 \times 10^{-4} LD_{50} - 0.75 \times 10^{-2}K_{cum}$$

$$-0.1 \times 10^{-6} LD_{50} + 2 \times 10^{-3} LD_{50} \cdot K_{cum} \qquad (\eta_m = 0.97) \tag{58}$$

where MAC is in milligrams per cubic meter, LD_{50} is in milligrams per kilogram, C_{chr} is the threshold concentration of the pesticide on chronic exposure (mg/m^3), C_{min} is the threshold concentration on single exposure (mg/m^3), r is the correlation coefficient, η is the correlation ratio, η_m is the correlation ratio for multiple regression, F_s is the safety factor, and K_{cum} is the cumulation coefficient. These authors also presented nomograms to facilitate the calculations.

In most cases the calculated values of the MAC and K_{cum} show satisfactory agreement with those found experimentally. Equations 55 and 57 cannot, in effect, be of predictive value because they include the threshold concentration from a chronic test, that is, the quantity which is the last to be obtained in such a test but has the greatest impact on the MAC. Nevertheless these two equations are useful in that they indicate the general relationship between the C_{chr} and the other indices. Equation 58 may apparently be simplified by deleting the terms with very small coefficients such as 10^{-4} and 10^{-6}.

As regards inorganic compounds, we have derived several equations; they give cruder approximations, however, than the equations for organic compounds.

The following equation may be used to estimate the MAC for inorganic gases or vapors:

$$MAC \ (mg/m^3) = 2.52 \ LC_{50} \ (mg/liter) \tag{59}$$

The equation proposed for aerosols of oxides or other slightly soluble metal compounds is

$$\log MAC \ (mg/m^3) = 0.85 \log LD_{50} - 3.0 + \log M - \log N \tag{60}$$

where LD_{50} is the intraperitoneal dose for mice expressed in milliatoms per kilogram of body weight,* M is the molecular weight, and N is the number of metal atoms in a molecule of the substance.

---

* To convert milligrams per kilogram to milliatoms per kilogram, the number of milligrams must be divided by the molecular weight of the compound, and the quotient multiplied by the number of metal atoms in a molecule.

7. CALCULATION OF LESS ACCESSIBLE PHYSICAL AND PHYSICOCHEMICAL CONSTANTS FROM THOSE MORE READILY ACCESSIBLE

In Chapter 7 the importance of obtaining information about such physico-chemical properties as the oil/water and water/air partition coefficients and water solubility was shown. Our experience with the statistical treatment of data on most diverse physical and physicochemical properties and various toxicity indices of 218 organic compounds (Filov and Liublina, 1965) has revealed that, while the above-mentioned coefficients and water solubility correlate well with one another, they show no significant correlations with the other properties studied, with one exception. The exception is the molar volume ($V_m = M/\rho$), which has a relatively close correlation ($r = 0.61$) with the oil/water partition coefficient (log K). However, the calculation of log K from V_m gave an $\bar{S}_{YX}$ of 1.5, which meant that the coefficients thus obtained could serve at best as very rough guides to the group in Lazarev's system of nonelectrolytes to which the substance belonged. Unfortunately, it is not always possible to calculate K from the molar volume for volatile organic compounds since their specific weights may be unknown. The molecular weight, however, is a cofactor in the formula for molar refraction:

$$R_m = \frac{n_D^2 - 1}{n_D^2 + 2} \cdot \frac{M}{\rho}$$

The value of R_m can be calculated with reasonable accuracy from the structural formula of an organic compound. It is convenient to use for this purpose bond refraction values, for example, those given by Vogel et al. (1952). When the refractive index and molar refraction are known, the molar volume can be readily calculated from a table of values of the function $(n_D^2 - 1)/(n_D^2 + 2)$ $\times 10^4$. The refractive index is often unknown, however. The molecular weight is usually known, and the molar refraction can be calculated from the structural formula. But a log K estimated from the molar volume, calculated in turn from the molar refraction, would be too inaccurate, since the deviations ($\bar{S}_{YX}$) would be about ± 1.8, that is, would amount to nearly two orders of magnitude. In this case it is better to use the correlation of log K directly with the R_m, given by the equation

$$\log K = 0.16 R_m - 2.43 \tag{61}$$

The values thus obtained will deviate from the true values no more than $\pm 1.27 (\bar{S}_{YX})$.

As for the water/air partition coefficient (λ), which allows one to judge the speed of saturation of the body with a volatile substance during inhalation, quite satisfactory results can be obtained from the generally known equation

$$\lambda = \frac{S \times 760 \times 22 \times 4T}{P \cdot M \times 273.1} \tag{62}$$

where S is the water solubility of the substance (in g/liter), T is the absolute temperature, P is the saturated vapor pressure at 20°C, and M is the molecular weight.

As already stated in Section 3, the saturated vapor pressure P for volatile organic compounds can be calculated from the boiling point of the compound by the equation (Levina, 1952)

$$\log P = 3.5 - 0.0202(t_{boil} + 3) \tag{63}$$

for which $r = -0.98$. The results agree well with the true values of P for t_{boil} values from 20° to 200°C and more or less satisfactorily for those between 200° and 280°C.*

Information on water solubility is often of a qualitative nature; to convert it at least into rough quantitative data, the following assumptions appear to be warranted. If the solubility of a substance miscible with water in any ratio is taken to be 100 g/100 ml of water, the following solubilities may be ascribed to other substances: 10 g/100 ml to substances described as readily soluble, 1 g/100 ml to those just soluble, 0.1 g/100 ml to those slightly or difficultly soluble, and 0.001 g/100 ml to insoluble substances. When no information is available on the water solubility of a substance, the oil/water and water/air partition coefficients of the substance are usually unknown as well.

The existence of correlations between physical and physicochemical properties led us to attempt a graphic representation of the more frequent correlations between the properties that are of particular importance from hygienic and toxicological points of view. Figure 53 is a diagram giving rough values of some physicochemical properties in relation to the boiling point and molar refraction—two of the most often known or most readily measurable physical constants for volatile organic compounds.

This diagram (in which all the lines for physicochemical constants were drawn through areas of maximum density of corresponding data points) provides some, if only rough, indication of the magnitudes of such distributive properties as the water solubility, oil/water and water/air partition coefficients, saturated vapor pressure for air, and saturation concentration. An attempt to construct a similar diagram with coordinates of molecular weight versus boiling point met with failure.

---

* Many equations for the calculation of saturated vapor pressure were presented by Zayeva (1964), who also gave some equations for calculating t_{boil}.

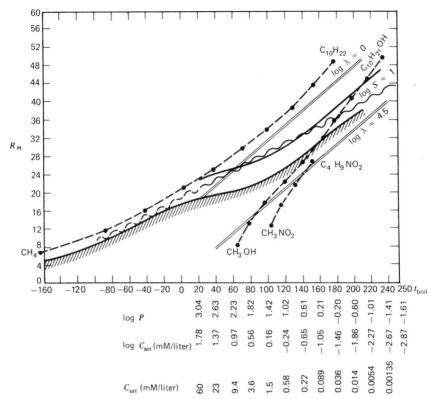

Figure 53. Diagram showing approximate positions of some physicochemical properties of substances in relation to their boiling point and molar refraction. Dashes connect points giving the position of consecutive members of homologous series. Double straight lines roughly correspond to water/air partition coefficients of volatile organic compounds: the upper line, to $\log \lambda = 0 \pm 1.5$; the lower line, to $\log \lambda = 4.5 \pm 1.5$. The continuous wavy line marks approximately a water solubility of about 10 mM/liter. The discontinuous wavy line denotes the water solubility of gases at the same level. The upper curved line roughly corresponds to the boundary between Groups VI and VII ($K = 10^3$) in Lazarev's system of nonelectrolytes; the lower curved line, to the boundary between Groups IV and V ($K = 10$) of that system; the hatched band corresponds roughly to Group IV ($K = 1 - 10$).

Correlations were calculated on a computer, separately for each class of compounds studied, between several physical constants (molecular weight, density, molar volume, refractive index, molar refraction, melting point, and boiling point) and the logarithms of three of the above-mentioned distribution constants ($\log K$, $\log \lambda$, and $\log S$), using all possible paired combinations of the constants considered. The smallest number of significant correlations was obtained for the $\log \lambda$ which correlated in a few cases with some one

Table 41. Reliability of Correlations and Equations for Calculating the Oil/Water Partition Coefficient ($\log K$) from the Molecular Weight (M), Molar Volume (V_m), and Molar Refraction (R_m)

Class of Compounds	n	r	p	$\bar{S}_{YX}$	Equation: $\log K =$
Hydrocarbons	37	0.81	<.001	0.68	$1.0 + 0.030M$
	35	0.90	<.001	0.47	$-0.04 + 0.032V_m$
	37	0.77	<.001	0.73	$1.00 + 0.088R_m$
Saturated alcohols	7	0.98	<.001	0.05	$-2.68 + 0.043M$
	7	0.87	<.02	0.47	$-3.60 + 0.040V_m$
	7	0.98	<.001	0.22	$-2.80 + 0.12R_m$
Aldehydes	7	0.99	<.001	0.33	$-3.95 + 0.063M$
	7	0.98	<.001	0.41	$-4.15 + 0.054V_m$
	7	0.97	<.001	0.53	$-3.79 + 0.22R_m$
Amines	13	0.80	<.001	1.04	$-3.30 + 0.042M$
	12	0.95	<.001	0.57	$-4.81 + 0.052V_m$
	13	0.83	<.001	0.98	$-4.25 + 0.16R_m$
Chlorinated	20	0.76	<.001	0.48	$0.33 + 0.014M$
hydrocarbons	19	0.83	<.001	0.42	$0.67 + 0.029V_m$
	20	0.83	<.001	0.41	$-0.15 + 0.088R_m$
Miscellaneous organic compounds	91	0.80	<.001	1.15	$-3.50 + 0.053V_m$

Table 42. Reliability of Correlations and Equations for Calculating the Water Solubility ($\log S$) from the Molecular Weight (M), Molar Volume (V_m), and Molar Refraction (R_m)

Class of Compounds	n	r	p	$\bar{S}_{YX}$	Equation: $\log S$ (mM/liter) $=$
Hydrocarbons	38	−0.46	<.01	0.69	$0.61 - 0.011M$
	36	−0.58	<.001	0.64	$1.52 - 0.016V_m$
	38	−0.45	<.01	0.69	$0.60 - 0.03R_m$
Alcohols	17	−0.81	<.001	1.59	$4.78 - 0.024M$
	13	−0.92	<.001	0.49	$6.30 - 0.035V_m$
	17	−0.82	<.001	1.00	$6.00 - 0.12R_m$
Nitro compounds	11	−0.74	<.01	1.05	$3.97 - 0.021M$
	11	−0.89	<.001	0.81	$6.15 - 0.046V_m$
	11	−0.89	<.001	0.24	$4.44 - 0.103R_m$
Amines	25	−0.58	<.01	1.09	$4.88 - 0.026M$
	23	−0.43	<.05	1.26	$4.68 - 0.020V_m$
	25	−0.61	<.001	0.35	$4.90 - 0.080R_m$

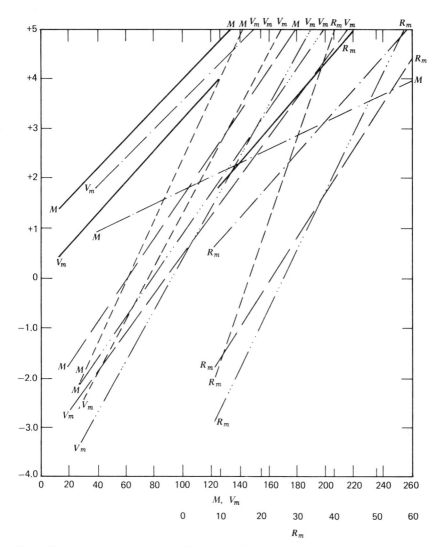

Figure 54. Approximate positions of oil/water partition coefficients (K) in relation to molecular weight (M), molar volume (V_m), and molar refraction (R_m). Solid lines refer to hydrocarbons; dashes with dots, to chlorohydrocarbons; long dashes, to alcohols; short dashes, to aldehydes; and dashes with three dots, to amines.

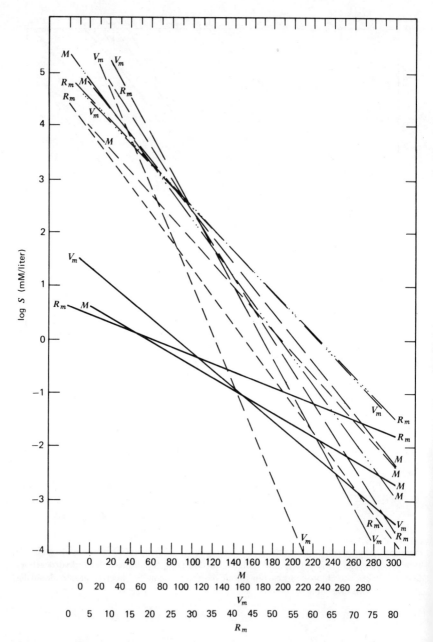

Figure 55. Approximate positions of water solubilities (S) in relation to molecular weight (M), molar volume (V_m), and molar refraction (R_m). Designations as in Figure 54, except that the short dashes refer to nitro compounds.

property only at $p > .001$. In contrast, log K and log S showed correlations with several constants, in many cases at $p < .001$.

Most suitable for the calculation of log K and log S were found to be correlations with molecular weight, molar volume, and molar refraction; the corresponding equations are presented in Tables 41 and 42.

The equations of Tables 41 and 42 are shown in graphic form in Figures 54 and 55, respectively. These figures make it possible to draw certain conclusions. Thus a substance with a molecular weight over 180 may be expected to belong to one of the last groups (VIII or IX) of Lazarev's system of nonelectrolytes and so to cause rapid, acute poisoning at high inspired concentrations, similar, for example, to the well-known intoxication resulting from the inhalation of gasoline vapors. A volatile organic substance having a molar volume above 160 may be expected to be a type II narcotic. A molar volume above 200 suggests that the substance is insoluble in water, while a molecular weight below 100 points to high solubility (unless the substance is a hydrocarbon). Two striking features are the low solubility of hydrocarbons (Figure 55) and the relatively high values of their log K (Figure 54).

Thus a number of methods are now available for the calculation of some toxicologically and hygienically important physical and physicochemical constants which are not to be found in the literature and are difficult to determine experimentally.

ADDENDUM: RECENT PROGRESS IN METHODS FOR THE CALCULATION OF TOXICITY PARAMETERS

This addendum discusses some new procedures for calculating toxicity parameters proposed in the USSR in the last few years.

A1. NONVOLATILE ORGANIC COMPOUNDS

Loit (1974) used his experimental data to construct a scheme showing variations in log LD_{50} with t_{boil} and t_{melt} in passing from vapors to aerosols (Figure A1). Substances with t_{boil} between 180° and 235°C and t_{melt} between 20° and 70° may be present in the air both as vapors and as aerosols. Within these ranges the linear correlation of log LD_{50} with both t_{boil} and t_{melt} changes from inverse to direct. Figure A1 shows an average log LD_{50} line with two parallel lines representing the confidence limits. The short horizontal line above the upper confidence limit serves to indicate that the scatter of LD_{50} values is greater within this temperature range. It can also be seen that

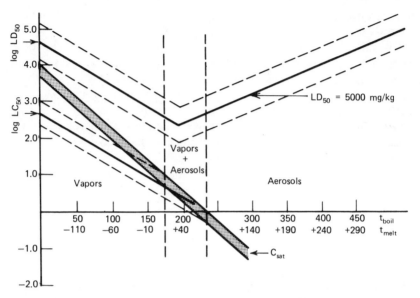

Figure A1. Schematic representation of variations in log LD_{50}, log LC_{50}, and C_{sat} (concentration saturating air at 20–25°C) with t_{boil} and t_{melt} for organic compounds. The upper solid line (which reverses its direction in the zone where both vapors and aerosols are present) gives approximate mean values of log LD_{50} (*per os*, for mice), the lower solid line (which ends in the same zone) gives such values for log LC_{50} (also for mice), and the dashed lines running parallel to the above two lines mark the upper and lower confidence limits of the respective mean log LD_{50} and log LC_{50} values. The hatched band represents C_{sat} values. To the left of the left vertical line, substances are present in air in the form of gas or vapor, and to the right of the right vertical line, in the form of aerosol. Between these vertical lines (i.e., at t_{boil} from 180° to 235°C and t_{melt} from 20° to 70°C, substances may be present in air both as vapors and as aerosols. C_{sat} and LC_{50} are in mg/liter and LD_{50} are in mg/kg.

no reversal occurs in correlations for the LC_{50} (the LC_{50} line in the figure). The hatched band denotes saturated concentrations.

Clearly, it is difficult to calculate toxicity indices from t_{boil}, t_{melt}, or other readily available constants for substances that may occur both as vapors and as aerosols.

It is very likely that the above-mentioned reversal in the correlation of log LD_{50} with the constants that continually increase as the homologous series is ascended will affect MAC values as well—not to the extent of reversing their correlations with such constants, but in that there will be a significantly smaller decrease in MAC for nonvolatile than for volatile compounds in ascending a series (see Table 36).

A2. NEW METHODS FOR CALCULATING TENTATIVE SAFE EXPOSURE LEVELS AND OTHER TOXICITY INDICES

In 1975 an index called the Tentative Safe Exposure Level (TSEL) was introduced into industrial toxicology in the USSR in addition to the MAC. The TSEL is a temporary MAC, valid for a period of 2 years and estimated from data of short-term tests and/or by calculation.

Sidorov and Shapiro (1977) have developed an original stepwise method for calculating the TSEL for harmful substances in the air of work areas (respiration zones) using the following information: (1) single-exposure threshold concentration; (2) the LC_{50} for mice or rats (the smaller value is used if LC_{50} values are available for both mice and rats); and (3) and (4) oral LD_{50} values for the species most and least sensitive, respectively, to a given poison.

In this method the logarithm of the tentative chronic action threshold (log C_{chr}) is first calculated by the following two equations, derived from data for 118 volatile organic compounds:

$$\log C_{chr} = 0.62 \log LC_{50} - 1.08$$
$$(r = 0.71 \pm 0.05, \bar{S} = \pm 0.69)$$

$$\log C_{chr} = 0.77 \log C_{min} - 0.56$$
$$(r = 0.81 \pm 0.03, \bar{S} = \pm 0.60)$$

Next, the safety factor is calculated, consisting of two cofactors; one of these is a score of degree of cumulation as determined from the LC_{50}/C_{chr} ratio (Table A1), while the other is a score of species differences in sensitivity as assessed from the ratio of the oral LD_{50} value for the least sensitive species to that for the most sensitive one (Table A2). (The rationale for selecting the safety factor is described in Sidorov, 1971.) Multiplying these two scores will give the safety factor, by which the calculated chronic action threshold concentration is divided to obtain the TSEL. If the LC_{50} is known, the cumulative

Table A1.   Degree of Cumulation as Estimated from the LC_{50}/C_{chr} Ratio

Degree of Cumulation	LC_{50}/C_{chr}	Score
Slight	≤ 10	2
Moderate	11–100	3
Strongly marked	101–1000	4
High	> 1000	5

Source.   Sidorov and Shapiro (1977).

Table A2. Degree of Species Difference in Sensitivity to Poisons

Species Difference in Sensitivity	$LD_{50\,max}/LD_{50\,min}$	Score
Slight	3	2
Medium	3.1–9	3
Large	9	4

Source. Sidorov and Shapiro (1977).

properties of the substance can be allowed for by calculating the C_{chr}, thus making the estimated TSEL much more reliable.

Kagan et al. (1976) have suggested calculating TSEL values for individual groups of pesticides not only from the oral LD_{50} and the cumulation coefficient (K_{cum}) but also from the LD_{50} for skin absorption. They have proposed the following equations for organophosphorus pesticides:

$$\ln TSEL = 0.517 \ln LD_{50\,per\,os} - 3.928$$

$$\ln TSEL = 0.299 \ln LD_{50\,per\,os} + 0.255 \ln LD_{50\,skin} - 4.458$$

$$\ln TSEL = 0.483 \ln LD_{50\,per\,os} + 0.086 K_{cum} - 4.347$$

$$\ln TSEL = 0.284 \ln LD_{60\,per\,os} + 0.237 \ln LD_{50\,skin} + 0.08 K_{cum} - 4.811$$

They have also derived similar equations for organochlorine pesticides and carbamates, as well as for pesticides as a whole. Separate calculation of the TSEL for each particular class of compounds has greatly reduced the discrepancies between calculated and experimentally found values.

That the LD_{50} for skin absorption might be of importance in calculating the TSEL was indicated by an analysis of variance: this LD_{50} was found to affect the TSEL to almost the same extent as the oral LD_{50}. As might have been anticipated, the TSELs calculated from physicochemical constants (molecular weight, solubility, volatility, boiling point, etc.) for the same three groups of pesticides were less reliable than those derived from experimentally determined indices.

For poisons with irritant action, Ivanov (1976) has calculated TSELs from irritant threshold concentrations for rats and for man, using in some of his equations also the irritant zone (Z_{irrit}), defined as C_{min}/C_{irrit}, where C_{min} is the single-exposure threshold concentration and C_{irrit} is the irritant threshold concentration. If this ratio is equal to or smaller than unity, the substance is regarded as not producing any specific (irritant) action. The following equations have been generated (all indices in mg/m^3):

$$\log \text{TSEL} = 0.892 \log C_{\text{irrit rat}} - 1.034 \text{ mg/m}^3$$
$$(n = 31, r = 0.88, p = .001, \bar{S} = 0.32)$$
$$\log \text{TSEL} = 1.024 \log C_{\text{irrit man}} - 0.742 \text{ mg/m}^3$$
$$(n = 31, r = 0.82, p = .001, \bar{S} = 0.36)$$
$$\log \text{TSEL} = 0.69 \log C_{\text{irrit rat}} + 0.18 \log C_{\text{irrit man}} - 0.7 \log Z_{\text{irrit}} - 0.51 \text{ mg/m}^3$$
$$(n = 27, R = 0.96, p < .001, \bar{S} = 0.21)$$
$$\log \text{TSEL} = 0.11 \log \text{LC}_{50} + 0.65 \log C_{\text{irrit rat}} - 0.72 \log Z_{\text{irrit}} - 0.65 \text{ mg/m}^3$$
$$(n = 14, R = 0.91, p < .001, \bar{S} = 0.27)$$

Although Ivanov has claimed that 95 % of the TSEL values generated by the last two (multiple regression) equations do not differ from the observed values more than 3.2-fold and 3.7-fold, respectively, the relatively small (-0.44) correlation coefficient between Z_{irrit} and TSEL casts doubt on the desirability of using this index in TSEL calculations.

A3. CORRELATIONS BETWEEN TOXICITY OF CHEMICALS AND THEIR INHIBITORY ACTIONS ON ISOLATED MITOCHONDRIA

Rotenberg (1974) has considered concentrations causing 50 % inhibition of mitochondrial respiration ($C_{50 \text{ inh}}$) in relation to the LC_{50} and LD_{50} values of the substances, as well as to their MACs in force for the air of work areas (MAC_{wa}) and the ambient air in residential areas (MAC_{aa}). Experimental $C_{50 \text{ inh}}$ values were determined by measuring ADP-stimulated respiration of rat liver mitochondria in the incubation medium. The LC_{50} and LD_{50} were stated in millimoles. Since the LC_{50}, LD_{50}, MAC, and $C_{50 \text{ inh}}$ values of different substances differed by several orders of magnitude, logarithms of these indices had to be used. Rotenberg used logarithms of reciprocals, that is, $\log(1/C_{50 \text{ inh}})$, $\log(1/\text{LD}_{50})$, $\log(1/\text{LC}_{50})$, $\log(1/\text{MAC}_{\text{wa}})$, and $\log(1/\text{MAC}_{\text{aa}})$. A total of 29 diverse substances, both organic and inorganic, were considered. The results are reproduced in Table A3.

Equations derived by Rotenberg for calculating toxicity at the four different levels are presented in Table A4, where the mean errors are deviations from observed values.

Disagreement between observed and calculated values was particularly large for methanol, ethanol, and dimethylaniline in the case of the LD_{50} and LC_{50}, and for cyanides and hydrogen sulfide in the case of the MAC_{wa} and MAC_{aa}. The deviation for ethanol is attributed by the author to its rapid oxidation to nontoxic products; that for methanol, to the formation of more toxic products than methanol; and those for aniline and dimethylaniline, to the formation of methemoglobin (the LD_{50} of aniline for rabbits, in which methemaglobin does not form, is 2.5 to 3 times higher than for rats).

Table A3. Values of Inhibiting Concentrations and of Toxicometric Parameters

Compound	$\log(1/C_{50\,inh})^a$	$\log(1/LD_{50})$	$\log(1/LC_{50})$	$\log(1/MAC_{wa})^a$	$\log(1/MAC_{aa})^a$
Phenol	2.00	2.27	4.37	7.28	9.98
4-Chlorophenol	2.85	2.75	4.60	8.11	—
2,4-Dichlorophenol	3.65	3.29	4.72	—	—
2,4,6-Trichlorophenol	3.40	3.29	—	8.29	—
Pentachlorophenol	4.40	3.68	—	9.42	—
Aniline	1.72	2.67	4.76	8.97	9.5
4-Methylaniline	2.2	—	—	7.55	—
N,N-Dimethylaniline	2.82	—	6.02	8.70	10.35
Methanol	−0.3	1.96	3.50	6.81	—
Ethanol	0.3	0.76	2.60	4.66	6.97
Butanol	0.65	1.41	3.57	6.87	—
2,4-Dinitrophenol	4.2	3.64	5.66	9.57	—
Butophen (2,4-dinitro-6-fluorobutylphenol)	4.75	3.86	—	9.68	—
Ethyl-β,β,β-trichloropropionate	3.15	2.75	—	—	—

Monochloroacetate	2.30	2.75	—	—	—
Monobromoacetate	3.30	3.14	—	—	—
Monoiodoacetate	4.30	3.44	—	—	—
Cyanides	5.70	4.51	6.43	7.94	9.43
Azides	4.26	3.81	6.34	—	—
Hydrogen sulfide	4.00	—	4.83	7.11	9.63
Sulfurous anhydride and sulfites	1.62	2.00	—	6.83	9.1
Formaldehyde	2.58	—	4.84	7.78	—
Mercury (divalent)	5.00	4.25	—	9.43	11.82
Arsenites	2.92	3.07	—	8.61	10.61
Lead	4.3	—	—	10.3	11.47
Hyperiz (hydroperoxide of isopropylbenzene)	3.0	—	—	8.18	—
Cadmium	4.75	—	6.45	9.11	—
Ethylbenzene	2.80	—	—	—	9.72
Acetone	0.3	1.08	2.60	5.46	8.22

Source. Rotenberg (1974).

[a] $C_{50\,inh}$ = concentration causing 50 % inhibition of mitochondrial respiration; MAC_{wa} = MAC for the air of work areas; MAC_{aa} = MAC for ambient air.

Table A4.   Equations for Calculating Toxicity at Different Levels

Number of Pairs from List in Table A3	Correlation Coefficient r	Inverse Probability p	Mean Error m (%)	Equation[a]
21	0.92	<.001	103	$\log(1/LD_{50})$ = $1.35 + 0.54C_{50\,inh}$
15	0.81	<.01	140	$\log(1/LC_{50})$ = $3.05 + 0.60C_{50\,inh}$
22	0.92	<.001	109	$\log(1/MAC_{wa})$ = $6.00 + 0.73C_{50\,inh}$
12	0.90	.01	129	$\log(1/MAC_{aa})$ = $7.70 + 0.91C_{50\,inh}$

Source.   Rotenberg (1974).
[a] Designations as in Table A3.

At the safe levels the large differences between calculated and experimentally derived MAC_{wa} and MAC_{aa} values (164-fold for cyanides and 144-fold for hydrogen sulfide) are believed by the author to be due to the fact that, while the risk of acute poisoning with these compounds is very high, their cumulative capacities are relatively low, and this has influenced their experimentally established MACs.

The finding that $C_{50\,inh}$ correlates with the more common indices of acute toxicity, as well as with indices of safe levels (concentrations in work areas and in ambient air) for widely different substances, calls for special attention to this index. Although the number of data points is still too small to permit any conclusions about the practical utility of the relationships noted by Rotenberg, it appears that further work in this direction might bring rewarding results both in the way of elucidating the mechanisms of action of various substances in relation to their toxicities and in the development of equations for calculating tentative indices of toxicity and safety.

A4.   PREDICTION OF SKIN-ABSORPTIVE PROPERTIES OF CHEMICALS

N. V. Lazarev wrote in 1938 that to penetrate the skin a substance must be soluble not only in lipids but also in water; this explains why the skin is more permeable for organic compounds (nonelectrolytes) belonging to Group IV of Lazarev's system of nonelectrolytes (see Chapter 7, p. 329).

Rumiantsev and Novikov (1975a) have demonstrated the possibility of calculating LD_{50} values for substances absorbed through the skin of animals from the octanol/water partition coefficient (P). They used this coefficient because it is now known for a very large number of organic compounds and, if unknown, can be calculated. They derived the equation

$$\log LD_{50} \text{ (rabbits via skin)} = 1.25 + 0.199P$$
$$(n = 72, r = 0.633, \bar{S} = \pm 0.376)$$

Moreover, they have correlated skin absorption LD$_{50}$ values for rats and rabbits with intragastric LD$_{50}$ values for rats and have derived a multiple regression equation relating the LD$_{50\,skin}$ for rabbits to the octanol/water partition coefficient P and to the LD$_{50}$ for rats with intragastric (ig) administration. The following three equations were generated (4-hr contact for rats and 24-hr contact for rabbits):

$$\log LD_{50} \text{ (rats via skin)} = 0.79 \log LD_{50} \text{ (rats ig)} + 0.77$$
$$(n = 107, r = 0.842)$$

$$\log LD_{50} \text{ (rabbits via skin)} = 0.77 \log LD_{50} \text{ (rats ig)} + 0.87$$
$$(n = 72, r = 0.809, \bar{S} = \pm 0.386)$$

$$\log LD_{50} \text{ (rabbits via skin)} = 0.645 + 0.54 \log LD_{50} \text{ (rats ig)} + 0.09\ P$$
$$(R = 0.849, \bar{S} = \pm 0.259)$$

Finally, they have presented an equation for passing from the LD$_{50}$ for rats via skin on 4-hr contact to the LD$_{50}$ for rabbits via skin on 24-hr contact:

$$\log LD_{50} \text{ (rabbits via skin)} = 0.7383 \log LD_{50} \text{ (rats via skin)} - 0.1945$$

A5. TRANSITION FROM LD$_{50}$ VALUES FOR ONE ROUTE OF ENTRY TO THOSE FOR ANOTHER ROUTE

In 1975 Rumiantsev and Novikov (1975b) published a paper on this subject containing several equations, being unaware of similar equations that had been published much earlier by Loit (1967) and had remained largely unknown. It may be useful to compare these two groups of equations. Rumiantsev and Nivikov write: "Interestingly, the regression equations relating median lethal doses with oral administration to those with other routes of absorption are practically the same for mice as for rats." This fact had been noticed by many authors before. Thus Loit (1967) presented the following two equations:

$$LD_{50} \text{ for mice (mg/kg)} = LD_{50} \text{ for rats (mg/kg) (orally, subcutaneously,}$$
$$\text{intraperitoneally, or intravenously)}$$

$$LD_{50} \text{ for mice (mg/kg)} = LD_{50} \text{ for rabbits (mg/kg) (intravenously)}$$

Loit used LD_{50} values rather than their logarithms, which tend to yield better correlations. Shown below are only those of his equations derived from a much larger data base (102 to 210 substances) or involving combinations of routes of entry other than those in Rumiantsev and Novikov's equations.

Loit's (1967) equations:

$$LD_{50\,per\,os} = 1.78\,LD_{50\,sc}$$
$$LD_{50\,iv} = 0.32\,LD_{50\,ip}$$
$$LD_{50\,iv} = 0.32\,LD_{50\,sc}$$
$$LD_{50\,ip} = 0.56\,LD_{50\,sc}$$
$$LD_{50\,iv} = 0.10\,LD_{50\,per\,os}$$

Rumiantsev and Novikov's (1975b) equations:

$$\log LD_{50\,ip} = 0.9 \log LD_{50\,per\,os}$$
$$(n = 104, r = 0.908)$$

$$\log LD_{50\,sc} = 1.17 \log LD_{50\,per\,os} - 0.80$$
$$(n = 45, r = 0.968)$$

$$\log LD_{50\,iv} = 0.6 \log LD_{50\,per\,os} + 0.03$$
$$(n = 58, r = 0.866)$$

$$\log LD_{50}\,(\text{rats via skin}) = 0.79 \log LD_{50\,per\,os} + 0.77$$
$$(n = 107, r = 0.842)$$

All these equations are of course fairly approximate. Neverthtless they prove to be very useful for practical purposes of preventive toxicology, especially as a guide in the experimental determination of LD_{50} values with different routes of administration.

A6. CALCULATION OF MAXIMUM ALLOWABLE CONCENTRATIONS IN AMBIENT AIR AND IN WATER

In recent years environmental protection has become the most pressing of all prophylactic problems. The accelerated development of industry, transportation, and energy resources and the increasing use of chemicals in agriculture and domestic life have led to ever larger quantities of chemicals being released daily to the atmosphere, bodies of water, and soil.

In the USSR the first to formulate this problem as a global environmental issue was N. V. Lazarev, in 1957. Later he published a book on this subject (Lazarev, 1966) entitled *Vvedeniye v Geogigiyenu (An Introduction to Environmental Hygiene).*

The need for standards setting limits to the ever-rising levels of various substances in the atmosphere, bodies of water, soils, and foods has led communal hygienists to follow industrial toxicologists and start work on the development of methods for estimating such standards by calculation. Here, as in the area of occupational hygiene, maximal permissible levels of toxic chemicals are set on the basis of threshold and subthreshold data.

Before proceeding to discuss the particular equations that have been proposed, a word should be said about the overall approach to establishing standards for ambient air and water (standards for food and soil will not be dealt with here) as distinct from those for the air of work areas.

Until very recently the only kind of standard for the air of work areas (respiration zones) was maximum allowable concentrations, that is, the concentrations not to be exceeded on even a single occasion. It was only for carbon monoxide that different (five) permissible values were specified for different exposure durations. In 1976 five more standards were introduced, prescribing average permissible concentrations per shift for mercury, copper, antimony, cadmium oxide, and lead (or its inorganic compounds). These average values are set 1.5- to 3.3-fold lower than the maximum single-occasion permissible concentrations.

As regards standards for atmospheric pollutants in residential areas, there are two kinds of MAC—maximal on one occasion (i.e., momentary or peak concentrations), and average over 24 hr (i.e., average daily concentrations). The former MACs are based on threshold concentrations of reflex action, such as thresholds of smell, of effect on the light sensitivity of the eye, and of change in bioelectric activity of the cerebral cortex. All maximal momentary concentrations in the ambient air must be lower than the respective threshold values for the most sensitive persons.

If, for example, a given substance has a strong smell but low toxicity, its average daily concentration is set equal to its maximal momentary concentration. If the threshold of toxic action as established in animal experiments with prolonged (usually no less than 3 months), continuous 24-hr exposure is found to be lower than the threshold of reflex action on man, the standard is set on the basis of the concentration which has proved ineffective in animals. For most substances standards for ambient air have been established using both these principles, and the average daily concentration is equal to the maximal momentary one in the majority of cases. For the remaining substances the average daily values are 1.5- to 10-fold lower than the maximal momentary ones.

In establishing standards on the basis of reflex-action subthreshold concentrations, the prime consideration is that even a very weak stimulus may become obtrusive and disagreeable if it acts long enough. For this reason the momentary MAC for, say, an odorous substance in the air of residential areas will be low even though the substance is virtually harmless. The average daily MAC of this substance will be the same as its momentary MAC.

For bodies of water used for domestic, public, and recreational purposes (these are termed "water bodies for sanitary-domestic uses") MACs are established on the basis of what is called the limiting index of harmfulness. This may be defined in terms of the effect that a given substance has on an organoleptic property of water (odor, taste, turbidity, or color) or on the general sanitary condition of water bodies (processes of self-purification from organic contaminants), or it may be derived from toxicological data. The largest number of MACs in force are based on limiting organoleptic indices; even such a substance as hexachloran has its MAC for water established in that way, even though it is treated as a very dangerous substance as far as its MAC (which is very low) for the environment of work areas is concerned.

The experimental determination of threshold and subthreshold concentrations of substances in water on the toxicological basis is a particularly costly, laborious, and time-consuming procedure—hence the importance of being able to establish tentative MAC values by calculation. Work along this line was started with attempts to establish correlations between MACs for the atmosphere and those for the air of work areas because most of the MACs in force were for work areas and were based on experimental findings.

The existence or orderly relationships between the physicochemical properties and toxicities of airborne substances determined the existence of such relationships between MACs for the air of work areas and those for the atmosphere (ambient air). Similar relationships could of course be expected to exist between MACs for work areas and MACs for water in cases where the latter had been established on a toxicological basis.

One of the first attempts to correlate MACs for work areas with those for ambient air and for water bodies was undertaken by Tolokontsev (1967). At that time the number of standards for vapors was small, and the collations done for 37 substances did not yield correlations significant enough to permit more or less reliable calculations ($.001 < p < .01$). Consideration of MACs for water as established on a toxicological basis in relation to those for work areas gave insignificant correlations ($n = 16, p > .05$). Somewhat later, Golubev and Subbotin (1968), who included in their analysis not only MACs in force but also those recommended for water bodies on a toxicological basis, succeeded in deriving a satisfactory equation ($n = 37$). In the following years, many authors have presented a number of equations relating MACs for ambient air or water both to those for work areas and to LC_{50}s, LD_{50}s, and some physicochemical constants. Moreover, correlations have been established between momentary MACs for ambient air and threshold concentrations for olfactory sensation and other reflex responses.

Table A5 presents equations of different authors relating average daily

MACs (MAC_{ad}) and maximal momentary MACs (MAC_{mm}) in the ambient air to MACs in work areas (MAC_{wa}), as well as to some other toxicological indices and to t_{boil}. It can be seen from this table that the equations of different authors based on MAC_{wa} (equations A1, A4, and A20) are not very different. If the calculated preliminary values of MAC are to be used for limited purposes (in a limited area) pending their experimental verification, (A1) is to be preferred as giving lower values. Equations A2 and A5, which relate MAC_{mm} to MAC_{wa}, have practically the same free terms, but the regression line in (A5) is much steeper. Equation A5 therefore yields higher values in the region of high MAC_{wa} and lower values in the region of low MAC_{wa} (i.e., for more dangerous substances) than does (A2). Accordingly, for preliminary practical calculations, (A2) may be employed when $MAC_{wa} > 0.6$, using a negative correction factor; when $MAC_{wa} \leq 0.6$, it is safer to use (A5).

Equations A3 and A6 are for calculating MAC_{ad} from MAC_{mm}. The difference between these equations is small, but (A3) is to be preferred because it gives lower values for more hazardous substances (i.e., those with low MAC_{wa} values).

For the same reason (A8) would seem preferable to (A21), but in view of considerable disagreement between the values calculated by these equations in the region of low LD_{50} values (as much as one order of magnitude even at $LC_{50} = 2.5$ mg/liter and progressively greater with lower LC_{50} values) it is better to use other indices for the calculations.

When MACs for work areas are not available, it is rather risky to calculate daily average MACs from LC_{50} or LD_{50} only; more satisfactory results are obtained from calculations based on olfactory threshold concentrations, that is, from (A19) and (A23).

As a rule, all the available indices should be used in the calculations, taking the mean logarithm of the obtained concentrations. When neither the MAC_{wa} nor any reflex action threshold concentration is available and one has to rely on much less accurate indices, preference must be given to the lowest calculated value.

Of the equations shown in Table A5, the correlation coefficients are highest and the mean square errors are lowest for Krotov's equations relating threshold concentrations of reflex action on man to momentary MACs.

Thus we can see that MAC_{mm} and MAC_{ad} can be calculated in various ways. It should be noted that (A14) (for calculations from t_{boil}) gives the least reliable results and should not be used when the calculation can be done by using some other equation.

Table A6 presents equations for calculating MACs for water on the toxicological basis. According to the author (Shigan, 1976a), (A7), (A11), and (A12), all based on the LD_{50}, require a correction for the cumulative properties of the substance. Thus (A7) can be used without a correction factor only for substances with weak cumulative properties; otherwise, correlation

Table A5. Equations Relating Daily Average MACs (MAC_{ad}) and Maximal Momentary MACs (MAC_{mm}) in the Air of Residential Areas with Each Other, to MACs in the Air of Work Areas (MAC_{wa}), and to Some Other Parameters[a] (MAC_{ad}, MAC_{mm}, MAC_{wa}, and threshold concentrations in mg/m^3, LC_{50} in $mg/liter$, and LD_{50} in mg/kg)

Equation	n	r	$\bar{S}$
Source: Spynu and Ivanova (1969)			
(A1) $\log MAC_{ad} = (-2.16 \pm 0.28) + (0.88 \pm 0.16)\log MAC_{wa}$	30	0.69	—
(A2) $\log MAC_{mm} = (-1.777 \pm 0.3) + (0.55 \pm 0.09)\log MAC_{wa}$	30	0.69	—
(A3) $\log MAC_{ad} = (-0.15 \pm 0.03) + (1.02 \pm 0.20)\log MAC_{mm}$	30	0.94	—
Source: Loit et al. (1971)			
(A4) $\log MAC_{ad} = -2.00 + 0.86 \log MAC_{wa}$	40	0.65	—
Source: Zaugolnikov et al. (1975)			
(A5) $\log MAC_{mm} = 1.78 + \log MAC_{wa}$ or $MAC_{mm} = 0.0166\, MAC_{wa}$	—	0.65	—
(A6) $\log MAC_{ad} = -0.47 + 0.86 \log MAC_{mm}$	40	0.88	—
(A7) $\log MAC_{mm} = 0.54 + 1.16 \log MAC_{ad}$	40	0.88	—
(A8) $\log MAC_{ad} = -3.16 + 1.72 \log LC_{50}$	—	0.66	—
(A9) $\log MAC_{ad} = -6.00 + 1.50 \log LD_{50}$	—	0.52	—

410

(A10) $\log \mathrm{MAC_{mm}} = -2.08 + 1.02 \log \mathrm{LC_{50}}$	—	0.55	—
(A11) $\log \mathrm{MAC_{mm}} = -5.73 + 1.39 \log \mathrm{LD_{50}}$	—	0.49	—
(A12) $\log \mathrm{MAC_{mm}} = -1.7 + 1.3 \log \mathrm{LC_{50}} \div 3.3 \log \mathrm{LD_{50}}$	27	0.68	—
(A13) $\log \mathrm{MAC_{ad}} = 0.7 + 1.7 \log \mathrm{LC_{50}} - 0.8 \log \mathrm{LD_{50}}$	27	0.74	—
(A14) $\log \mathrm{MAC_{ad}} = 0.5 - 0.013 t_{\mathrm{boil}}$	—	−0.48	—

Source: Krotov (1971, 1975)

(A15) $\log \mathrm{MAC_{mm}} = 0.96 \log C_{\mathrm{min\,odor}} - 0.51$	82	0.957	±0.249
(A16) $\log \mathrm{MAC_{mm}} = 0.93 \log C_{\mathrm{min\,eye\,l.\,sens.}} - 0.45$	54	0.944	±0.276
(A17) $\log \mathrm{MAC_{mm}} = 0.97 \log C_{\mathrm{min\,bioel.\,act.}} - 0.23$	66	0.948	±0.105
(A18) $\log \mathrm{MAC_{mm}} = \log C_{\mathrm{min}}$ from (A15), (A16), and (A17) $- 0.21$ or	82	0.992	±0.139
$\quad \mathrm{MAC_{mm}} = 0.617 C_{\mathrm{min}}$ from (A15), (A16), and (A17)			

(A19) $\log \mathrm{MAC_{ad}} = 0.86 \log C_{\mathrm{min\,odor}} - 0.79$ (for low-toxic substances)	—	0.91	±0.398
(A20) $\log \mathrm{MAC_{ad}} = 0.62 \log \mathrm{MAC_{wa}} - 1.77$	75	0.70	±0.692
(A21) $\log \mathrm{MAC_{ad}} = 0.58 \log \mathrm{LC_{50}} - 1.6$	59	0.68	±0.68
(A22) $\log \mathrm{MAC_{ad}} = 0.72 \log C_{\mathrm{min\,odor}} + 0.22 \mathrm{MAC_{wa}} - 1.05$	—	—	±0.324
(A23) $\log \mathrm{MAC_{ad}} = 0.81 \log C_{\mathrm{min\,odor}} + 0.1 \log \mathrm{LC_{50}} - 0.86$	—	—	±0.370

[a] $C_{\mathrm{min\,odor}}$, $C_{\mathrm{min\,eye\,l.\,sens.}}$, and $C_{\mathrm{min\,bioel.\,act.}}$ are threshold concentrations for odor, light sensitivity of the eye, and bioelectric activity of the cerebral cortex, respectively.

Table A6. Equations Relating MACs in Bodies of Water (for Substances Whose MACs for Water Are Established on a Toxicological Basis) to MACs in the Air of Work Areas (MAC_{wa}), LD_{50}, t_{melt}, t_{boil}, and TLV (U.S. Threshold Limit Values)

Equation[a]	n	r	Note
Source: Ivanova (1971) (for pesticides)			
(A1) $\log MAC_{water} = -3.90 + 0.55 \log LD_{50} + 0.06 \log M + 0.74 \log t_{melt}$	—	—⎫	Threefold difference from
(A2) $\log MAC_{water} = 5.20 + 0.5 \log LD_{50} - 3.31 \log M + 0.15 \log t_{boil}$	—	—⎭	observed values, on average
Source: Zaugolnikov et al. (1975)			
(A3) $\log MAC_{water} = -4.76 + 1.39 \log LD_{50}$	—	0.62	
(A4) $\log MAC_{water} = -0.45 + 0.007 t_{melt}$	—	0.52	For nonvolatile substances
(A5) $\log MAC_{water} = 0.85 - 0.01 t_{melt}$	—	-0.47	For volatile substances
Source: Shigan (1976a, 1976b)			
(A6) $\log MAC_{water} = 0.47 \log MAC_{wa} - 1.4$	140	0.79	
(A7) $\log D_{chr} = 0.923 \log LD_{50} - 2.89$	286	0.53	
(A8) $\log MAC_{water} = 1.1 \log MAC_{wa} - 0.60$	14	0.68 ⎫	For organophosphorus
(A9) $\log MAC_{water} = 0.99 \log TLV - 1.05$	9	0.998 ⎬	compounds
(A10) $\log D_{chr} = 0.99 \log MAC_{wa} + 0.60$	17	0.63 ⎭	
(A11) $\log MAC_{water} = 0.89 \log LD_{50} - 3.60$	30	0.97 ⎫	For nitro compounds
(A12) $\log D_{chr} = 0.68 \log LD_{50} - 2.04$	27	0.98 ⎬	
(A13) $\log MAC_{water} = 1.23 \log TLV - 2.14$	11	0.97	For aldehydes and ketones

[a] MAC_{water} in mg/liter; MAC_{wa} in mg/m^3; LD_{50} in mg/kg; D_{chr} = threshold dose on chronic exposure in mg/liter; M = molecular weight.

factors are needed. These are -3 for substances showing supercumulation, -2 for those with high cumulation, -0.5 for those with medium cumulation, and $+0.5$ for those that do not cumulate at all. Equation A7 can therefore be made more generally applicable by adding a quantity K to take account of cumulative properties:

(A7a) $$\log D_{chr} = 0.923 \log LD_{50} - 2.89 + K$$

Similar correction factors are required for (A11) and (A12).

Shigan's equations were tested using MAC and D_{chr} values adopted or proposed on the basis of experimental studies. In the case of MACs, the disagreement was found to be 2- to 5-fold (or even less) for 15 substances, up to 10-fold for 6, and more than 10-fold for 2. In the case of D_{chr} it was not more than one order of magnitude for most substances.

As is indicated by Table A6, some authors have already begun deriving equations for particular classes of compounds, and separately for volatile and nonvolatile compounds, to calculate their MACs for bodies of water.

That separate treatment of data for individual classes of compounds can give better correlations is attested by the equations for nitro compounds and for aldehydes and ketones (see Table A6) where $r > 0.96$. Particularly high correlation coefficients are seen with TLVs, but it should be noted that in both cases (Equations A9 and A13) the number of data points used to derive the equations for Soviet MACs is smaller than elsewhere.

Unfortunately it is hard to say anything definite about the MAC_{water} values as calculated from t_{boil}, since no data apart from the correlation coefficients are given by the authors. The coefficients for volatile compounds (Equation A14 in Table A5 and Equation A5 in Table A6) are very close (-0.48 and -0.47). Liublina (1976) has derived a similar equation for the average daily MAC, stated in millimoles per cubic meter rather than milligrams per liter:

$$\log MAC_{ad} = -0.01 t_{boil} - 1.99$$
$$(n = 46, r = -0.64, p = <.001, \bar{S} = \pm 0.86)$$

Calculations in millimoles have yielded better correlations. For calculating concentrations in air (whether for work areas or for the atmosphere) the use of millimoles generally gives closer correlations, probably on account of millimoles being more informative than milligrams because equal volumes are occupied by molecules of vapors and gases. A comparison was then made of regression lines for the above equation and two other equations, designed for the calculation of the LC_{50} and MAC_{wa}, respectively, and derived from a much larger data base. It should be noted that the slopes of regression lines cannot be compared from analytically derived equations. Indeed, to obtain the regression coefficient b, the ratio of mean square deviations is multiplied

Table A7.   Analytical Equations of Regression Lines (all indices in mM/m^3)

Equation	n	r	Recalculated Regression Coefficients
$\log LC_{50} = 2.98 - 0.009 t_{boil}$	245	-0.62	-0.0145
$\log MAC_{wa} = -0.40 - 0.006 t_{boil}$	241	-0.45	-0.0133
$\log MAC_{ad} = -1.99 - 0.01 t_{boil}$	46	-0.64	-0.0156

by the correlation coefficient: $b = \sigma_y/\sigma_x \cdot r$. Since the equations being compared have different values of r, the true slope of the regression line will be less steep the smaller is r. If, instead, the calculated regression coefficient is divided by the corresponding r, a regression coefficient closer to reality will result.

Table A7 gives the three equations and their regression coefficients recalculated in this way. As this table shows, the difference between the regression coefficients is now not more than 16 % (taking the highest coefficient as 100 %), as compared to a difference of about 40 % before. For practical purposes the changes in the MACs of the different levels and in the LC_{50}s (for mice) may be considered to be, on the average, equally related to changes in t_{boil}. This of course applies only to the t_{boil} range where the toxicity of vapors rather than aerosols is the prime consideration for a given index. For instance, this range is much narrower for $\log LC_{50}$ than for MAC_{wa} or MAC_{ad} because of the impossibility of attaining a lethal effect, since the saturation concentrations of substances decrease much more rapidly than their toxicities with rising t_{boil}. The similarity of the slopes of regression lines brings out the importance of calculating effective concentrations from t_{boil}.

The equations for calculating the MACs in water and in air of work areas (MAC_{wa}) when they are expressed as fractions of the saturation concentrations (C_{sat}) for water and for air, respectively, are very similar:

$$\log MAC_{water} = -0.74 \log C_{sat} - 1.79$$
$$(n = 58, r = -0.88, \bar{S} = \pm 0.74)$$

$$\log MAC_{wa} = -0.71 \log C_{sat} - 1.69$$
$$(n = 252, r = -0.71, \bar{S} = \pm 0.96)$$

This example illustrates the advantages of using effective concentrations stated as fractions of the saturation concentrations (i.e., in terms of thermodynamic activities; see Chapter 3), for changes in the toxicity of a substance then do not depend on the medium in which it is present.

It should be pointed out that, if the MAC for the air of work areas is available for a given substance, a tentative momentary MAC for that substance may be calculated from its experimentally found olfactory threshold concentration, since the correlations established between such concentrations and the MAC_{wa} are sufficiently reliable ($r > 0.95$).

As for the calculation of MACs for water when these are based, as they often are, on organoleptic indices, the most promising line of work appears to be the development of equations based on threshold concentrations that cause a change in the turbidity, color, odor, or taste of water.

In conclusion it must be recognized that considerable success has been achieved in the development of methods for the rapid determination by calculation of maximum allowable concentrations in water and in the atmosphere.

ADDENDUM REFERENCES

Golubev, A. A., and V. G. Subbotin, Possible uses of computing methods for establishing tentative maximum allowable concentrations of harmful substances in bodies of water, in *Gigiyena Primeneniya, Toksikologiya Pestitsidov i Klinika Otravleniy*, No. 6, pp. 284–287, Institut Gigiyeny i Toksikologii Pestitsidov, Polimernykh i Plasticheskikh Mass, Kiev, 1968.

Ivanov, N. G., A rapid method for determining safe levels of poisons by recording specific manifestations of intoxication, in *Primeneniye Matematicheskikh Metodov dlya Otsenki i Prognozirovaniya Realnoi Opasnosti Nakopleniya Pestitsidov vo Vneshnei Srede i Organizme. Materialy Vtorogo Simpoziuma*, pp. 83–85, Institut Gigiyeny i Toksikologii Pestitsidov, Polimernykh i Plasticheskikh Mass, Kiev, 1976.

Ivanova, L. N., Possible uses of mathematical models in establishing maximum allowable concentrations for pesticides in bodies of water, in *Gigiyena Primeneniya, Toksikologiya Pestitsidov i Klinika Otravleniy*, No. 9, pp. 83–86, Institut Gigiyeny i Toksikologii Pestitsidov, Polimernykh i Plasticheskikh Mass, Kiev, 1971.

Kagan, Yu. S., L. M. Sasinovich, and G. I. Ovseenko, A differential approach to establishing tentative safe exposure levels for individual groups of pesticides by calculation, in *Primeneniye Matematicheskikh Metodov dlya Otsenki i Prognozirovaniya Realnoi Opasnosti Nakopleniya Pestitsidov vo Vneshnei Srede i Organizme, Materialy Vtorogo Simpoziuma*, pp. 78–81, Institut Gigiyeny i Toksikologii Pestitsidov, Polimernykh i Plasticheskikh Mass, Kiev, 1976.

Krotov, Yu. A., Use of computing methods for establishing tentative maximal momentary concentrations of atmospheric pollutants, *Gig. Sanit.*, **12**, 8–12 (1971).

Krotov, Yu. A., Ed., *Predelno Dopustimiye Kontsentratsii Vrednykh Veshchestv v Vozdukhe i Vode. Spravochnoye Posobiye dlya Vybora i Gigiyenicheskoi Otsenki*

Metodov Obezvrezhivaniya Promyshlennykh Otkhodov [*Maximum Allowable Concentrations of Harmful Substances in the Air and in Water: Guidelines for the Selection and Hygienic Evaluation of Methods for Decontaminating Industrial Wastes*], pp. 94–99, Khimiya, Leningrad, 1975.

Lazarev, N. V., Problems in environmental hygiene and their relation to searches for new insecticides, fungicides, and herbicides, in *Pervaya Vsesoyuznaya Konferentsiya po Gigiyene i Toksikologii Insektofungitsidov*, pp. 76–78, Meditsinskoye Izdatelstvo Ukrainskoi SSR, Kiev, 1957.

Lazarev, N. V., Ed., *Vvedeniye v Geogigiyenu* [*An Introduction to Environmental Hygiene*], Nauka, Moscow and Leningrad, 1966.

Liublina, E. I., Physicochemical constants of harmful substances and their maximum allowable concentrations in ambient air, workroom air, and water: some general relationships, *Gig. Sanit.*, **8**, 88–92 (1976).

Loit, A. O., Some correlations between toxicity of chemicals and their route of entry into the body, in P. M. Komo, Ed., *Voprosy Gigiyeny, Profpatologii i Onkologii v Sibiri*, Vol. 2, pp. 34–35, Angarskii Institut Truda i Profzabolevaniy, Angarsk, 1967.

Loit, A. O., "Predvaritelnaya Toksikologicheskaya Otsenka Organicheskikh Soyedineniy" ["Preliminary Toxicological Evaluation of Organic Compounds"], unpublished doctoral dissertation, Leningrad, 1974.

Loit, A. O., M. M. Kochanov, and S. D. Zaugolnikov, On correlations between maximum allowable concentrations of some chemicals in workroom air and in the atmosphere of inhabited areas, *Gig. Tr. Prof. Zabol.*, **5**, 15–17 (1971).

Rotenberg, Yu. S., On the correlation between toxicity of chemical agents and their inhibitory action on isolated mitochondria, *Biull. Eksp. Biol. Med.*, **7**, 65–68 (1974).

Rumiantsev, G. I., and S. M. Novikov, Predicting skin-absorptive properties of new chemicals, *Gig. Sanit.*, **4**, 9–95 (1975a).

Rumiantsev, G. I., and S. M. Novikov, Toxicity of substances in relation to their route of entry into the body, *Gig. Sanit.*, **2**, 25–27 (1975b).

Shigan, S. A., Role of computing methods in the establishment of standards for chemical water pollutants, *Gig. Sanit.*, **11**, 15–19 (1976a).

Shigan, S. A., Methods for predicting chronic toxicity parameters of substances in the area of water hygiene, *Environ. Health Perspect.*, **13**, 83–89 (1976b).

Sidorov, K. K., Calculation of the safety factor in establishing MACs for harmful substances in the air of work areas, *Gig. Tr. Prof. Zabol.*, **6**, 54–56 (1971).

Sidorov, K. K., and A. B. Shapiro, A method for calculating tentative safe exposure levels of substances in the air of working areas, in *Primeneniye Matematicheskikh Metodov dlya Otsenki i Prognozirovaniya Realnoi Opasnosti Nakopleniya Pestitsidov vo Vneshnei Srede i Organizme. Materialy Vtorogo Simpoziuma*, pp. 81–83, Institut Gigiyeny i Toksikologii Pestitsidov, Polimernykh i Plasticheskikh Mass, Kiev, 1976.

Sidorov, K. K., and A. B. Shapiro, Establishment of tentative safe exposure levels of harmful substances in the air of working areas, *Vrach. Delo*, **3**, 131–133 (1977).

Spynu, E. I., and L. N. Ivanova, Prediction of maximum allowable concentrations for some chemicals present in the air, *Gig. Tr. Prof. Zabol.*, **7**, 18–21 (1969).

Tolokontsev, N. A., Prospects for the application of mathematical methods in toxicology, in *Obshchiye Voprosy Promyshlennoi Toksikologii*, pp. 96–100, Institut Gigiyeny Truda i Profzabolevaniy, Moscow, 1967.

Zaugolnikov, S. D., M. M. Kochanov, A. O. Loit, and I. I. Stavchansky, Rapid methods of estimating toxicity and MACs and the evaluation of hazards presented by environmental chemicals, *Vestn. Akad. Nauk SSSR*, **3**, 75–83 (1975).

CONCLUSION

In these concluding paragraphs an attempt is made to summarize briefly and to put into perspective some of the problems dealt with in the book as they are seen by the authors, taking into consideration the practical needs of toxicology today and tomorrow.

Chapters 1, 2, and 6 and the addenda to them emphasize that the toxic effect of any chemical substance is, and must be viewed as, the result of interaction between that substance and a given living organism and is subject to considerable variation, depending on exposure time and environmental conditions. By far the most complex and least constant of these four determinants of the toxic effect is of course the organism, but none of the other three is invariant, either. The toxic effect is therefore a function of many uncontrollable variables. It follows from this basic truth that a statistical, probabilistic approach is necessary in any quantitative estimation of the magnitude of toxic effect. Such an approach has been adopted in discussing the parameters and criteria of toxicity in this book.

The main achievements of quantitative toxicology in the calculation and evaluation of toxicity parameters are associated with the classical work of Bliss, where dose-effect and time-effect relationships are treated as curves governed by the normal distribution law. The concept of normality of dose-effect curves underlies most of the parameters of effective doses and concentrations and magnitudes of toxicity zones established for various poisons, as well as the attempts (made in Chapter 2) to apply Gaddum's principle to defining ineffective (permissible) values for these doses, concentrations, and zones.

In some cases dose-effect and time-effect relationships cannot be satisfactorily approximated by equations of a normal distribution curve. This means that the actual hazards presented by poisons cannot always be reliably characterized by toxicity parameters such as median (mean) effective values and their standard errors ($ED_{50} \pm S_{ED_{50}}$) and similar statistical indices. For this reason the possibility of applying nonparametric tests was considered in Chapter 2. However, although the use of nonparametric statistics as criteria of toxicity remains a possibility, further purposive efforts are necessary to gather more information about the pattern of the above curves. It would be desirable especially to study toxicity curves in relation, on the one hand, to the mechanism of action and, on the other, to the physicochemical and other properties of poisons. Such studies, apart from their obvious toxicological value, should provide further insights into the structures and functions of biological substrates and biological systems.

The increasing need to establish maximum permissible values of toxic substances in the environment for combined and complex exposures, as well as exposures involving physical agents, mandates the development of adequate methods of experimental design that would permit, in particular, assessment of the contribution to the toxic effect of each factor involved, including the biological characteristics of the organism.

An important line of work in quantitative toxicilogy is represented by toxicity studies giving full consideration to the time factor, including both the "external" and the "internal" (biorhythms of various periods and amplitudes) time. Research into time-effect relationships is of great theoretical significance for the development of work on several complex problems of current interest, primarily cumulation and adaptation.

There is continued and, indeed, growing concern with the problem of animal data extrapolation to man. The progress attained so far by quantitative toxicology in this area cannot be considered satisfactory.

Chapter 3 sets forth the general theory of equilibrium distribution of non-electrolytes between the environment and the living organism. For all practical purposes this theory may be regarded as complete. Some of its possible applications are exemplified in the last section of the chapter; if required, it can be similarly applied to other practical situations.

Chapter 4 *and the long addendum to it* are devoted to toxicokinetics, one of the most dynamic and rapidly evolving areas of toxicology. Its tasks and prospects were outlined in Section A7. Here it may be noted that toxicokinetics, possessing as it does a rather well-developed theory, can find many more practical applications than are known today. Undoubtedly it will not be long before toxicokinetic methods are put to wide practical use. This concerns not only individual but also—and especially—ecological toxicokinetics.

Chapter 5 *and its addendum* are concerned with the quantitative evaluation of cumulation, where a relatively new development is the study of cumulative action at the threshold level. The prospects and potentials of such studies were mentioned in Chapter 5. Here it is appropriate to note the following.

In current practice the degree of cumulation is assessed by the cumulation coefficient as determined from results of daily exposures to a constant concentration or dose. Although this procedure simulates more or less the actual industrial exposures, it may be inadequate to represent other situations such as those encountered, for example, in agriculture, where several days of close contact with a poison may be followed by a period free from exposure, so that the overall toxicity may well be different from that with continuous exposure, even though the total dose is the same. For instance, daily exposures to trichlorfon were found to result in much more severe effects than exposures interrupted by nonexposure periods; the reverse was true in the case of dicresyl ester of methylcarbamic acid (Burkatskaya and Matiushina, (1968).

These and other, similar facts suggest the desirability of constructing mathematical and other models to simulate various exposure regimens with the aim of assessing the effects of cumulation, both material and functional. Important parameters of such models should be the physicochemical properties of toxic substances. It should then be possible to specify optimal and unfavorable exposure regimens for different poisons.

Chapters 7 and 8 and their addenda are closely interrelated. Quantitation of structure-toxicity relationships makes it possible to work out methods for calculating toxicity parameters. Research into structure-biological activity relationships, which have become a subject of major interest in biochemistry, will undoubtedly be pursued in toxicology also, although it is risky to indulge in forecasts of further developments. It is much safer and easier to speak about the prospects for methods of determining toxicity indices by calculation.

Searches are now underway for relationships between MAC or TSEL (tentative safe exposure level) values in various chemical classes by considering log MAC in relation to the difference between log LC_{50} and log MAC for volatile organic compounds and between log LD_{50} and log MAC for slightly volatile or nonvolatile ones.

Research is expanding into the relationship between biochemical reactions determining the toxicity of a group of substances (e.g., cholinesterase inhibition by organophosphorus compounds) and quantum-chemical constants of the same substances. Classifying sets of substances in terms of their predominant toxic actions may be expected to permit much more accurate predictions. Attempts may be made to relate the toxicity indices of polymeric materials and some of their physicochemical characteristics. It is desirable to establish relationships between toxicity and MAC in the air of work areas for industrial poisons having some common predominant type of toxic action (e.g., irritant, narcotic, or hepatotropic).

The potential and importance of toxicity predictions based on correlations with physicochemical properties should not be overestimated. Nor, on the other hand, should they be underrated. Several instances may be cited where such correlations have proved very useful.

Calculations can provide information as to the dose or concentration with which to begin an experimental toxicity study of a new substance, resulting in reduced duration and lower cost of the experiment.

Calculation is the simplest and most rapid means of obtaining toxicity data in hygienic surveys of industrial environments where new compounds are likely to occur. Of great importance here is the possibility of calculating tentative MACs in the air, in particular for substances whose ranges of application are so limited that it would not make much sense to undertake laborious experimental determinations. Calculations may be used to advantage to determine temporary MACs of substances in work environments, to be adopted pending the completion of long-term chronic tests.

Recently, the establishment of correlations between MACs for workroom air and those for the atmosphere and water has increased the importance of MAC determinations by calculation.

While industrial toxicology was still taking its first steps, Nikolai V. Lazarev, a teacher of the present authors, insisted that a quantitative approach be used to assess research results, rightly believing that even very rough calculations can afford a much better understanding of an observed phenomenon than a purely qualitative description. Our generation is witnessing the triumphant march of mathematical methods into biology and medicine. Toxicology, and industrial toxicology in particular, is in a favorable position in this regard, for mathematical methods have already led to appreciable success.

REFERENCES

Abasov, D. M., "Toksikologicheskaya Kharacteristika Bakinskikh Benzinov i Deistviye ikh pri Razlichnykh Temperaturnykh Usloviyakh " ["Toxicological Characteristics of Gasolines from Baku Oil and Their Effects at Different Temperatures"], unpublished candidate's dissertation, Baku, 1967.

Abshagen, U., and N. Rietbrock, Kinetic der Elimination von 2-Propanol und seines Metaboliten Aceton bei Hund und Ratte, *Arch. Pharm.*, **26**, 110–118 (1969).

Agadzhanian, N. A., *Biologischeskiye Ritmy* [*Biological Rhythms*], Meditsina, Moscow, 1967.

Aivazian, S. A., *Statisticheskoye Issledovaniye Zavisimostei* [*Statistical Study of Relationships*], Metallurgiya, Moscow, 1968.

Albert, A., The relationship between structure and biological activity, *Ergeb. Physiol., Biol. Chem. Exp. Pharmakol.*, **49**, 425–461 (1957).

Albert, A., *Selective Toxicity and Related Topics*, 4th ed., Methuen, London, 1968.

Albert, A., *Selective Toxicity*, 5th ed., Chapman and Hall, London, 1973.

Anichkov, S. V., and M. L., Belenky, *Uchebnik Farmakologii* [*Textbook of Pharmacology*], Medgiz, Leningrad, 1954.

Atkins, G. C., *Multicompartment Models for Biological Systems*, Methuen, London, 1969.

Averianov, A. G., Evaluating the ambient air containing several harmful components, *Gig. Sanit.*, **8**, 64–67 (1957).

Badger, G. M., Biological activity of compounds in homologous series, *Nature*, **158**, 585 (1946).

Badger, G. M., *The Chemical Basis of Carcinogenic Activity*, Charles C. Thomas, Springfield, Ill., 1962. (Russian translation published in 1966 by Meditsina, Moscow.)

Baily, N. T. J., *Statistical Methods in Biology*, English Universities Press, London, 1959.

Ball, W. L., The toxicological basis of threshold limit values. 4. Theoretical approach to prediction of toxicity of mixtures, *Am. Ind. Hyg. Assoc. J.*, **20**, 357–363 (1959).

Barlow, R. B., *Introduction to Chemical Pharmacology*, 2nd ed., John Wiley, New York, 1964.

Belenky, M. L., On the quantitative assessment of the range of therapeutic action, *Farmakol. Toksikol.*, **22**(6), 566–568 (1959).

Belenky, M. L., *Elementy Kolichestvennoi Otsenki Farmakologicheskogo Effekta* [*Elements of the Quantitative Evaluation of Pharmacological Effects*], Medgiz, Leningrad, 1963.

Belenky, M. L., S. K. Germane, A. K. Aren, and G. Ya. Vanag, A new class of pharmacologically active substances with marked effects on the central nervous system, *Dokl. Akad. Nauk SSSR*, **134**, 217–220 (1960).

Bienvenu, P., C. Nofre, and A. Cier, Toxicité générale comparée des ions métalliques, *C.R. Acad. Sci.*, **256**, 1043–1044 (1963).

Biological Clocks, Cold Spring Harbor Symposia on Quantitative Biology, Vol. XXV, New York, 1961.

Biological Rhythms in Psychiatry and Medicine, Government Printing Office, Washington, D.C., 1970.

Bliss, C. J., The comparison of dosage-mortality data, *Ann. Appl. Biol.*, **22**, 307–333 (1935).

Bliss, C. J., The comparison of dosage-mortality data, *Ann. Appl. Biol.*, **24**, 815–852 (1937).

Bliss, C. J., Toxicity of poisons applied jointly, *Ann. Appl. Biol.*, **26**, 585–615 (1939).

Boček, K., J. Kopecký, M. Krivucova, and D. Vlachova, Biological activity and chemical structure, *Experientia*, **20**, 667–668 (1964).

Boček, K., J. Kopecký, M. Krivucova, and D. Vlachova, Chemical structure-biological activity correlations of disubstituted benzene derivatives, in *21st International Congress on Pure and Applied Chemistry, Prague, 1967, Abstracts of Papers: Toxicological Chemistry*, Prague, 1967.

Bolanowska, W., J. Piotrowski, and B. Trojanowska, Kinetika rozmieszczania i wydalania olowiu (Pb-210) u szczurów, *Med. Pr.*, **18**, 29–41 (1967).

Borodin, A., "Ob Analogii Myshiakovoi Kisloty s Fosfornoyu v Khimicheskom i Toksicheskom Otnosheniyakh" ["Concerning the Analogy between Arsenic and Phosphoric Acids in Chemical and Toxicological Respects"], dissertation, St. Petersburg, 1858.

Boyland, E., The biochemical mechanisms of induction of bladder cancer, in G. E. W. Wolstenholme and M. O'Connor, Eds., *CIBA Foundation Symposium on Carcinogenesis. Mechanisms of Action*, pp. 218–232, Churchill, London, 1959.

Bradbury, F. R., and G. Armstrong, A method for measuring the narcotic action of chemicals using the grain weevil, *Ann. Appl. Biol.*, **41**, 65–76 (1954).

Bradbury, F. R., and G. Armstrong, Chemical structure and narcotic potency to grain weevils, *Ann. Appl. Biol.*, **43**, 203–212 (1955).

Brakhnova, I. T., and G. V. Samsonov, The toxicity of some substances as related to their electronic structure, *Poroshk. Metall.*, **9**, 101–109 (1966).

Bray, H. G., and K. White, *Kinetics and Thermodynamics in Biochemistry*, 2nd ed., Academic Press, New York and London, 1966.

Bray, H. G., W. V. Thorpe, and K. White, Kinetic studies of the metabolism of foreign organic compounds. I. The formation of benzoic acid from benzamide, toluene, benzyl alcohol, and benzaldehyde and its conjugation with glycine and glucuronic acid in the rabbit, *Biochem. J.*, **48**, 88–96 (1951).

Bray, H. G., Z. Hybs, S. P. James, and W. V. Thorpe, The metabolism of 2:3:5:6- and

2:3:4:5-tetrachloronitrobenzenes in the rabbit and the reduction of aromatic nitro compounds in the intestine, *Biochem. J.*, **53**, 266–273 (1953).

Brink, F., and J. M. Posternak, Thermodynamic analysis of the relative effectiveness of narcotics, *J. Cell Comp. Physiol.*, **32**, 211–233 (1948).

Broitman, A. Ya., The toxicity of some classes of stabilizers for plastics, in E. F. Burmistrov, Ed., *Sintez i Issledovaniye Effektivnosti Stabilizatorov dlya Polimernykh Materialov*, pp. 228–234, Tsentralno-Chernozemnoye Knizhnoye Izdatelstvo, Voronezh, 1964.

Broitman, A. Ya., V. E. Gavrilova, L. V. Putilina, and E. G. Robachevskaya, Toxic properties of stabilizers for plastics, in S. L. Danishevsky, Ed., *Toksikologiya Vysokomolekulyarnykh Materialov i Khimicheskogo Syriya dlya ikh Sinteza*, p. 207, Khimiya, Moscow and Leningrad, 1966.

Brzezicka-Bak, M., and A. Bojanowska, Toksyczność podostra insektycydów fosforo-organicznych: naledu, etoudu, metylowego i supracida, *Rocz. Państw. Zakl. Hig.*, **20**(4), 463–469 (1969).

Bünning, E., *The Physiological Clock*, Springer-Verlag, Berlin, 1964.

Bürgi, E., *Die Arzneikombinationen*, Springer, Leipzig, 1938.

Burkatskaya, E. N., and V. I. Matiushina, The intermittent action of some pesticides, *Gigiyena Primeneniya. Toksikologiya Pestitsidov i Klinika Otravleniy*, No. 6, pp. 698–703, Institut Gigiyeny i Toksikologii Pestitsidov, Polimernykh i Prasticheskikh Mass, Kiev, 1968.

Burtt, E. T., The mode of action of sheep dips, *Ann. Appl. Biol.*, **32**, 247–260 (1945).

Byrde, R. J. W., D. R. Clifford, and D. Woodcock, Fungicidal activity and chemical constitution, *Ann. Appl. Biol.*, **46**, 167–177 (1958).

Cammarata, A., Interrelationship of the regression models used for structure-activity analyses, *J. Med. Chem.*, **15**(6), 573–577 (1972).

Cherkinsky, S. N., Studies on the establishment of hygienic standards for bodies of water: results and tasks for the future, *Sanitarnaya Okhrana Vodoyemov ot Zagriazneniya Promyshlennymi Stochnymi Vodami*, No. 6, pp. 7–28, Meditsina, Moscow, 1964.

Cherkinsky, S. N., Studies in water hygiene: current and possible future trends, *Gig. Sanit.*, **12**, 8–12 (1969).

Cherkinsky, S. N., G. N. Krasovsky, and V. N. Tugarinova, Methodological aspects of sanitary-toxicological studies on the establishment of hygienic standards, *Sanitarnaya Okhrana Vodoyemov ot Zagriazneniya Promyshlennymi Stochnymi Vodami*, No. 6, pp. 290–300, Meditsina, Moscow, 1964.

Chernukh, A. M., and Aleksandrov, P. N., *O Teratogennom Deistvii Khimicheskikh Veshchestv [Teratogenic Actions of Chemicals]*, Meditsina, Moscow, 1969.

Clark, A. J., *The Mode of Action of Drugs on Cells*, Arnold, London, 1933.

Clark, A. J., *General Pharmacology*, Springer-Verlag, Berlin, 1937.

Clayton, J. M., and W. P. Purcell, Hansch and Free-Wilson analyses of inhibitory potencies of some 1-decyl-3-carbamoylpiperidines against butyrylcholinesterase and comparison of the two methods, *J. Med. Chem.*, **12**, 1087–1088 (1969).

Cornfield, J., Comparative bioassays and the role of parallelism, *J. Pharmacol. Exp. Ther.*, **144**, 143–149 (1964).

Craig, P., Comparison of Hansch's and Free-Wilson's methods for structure-activity correlation, *Cancer Chemother. Rep.*, Part 2, **4**(4), 39 (1974).

Crisp, D. J., and D. H. A. Marr, Energy relationships in physical toxicity, in T. H. Schulman, Ed., *Solid–Liquid Interface and Cell–Water Interface*, pp. 310–320, 350–351, Butterworths Scientific Publications, London, 1957.

Cullen, S. C., and E. G. Gross, The anesthetic properties of xenon in animals and human beings, with additional observations on krypton, *Science*, **113**, 580–582 (1951).

Cummings, A. L., and B. K. Martin, Excretion and the accrual of drug metabolites, *Nature*, **200**, 1296–1297 (1963).

Cummings, A. L., B. K. Martin, and G. S. Park, Kinetic considerations relating to the accrual and elimination of drug metabolites, *Br. J. Pharm. Chemother.*, **29**, 136–149 (1967).

Denisenko, P. P., M. M. Ostrovsky, and K. A. Lisitsina, The toxicity of Chlorophos (Trichlorfon) for mice under various conditions of exposure to heat and physical exercise, *Gig. Sanit.*, **8**, 14–18 (1968).

Dettli, L., and P. Spring, Factors influencing drug elimination in man, *Farmaco, Ed. Sci.*, **23**, 795–812 (1968).

Discussion on the chemical and physical basis of pharmacological action, 12 Nov. 1936, *Proc. Roy. Soc., Ser. B*, **121**, 580–609 (1937).

Dobrynina, V. V., Variations in blood levels of acetone in animals during habituation to this compound, in E. I. Liublina and M. A. Elkin, Eds., *Materialy Vtoroi Konferentsii Molodykh Nauchnykh Rabotnikov*, pp. 46–49, Institut Gigiyeny Truda i Profzabolevaniy, Leningrad, 1968.

Dobrynina, V. V., and E. I. Liublina, Toxicological and hygienic characterization of ethylidene norbonane, vinyl norbornane, and tetrahydroindene, *Gig. Tr. Prof. Zabol.*, **10**, 52–54 (1974).

Dominguez, R., Kinetics of elimination, absorption and volume of distribution in the organism, *Med. Phys.*, **2**, 476–489 (1950).

Doskin, V. A., The sensitivity of adolescents and young people to industrial poisons, *Gig. Sanit.*, **9**, 99–103 (1969).

Dost, F. H., *Der Blutspiegel: Kinetik der Konzentrationsabläufe in der Kreislaufflüssigkeit*, Georg Thieme, Leipzig, 1953.

Dost, F. H., and G. Medgyesi, Zur Bestimmung der Parameter von Bateman Funktionen, *Z. Naturforsch.*, **19b**, 174–176 (1964).

Druckrey, H., Grundlagen der toxikologischen Methodik, *Arzneimittelforsch.*, **7**, 449–456 (1957).

Dvorkin, E. A., The toxicity of substituted esters of phosphoric acid, in V. E. Kovshillo Ed., *Materialy Nauchnoi Sessii, Posviashchennoi Itogam Raboty Instituta za 1968–1969 Gody*, Institut Gigiyeny Truda i Profzabolevaniy, Leningrad, 1970.

Elizarova, O. N., *Opredeleniye Porogovykh Doz Promyshlennykh Yadov pri Peroralnom*

Vvedenii [*Determination of Threshold Doses of Industrial Poisons Administered* per os], Meditsina, Moscow, 1971.

Emme, A. M., *Chasy Zhivoi Prirody* [*Clocks of the Living Nature*], Sovetskaya Rossiya, Moscow, 1962.

Emme, A. M., *Biologocheskiye Chasy* [*Biological Clocks*], Nauka, Novosibirsk, 1967.

Ermakov, N. V., Medical properties of some film-forming agents and their mixtures, *Med. Parazitol.*, **3**, 42–54 (1943).

Ezekiel, M., and K. A. Fox, *Methods of Correlation and Regression Analysis*, 3rd ed., John Wiley, New York, 1959.

Fairhall, L. T., *Industrial Toxicology*, 2nd ed., Williams and Wilkins, Baltimore, 1957.

Fedorov, E. A., Patterns of distribution and elimination of ether during anesthesia, *Klin. Khir.*, **8**, 60–64 (1963).

Ferguson, J., The use of chemical potentials as indices of toxicity, *Proc. Roy. Soc., Ser. B*, **127**, 387–404 (1939).

Ferguson, J., Relations between thermodynamic indices of narcotic potency and the molecular structure of narcotics, in *CNRS, 26, Méchanisme de la Narcose*, pp. 25–39, Paris, 1951.

Ferguson, J., and S. W. Hawkins, Toxic action of some simple gases at high pressure, *Nature*, **164**, 963–964 (1949).

Ferguson, J., and H. Pirie, The toxicity of vapors to the grain weevil, *Ann. Appl. Biol.*, **35**, 532–550 (1948).

Ferguson, J., S. W. Hawkins, and D. Doxey, c-Mitotic action of some simple gases, *Nature*, **165**, 1021–1022 (1950).

Filov, V. A., Determination of solubility coefficients for vapors of some esters, in N. V. Lazarev and I. D. Gadaskina, Eds., *Materialy po Toksikologii Veshchestv, Primeniayemykh v Proizvodstve Plasticheskikh Mass i Sinteticheskikh Kauchukov*, pp. 61–62, Institut Gigiyeny Truda i Profzabolevaniy, Leningrad, 1957a.

Filov, V. A., The thermodynamic activity and two-phase toxicity, in *Tesizy Vsesoiuznogo Soveshchaniya po Probleme Mekhanizmov Farmakologicheskikh Reaktsiy*, pp. 120–122, Akad. Nauk Latviyskoi SSR, Riga, 1957b.

Filov, V. A., The thermodynamic activity of some industrial poisons, in Z. E. Grigoriev, Ed., *Trudy Nauchnoi Sessii, Posviashchennoi Itogam Raboty Instituta Gigiyeny Truda za 1958 God*, pp. 223–231, Institut Gigiyeny Truda i Profzabolevaniy, Leningrad, 1959a.

Filov, V. A., On the fate of vinyl esters and fatty acids in the body, *Gig. Tr. Prof. Zabol.*, **5**, 42–46 (1959b).

Filov, V. A., Retention and transformation of low-molecular weight esters in the body, *Gig. Tr. Prof. Zabol.*, **3**, 14–19 (1961a).

Filov, V. A., On the fate of methyl acetate in the body, *Farmakol. Toksikol.*, **24**(2), 224–226 (1961b).

Filov, V. A., The thermodynamic activity of volatile organic compounds acting on mammals, *Biofizika*, **7**(1), 73–79 (1962).

Filov, V. A., Toxic action of industrially used organic compounds and the thermodynamic activity, *Trudy Ufimskogo NII Gigiyeny Truda i Profzabolevanii*, Vol. 2, pp. 281–289, Ufa, 1963a.

Filov, V. A., Esterase activity in the blood of animals of various species, *Biull. Eksp. Biol. Med.*, **51**(4), 45–46 (1963b).

Filov, V. A., The absorption kinetics of substances freely penetrating into and undergoing degradation in biological systems, *Dokl. Akad. Nauk SSSR*, **157**(4), 1006–1009 (1964a).

Filov, V. A., Comparative narcotic potency of methyl and ethyl acetate and their metabolic products, *Farmakol. Toksikol.*, **27**(4), 492–493 (1964b).

Filov, V. A., Kinetic aspects of the absorption, distribution, metabolism, and elimination of extraneous chemical agents, in G. A. Stepansky, Ed., *Farmakologiya. Toksikologiya, Problemy Toksikologii*, pp. 45–92, VINITI, Moscow, 1967.

Filov, V. A., A study on the behavior of cyclohexylamine and dicyclohexylamine in the body, *Gig. Tr. Prof. Zabol.*, **7**, 29–33 (1968).

Filov, V. A., A kinetic model for the accumulation in the body of gaseous substances which are inhaled periodically, *Dokl. Akad. Nauk SSSR*, **184**(6), 1458–1460 (1969).

Filov, V. A., Mathematical aspects of pharmacokinetics and toxicokinetics, in *Farmakologiya. Khimioterapevticheskiye sredstva. Toksikologiya. Problemy Farmakologii*, Vol. 5, pp. 9–80, VINITI: *Itogi Nauki i Tekhniki* Series, Moscow, 1973.

Filov, V. A., and I. D. Gadaskina, Some prospects for the development of analytical toxicology, in N. V. Lazarev, A. A. Golubev, and E. T. Lykhina, Eds., *Aktualniye Voprosy Promyshlennoi Toksikologii*, pp. 161–168, Institut Gigiyeny Truda i Profzabolevaniy, Leningrad, 1970.

Filov, V. A., and E. I. Liublina, Relation of the toxic action of volatile organic compounds to their physicochemical properties, *Biofizika*, **10**(4), 602–608 (1965).

Filov, V. A., and E. S. Mironos, Calculation of the main parameters characterizing fatty tissues as a depot for benzene and carbon disulfide, in V. E. Kovshillo, Ed., *Voprosy Gigiyeny Truda i Professionalnoi Patologii*, pp. 155–158, Institut Gigiyeny Truda i Profzabolevaniy, Leningrad, 1967.

Finney, D. J., *Probit Analysis: A Statistical Treatment of the Sigmoid Response Curve*, 2nd ed., Cambridge University Press, London, 1952.

Finney, D. J., *Probit Analysis*, 3rd ed., Cambridge University Press, Cambridge, 1971.

Fisher, R. A., *Statistical Methods for Research Workers*, 12th ed., Oliver and Boyd, Edinburgh and London, 1954.

Flury, F., and W. Wirth, Zur Toxikologie der Lösungsmittel, *Arch. Gewerbepathol. Gewerbehyg.*, **5**, 1–90 (1933).

Flury, F., and F. Zernik, *Schädliche Gase*, Springer, Berlin, 1931.

Fomenko, V. N., Genetic implications of exposure to industrial substances, in *Otdalenniye Posledstviya Vliyaniya na Cheloveka Khimicheskikh Veschestv, Primeniayemykh v Promyshlennosti i Selskom Khoziaystve. Nauchniy Obsor*, pp. 66–100, Vsesoyuzniy Institut Meditsinskoi i Mediko-Tekhnicheskoi Informatsii, Moscow, 1969.

428   References

Free, S. M., and J. W. Wilson, A mathematical contribution to structure-activity studies, *J. Med. Chem.*, **7**, 395–399 (1964).

Fridliand, I. G., Some aspects of occupational hygiene for women and adolescents, in Z. I. Izraelson and Z. B. Smeliansky, Eds., *Rukovodstvo po Gigiyene Truda*, Vol. 2, pp. 608–635, Medgiz, Moscow, 1963.

Frolkis, V. V., *Regulirovaniye, Prisposobleniye i Stareniye* [*Regulation, Adaptation, and Aging*], Nauka, Leningrad, 1970.

Fühner, H., Über die Einwirkung verschiedener Alkohole auf die Entwicklung der Seeigel, *Arch. Exp. Pathol. Pharmakol.*, **51**, 1–10 (1904).

Fühner, H., Pharmakologische Studien an Seeigeleiern, *Arch. Exp. Pathol. Pharmakol.*, **52**, 69–82 (1905).

Fühner, H., Die Wirkungsstärke der Narkotika. I, *Biochem. Z.*, **120**, 143–163 (1921).

Fühner, H., Die Wirkungsstärke der Narkotika. II, *Biochem. Z.*, **139**, 216–224 (1923).

Gadaskina, I. D., Absorption of irritant gases in the respiratory tract, *Fiziol. Zh. SSSR*, **23**(6), 782–790 (1937).

Gadaskina, I. D., The retention of vapors of some narcotics in the upper respiratory tract, *Farmakol. Toksikol.*, **12**(4), 26–29 (1949).

Gadaskina, I. D., E. I. Liublina, N. A. Minkina, and M. L. Rylova, The effect of carbon monoxide on animals in chronic experiments, in *Materialy Nauchnoi Sessii, Posviashchennoi Itogam Raboty Instituta za 1959–1960 Gody*, pp. 42–43, Institut Gigiyeny Truda i Profzabolevaniy, Leningrad, 1961.

Gaddum, J. H., Reports on biological standards. III. Methods of biological assay depending on a quantal response, *Medical Research Council Special Report Series*, No. 183, pp. 1–46, London, 1933.

Gaddum, J. H., The estimation of the safe dose, *Br. J. Pharmacol.*, **11**, 156–160 (1956).

Garrett, E. R., and C. D. Alway, Drug distribution and dosage: complex pharmacological models and the analog computer, in *Proceedings, 3rd International Congress on Chemotherapy, Stuttgart, 1963*, Vol. 2, pp. 1666–1686, Georg Thieme Verlag, Stuttgart, 1964.

Gary-Bobo, C., and B. A. Lindenberg, Concentration thermodynamique liminaire des hydrocarbures et derivés polaires au seuil de leur action physiologique sur le poisson, *C.R. Acad. Sci.*, **234**, 2111–2113 (1952).

Gavaudan, P., *Pharmacodynamie de l'Inhibition de la Caryocinèse*, Libr. Le François, Paris, 1947.

Gavaudan, P., and H. Poussel, Le méchanisme de l'action insecticide du dichlorodiphenyl-trichloroéthane, *C.R. Acad. Sci.*, **224**, 683–685 (1947).

Gavaudan, P., H. Poussel, and M. Dode, Comparison du pouvoir mito-inhibiteur des substances de la série aromatique, *C.R. Soc. Biol.*, **138**, 267–268 (1944a).

Gavaudan, P., M. Dode, and H. Poussel, La toxicité générale et la notion d'activité thermodynamique, *Mem. Serv. Chim. État*, **31**, 384–423 (1944b).

Gizatullina, N. S., Identification of the cumulative effect, in N. V. Lazarev, A. A. Golubev, and E. T. Lykhina, Eds., *Aktualniye Voprosy Promyshlennoi Toksikologii*, pp. 202–208, Institut Gigiyeny Truda i Profzabolevanii, Leningrad, 1970.

Gizatullina, N. S., Quantitative evaluation of cumulation at the threshold level, in *Primeneniye Matematicheskikh Metodov dlya Otsenki i Prognozirovaniya Realnoi Opasnosti Nakopleniya Pestitsidov vo Vneshnei Srede i Organizme. Materialy Pervogo Simpoziuma*, pp. 67–71, Institut Gigiyeny i Toksikologii Pestitsidov, Polimernykh i Plasticheskikh Mass i Institut Kibernetiki Akad. Nauk. Ukr. SSR, Kiev, 1971.

Golikov, P. P., *Vremena Goda, Organizm i Lecheniye* [*The Seasons, the Organism and Medication*], Dalnevostochnoye Knizhnoye Izdatelstvo, Vladivostok, 1968.

Golubev, A. A., "K Toksikologii Nekotorykh Slozhnykh Efirov Vinilovogo Spirta" ["The Toxicology of Some Vinyl Esters"], unpublished candidate's dissertation, Leningrad, 1956.

Golubev, A. A., The toxicology of some vinyl esters. The relative toxicities in the homologous series of esters, in N. V. Lazarev and I. D. Gadaskina, Eds., *Materialy po Toksikologii Veshchestv, Primenyayemykh v Proizvodstve Plasticheskikh Mass i Sinteticheskikh Kauchukov*, pp. 66–75 and 82–87, Institut Gigiyeny Truda i Profzabolevaniy, Leningrad, 1957.

Golubev, A. A., The application in industrial toxicology of computing methods for estimating approximate values of some constants and indices, in N. V. Lazarev, Ed., *Voprosy Obshchei Promyshlennoi Toksikologii*, pp. 23–31, Institut Gigiyeny Truda i Profzabolevaniy, Leningrad, 1963.

Golubev, A. A., Use of computing methods for establishing maximum allowable concentrations for irritant gases, in N. V. Lazarev, A. A. Golubev, and E. T. Lykhina, Eds., *Aktualniye Voprosy Promyshlennoi Toksikologii*, pp. 72–82, Institut Gigiyeny Truda i Profzabolevaniy, Leningrad, 1970.

Golubev, A. A., and V. Ya. Rusin, The relationship between toxicity and chemical structure, in Z. I. Izraelson and Z. B. Smeliansky, Eds., *Rukovodstvo po Gigiyene Truda*, Vol. 2, pp. 109–121, Medgiz, Moscow, 1963.

Gorn, L. E., Individual differences in sensitivity to methemoglobin-forming agents: causes and methods of detection, *Gig. Tr. Prof. Zabol.*, **8**, 21–25 (1966).

Gramenitsky, M. I. *Obshchaya Farmakologiya* [*General Pharmacology*], OGIZ, Moscow and Leningrad, 1931.

Guseinov, T. A., "Sravnitelnaya Toksikologicheskaya Kharakteristika Propilaminov" ["Comparative Toxicological Characteristics of Propylamines"], unpublished candidate's dissertation, Moscow, 1967.

Gusev, M. I., A practical approach to the study of joint action of toxic substances present in the air in low concentrations, *Gig. Sanit.*, **8**, 99–102 (1970).

Hadaway, A. B., and F. Barlow, Some aspects of the effect of the solvent on the toxicity of solutions of insecticide, *Ann. Appl. Biol.*, **46**, 133–148 (1958).

Hammett, L. P., *Physical Organic Chemistry*, McGraw-Hill, New York and London, 1940; 2nd ed., 1970.

Hansch, C., The use of substituent constants in structure-activity studies, in *Proceedings, 3rd International Pharmacological Meeting, São Paulo, 1966*, Vol. 7, pp. 141–167, Pergamon, New York, 1968.

Hansch, C., A quantitative approach to biochemical structure-activity relationships, Acc. Chem. Res., **2**, 232–239 (1969).

Hansch, C., E. J. Lien, and F. Helmer, Structure-activity correlations in the metabolism of drugs, Arch. Biochem. Biophys., **128**, 319–330 (1968).

Hassal, K. A., Toxicity to the grain weevil of some alkyl compounds applied as vapors, Ann. Appl. Biol., **40**, 688–704 (1953).

Hassal, K. A., Relationships between the chemical constitution and fumigant toxicity of the alkyl iodides, Ann. Appl. Biol., **43**, 615–629 (1955).

Henderson, Y., and H. Haggard, Noxious Gases, Reinhold, New York, 1927.

Horsfall, J. G., Fungicides and Their Action, Chronica Botanica, Waltham, Mass., 1945.

Horsfall, J. G., Principals of Fungicidal Action, Chronica Botanica, Waltham, Mass., 1956.

Hurst, H., Principles of insecticidal action as a guide to drug reactivity-phase distribution relationships, Trans. Faraday Soc., **39**, 390–412 (1943).

Hurst, H., Biophysical factors in drug action, Brit. Med. Bull., **3**, 132–137 (1945).

Ivens, G. W., The phytotoxicity of mineral oils and hydrocarbons, Ann. Appl. Biol., **39**, 418–422 (1952).

Johnson, F. H., E. A. Flagler, R. Simpson, and K. McGeer, The inhibition of bacterial luminescence by a homologous series of carbamates, J. Cell. Comp. Physiol., **37**, 1–13 (1951).

Kagan, Yu. S., Toksikologiya Fosforoorganicheskikh Insektitsidov i Gigiyena Truda pri ikh Primenenii [The Toxicology of Organophosphorus Insecticides and Occupational Hygiene during Their Use], Medgiz, Moscow, 1963a.

Kagan, Yu. S., The toxicity of some organophosphorus insecticides acting jointly, in Gigiyena i Fiziologiya Truda, Proizvodstvennaya Toksikogiya, Klinika Professionalnykh Zabolevanii, pp. 59–62, Gosmetizdat USSR, Kiev, 1963b.

Kagan, Yu. S., Quantitative criteria of hazards from chemicals, in L. I. Medved, Ed., Gigiyena i Toksikologiya Pestitsidov i Klinika Otravleniy, pp. 46–59, Zdoroviye, Kiev, 1965.

Kagan, Yu. S., Toward a comprehensive quantitative approach to the study of hazards from pesticides, Gigiyena Primeneniya, Toksikologiya Pestitsidov i Klinika Otravleniy, No. 6, pp. 81–93, Institut Gigiyeny i Toksikologii Pestitsidov, Polimernykh i Plasticheskikh Mass, Kiev, 1968.

Kagan, Yu. S., Cumulation: criteria and methods of evaluation. Prediction of chronic intoxications, in A. A. Letavet and I. V. Sanotsky, Eds., Printsipy i Metody Ustanovleniya Predelno Dopustimykh Kontsentratsii Vrednykh Veshchestv i Vozdukhe Proizvodstvennykh Pomeshchenii, pp. 49–65, Meditsina, Moscow, 1970.

Kagan, Yu. S., and V. V. Stankevich, The coefficient of cumulation as a quantitative criterion, in G. M. Mukhametova, Ed., Aktualniye Voprosy Gigiyeny Truda, Promyshlennoi Toksikologii i Professionalnoi Patologii v Neftianoi i Neftekhimicheskoi Promyshlennosti, pp. 48–49, Ufimskiy Institut Gigiyeny Truda i Profzabolevaniy, Ufa, 1964.

Kagan, Yu. S., T. N. Panshina, and E. A. Antonovich, Guidelines for the study of cumulation of pesticides, *Gigiyena Primeneniya, Toksikologiya Pestitsidov i Klinika Otravleniy*, No. 6, pp. 691–697, Institut Gigiyeny i Toksikologii Pestitsidov, Polimernykh i Plasticheskikh Mass, Kiev, 1968.

Kagan, Yu. S., L. M. Sasinovich, and G. I. Ovseenko, The application of correlation analysis to indices of toxicity and of cumulation in establishing hygienic standards for pesticides in the air of workplaces, *Gig. Tr. Prof. Zabol.*, **8**, 21–25 (1972).

Kaminsky, L. S., *Izmereniye Sviazi (Korreliatsiya) [Measurement of Relationships (Correlation)]*, Leningradskiy Universitet, Leningrad, 1962.

Kapkayev, E. A., and V. A. Sukhanova, The effect of a-methylstyrene on the organism at elevated temperatures, *Gig. Tr. Prof. Zabol.*, **5**, 11–15 (1968).

Karasik, V. M., Curves of individual sensitivity to pharmacological action, *Usp. Sovrem. Biol.*, **17**(I), 71–86 (1944).

Katsnelson, B. A., Deposition, elimination, and retention of dust in the lungs, in G. A. Stepansky, Ed., *Itogi Nauki i Tekniki. Toksikologiya*, Vol. 7, pp. 7–23, VINITI, Moscow, 1976.

Katsnelson, B. A., and L. G. Babushkina, Sex differences in susceptibility to silicosis, *Gig. Sanit.*, **3**, 29–32, (1969).

Kaye, G. W. C., and T. H. Laby, *Tables of Physical and Chemical Constants and Some Mathematical Functions*, 11th ed., Longmans, Green, London, 1957.

Khadzhai, Ya. I., On graphic methods of determining the effective dose and its confidence limits in graded response assays, *Farmakol. Toksikol.*, **28**(1), 118–122 (1965).

Khalepo, A. I., "Toksikologicheskaya Kharakteristika Toluola v Zavisimosti ot Vvedeniya v ego Molekulu Razlichnykh Zamestitielei" ["Toxicological Characteristics of Toluene Depending on the Introduction of Different Substituents into Its Molecule"], unpublished candidate's dissertation, Moscow, 1969.

Khokhlov, V. A., and A. Ya. Broitman, Estimating the index of cumulative hazard, in *Primeneniye Matematicheskikh Metodov dlya Otsenki i Prognozirovaniya Realnoi Opasnosti Nakopleniya Pestitsidov vo Vnesnei Srede i Organizme. Materialy Pervogo Simpoziuma*, pp. 53–56, Institut Gigieny i Toksikologii Pestitsidov, Polimernykh i Plasticheskikh Mass i Institut Kibernetiki Akad. Nauk Ukr. SSR, Kiev, 1971.

Kist, A. A., Relationships between the toxicity of elements and their body contents, in *Aktivatsionniy Analiz Biologicheskikh Obiektov*, pp. 87–91, Fan, Tashkent, 1967.

Klenova, E. V., Discontinuous (intermittent) exposure to industrial poisons, *Gig. Sanit.*, **2**, 27–31 (1949).

Klinskaya, K. S., Relationship between the chemical structure of substances and their capacity to be concentrated by the kidneys, in G. Ya. Kingisepp, Ed., *Tezisy Dokladov Soveshchaniya po Probleme Sviazi mezhdu Strukturoi i Deistviyem Lekarstvennykh Veshchestv*, p. 46, Tartusskiy Universitet, Tartu, 1956.

Kobozev, N. I., Catalysts and enzymes, *Uch. Zap. Mosk. Gos. Univ.*, **174**, 125–154 (1955).

Kodama, J. K., H. H. Anderson, M. K. Dunlop, and C. H. Hine, Toxicity of organophosphorus compounds. I. Structure-action relationships, *Arch. Ind. Health*, **11**, 487–493 (1955).

Komarov, F. I., L. V. Zakharov, and V. A. Lisovsky, *Sutochniy Ritm Fiziologicheskikh Funktsii u Zdorovogo i Bolnogo Cheloveka [Diurnal Rhythms of Physiological Functions in Man in Health and Disease]*, Meditsina, Leningrad, 1966.

Kopecký, J., and K. Boček, A correlation between constants used in structure-activity relationships, *Experientia*, **23**, 125–129 (1967).

Kopecký, J., Boček, and D. Vlachova, Chemical structure and biological activity of *m*- and *p*-disubstituted derivatives of benzene, *Nature*, **207**, 981 (1965).

Korbakova, A. I., Establishing standards for new chemicals in the air of working premises: some problems of current interest, *Vestn. Akad. Med. Nauk SSSR*, **7**, 17–23 (1964).

Korbakova, A. I., G. N. Zayeva, S. N. Kremneva, L. A. Timofievskaya, and N. G. Ivanov, Evaluation of the joint action of products of thermo-oxidative destruction and some aspects of air quality monitoring in industry, *Toksikologiya Novykh Promyshlennykh Khimicheskikh Veshchestv*, No. 11, pp. 24–33, Meditsina, Moscow, 1969.

Korbakova, A. I., N. G. Ivanov, and S. N. Kremneva, Maximum allowable concentrations of mixtures, in A. A. Letavet and I. V. Sanotsky, Eds, *Printsipy i Metody Ustanovleniya Predelano Dopustimykh Kontsentratsii Vrednykh Veshchestv v Vozdukhe Proizvodstvennykh Pomeshchenii*, pp. 120–129, Meditsina, Moscow, 1970.

Krasovsky, G. N., Comparative sensitivity of man and laboratory animals to toxic agents, in A. V. Roshchin and I. V. Sanotsky, Eds., *Obshchiye Voprosy Promyshlennoi Toksikologii, Institut Gigiyeny Truda i Profzabolevaniy*, pp. 59–62, Moscow, 1967.

Krasovsky, G. N., "Modelirovaniye Intoksikatsii i Obosnovaniye Usloviy Ekstrapoliatsii Eksperimentalnykh Dannykh s Zhivotnykh na Cheloveka pri Reshenii Zadach Gigiyenicheskogo Normirovaniya" ["Simulation of Intoxications and Extrapolation of Animal Data to Man in Solving Problems Involved in the Establishment of Hygienic Standards"], unpublished doctoral dissertation, Moscow, 1973.

Krasovsky, G. N., and A. A. Korolev, Some observations on studies into the state of adaptation, *Gig. Sanit.*, **2**, 23–26 (1969).

Krasovsky, G. N., and S. A. Shigan, Evaluation of the mechanism of cumulative action by toxic substances, *Gig. Sanit.*, **1**, 17–21 (1970).

Krasovsky, G. N., and S. A. Shigan, Designing an optimum procedure for studying the cumulative properties of substances, in S. N. Cherkinsky, Ed., *Nauchno-Tekhnicheskiy Progress i Profilakticheskaya Meditsina*, Part I, pp. 84–88, Perviy Moskovskiy Meditsinskiy Institut, Moscow, 1971.

Krasovsky, G. N., and O. R. Sobiniakova, The comparative sensitivity of man and animals to various substances as assessed from indices of acute toxicity, *Gig. Sanit.*, **4**, 29–34 (1970).

Krasovsky, G. N., A. A. Korolev, N. T. Beliayeva, S. P. Varshavskaya, K. V. Kutakov, R. T. Malikova, and M. B. Trakhtman, Comparative sensitivity of man and laboratory animals to chemical agents, *Gig. Sanit.*, **1**, 45–49 (1969).

Krasovsky, G. N., A. A. Korolev, and S. A. Shigan, On methods for studying cumulative properties of toxic substances, *Gig. Sanit.*, **3**, 83–88 (1970a).

Krasovsky, G. N., A. A. Korolev, and S. A. Shigan, Relevance of adaptation for the study of cumulative properties of substances, in S. N. Cherkinsky, Ed., *Organizm i Sreda*, Part I, p. 75, Perviy Moskovskiy Meditsinskiy Institut, Moscow, 1970b.

Krasovsky, G. N., S. A. Shigan, B. R. Vitvitskaya, and M. V. Arsenieva, A method for the study of cumulative properties of substances by calculating their effective doses using body function tests, in *Primeneniye Matematicheskikh Metodov dlya Otsenki i Prognozirovaniya Realnoi Opasnosti Nakopleniya Pestitsidov vo Vneshnei Srede i Organizme. Materialy Pervogo Simpoziuma*, pp. 47–51, Institut Gigiyeny i Toksikologii Pestitsidov, Polimernykh i Plasticheskikh Mass i Institut Kibernetiki Akad. Nauk Ukr. SSR, Kiev, 1971

Kritsman, M. G., and A. S. Konikova, *Induktsiya Fermentov v Norme i Patologii [Enzyme Induction in Health and in Disease]*, Meditsina, Moscow, 1968.

Krolenko, S. A., and N. N. Nikolsky, Cell permeability for nonelectrolytes, in *Trudy XI Siezda Vsesoiuznogo Fiziologicheskogo Obshchestva im. I. P. Pavlova*, Vol. 1, pp. 3–7, Nauka, Leningrad, 1970.

Krotkov, F. G., and G. I. Sidorenko, A tentative forecast of research trends in the field of general and communal hygiene for the next 10 to 15 years, *Gig. Sanit.*, **1**, 11–15 (1970).

Krüger-Thiemer, E., Die Lösung chemotherapeutischer Probleme durch programmgesteuerte Ziffernrechenautomaten, *Arzneimittelforsch*, **14**, 1334–1343 (1964).

Krüger-Thiemer, E., W. Diller, L. Dettli, and P. Bünger, Demonstration des Einflusses der Eiweissbindung und der Ionisation auf die Pharmakokinetik am kombinierten gaskinetischen Modell nach Van Hoff und Langmuir, *Antibiot. Chemother.*, **12**, 171–193 (1964).

Kudrin, A. N., and G. T. Ponomareva, *Primeneniye Matematiki v Eksperimentalnoi i Klinicheskoi Meditsine [The Application of Mathematics in Experimental and Clinical Medicine]*, Meditsina, Moscow, 1967.

Kulagina, N. K., and T. A. Kochetkova, Comparative toxicological characteristics of organosilicon monomers and polymers, *Toksikologiya Novykh Promyshlennykh Khimicheskikh Veshchestv*, No. 10, pp. 82–90, Meditsina, Moscow, 1968.

Kulagina, N. K., A. I. Korbakova, and T. A. Kochetkova, Comparative toxicity of some organosilicon monomers, *Toksikologiya Novykh Promyshlennykh Khimicheskikh Veshchestv*, No. 3, pp. 81–101, Medgiz, Moscow, 1961.

Kulikov, M. A., and Yu. R. Malashenko, A simplified method for evaluating the accuracy of theoretical mortality curves, *Farmak. Toksikol.*, **29**(5), 621–624 (1966).

Kustov, V. V., and L. A. Tiunov, Evaluation of ambient air containing several harmful agents, *Gig. Sanit.*, **7**, 92–93 (1960).

Laffort, P., Efficacité odorante et activité thermodynamique, *Fr. Parfums*, **9**, 75–86 (1966).

Larrabee, M. G., and D. A. Holaday, Depression of transmission through sympathetic ganglia during general anesthesia, *J. Pharmol. Exp. Ther.*, **105**, 400–408 (1952).

Larrabee, M. G., and J. M. Posternak, Selective action of anesthetics on synapses and axons in mammalian sympathetic ganglia, *J. Neurophys.*, **15**, 91–114 (1952).

Larson, P. S., T. K. Finnegan, and H. B. Haag, Observations on the effect of chemical configuration on the edema-producing potency of acids, aldehydes, ketones, and alcohols, *J., Pharmol. Exp. Ther.*, **116**, 119–122 (1956).

Lawrence, J. H., W. F. Loomis, C. A. Tobias, and F. H. Turpin, Preliminary observations on the narcotic effect of xenon with a review of values for solubilities of gases in water and oils, *J. Physiol.*, **105**, 197–204 (1946).

Lazarev, N. V., *Obshchiye Osnovy Promyshlennoi Toksikologii* [*General Principles of Industrial Toxicology*], Medgiz, Moscow and Leningrad, 1938.

Lazarev, N. V., *Narkotiki* [*Narcotics*], Institut Gigiyeny Truda i Profzabolevaniy, Leningrad, 1940a.

Lazarev, N. V., The problem of maximum allowable concentrations of harmful substances in the air of working premises, in Z. E. Grigoryev and I. T. Fridliand, Eds., *Sbornik Rabot po Gigiyene Truda, Professionalnym Bolezniam i Ekspertize Trudosposobnosti*, pp. 7–38, Institut Vrachebno-Trudovoi Ekspertizy, Leningrad, 1940b.

Lazarev, N. V., *Biologicheskoye Geistviye Gazov pod Davleniyem* [*The Biological Action of Gases under Pressure*], Voyenno-Morskaya Meditsinskaya Akademiya, Leningrad, 1941.

Lazarev, N. V., *Neelektrolity* [*Nonelectrolytes*], Voyenno-Morskaya Meditsinskaya Akademiya, Leningrad, 1944.

Lazarev, N. V., *Obshchee Ucheniye o Narkotikakh i Narkoze* [*A General Theory of Narcotics and Narcosis*], Voenno-Morskaya Meditsinskaya Akademiya, Leningrad, 1958.

Lazarev, N. V., and V. A. Filov, The importance of "two-phase toxicity" and "thermodynamic activity" for toxicology, *Gig. Tr. Prof. Zabol.*, **4**, 19–24 (1964).

Lazarev, N. V., and M. A. Rozin, Nonspecific adaptive responses, in *Voprosy Tsitologii i Obshchei Fiziologii*, pp. 237–248, Izdatelstvo Akad. Nauk SSSR: Leningradskoye Otdeleniye, Leningrad, 1960.

Lazarev, N. V., and T. V. Staritsina, Experience with the consideration of physicochemical properties of organic poisons in relation to products of their transformation in the body, *Fiziol. Zh. SSSR*, **18**(5), 834–846 (1935).

Lazarev, N. V., A. I. Brusilovskaya, and I. N. Lavrov, On methods for the comparative study of penetration of organic substances through the skin, *Russ. Fiziol. Zh.*, **14**, No. 2–3, 284–289 (1931).

Lazarev, N. V., A. I. Brusilovskaya, and I. N. Lavrov, A quantitative study on the absorption of some organic substances into the blood through the skin, *Gig. Bezop. Tr.*, **2**, 52–62 (1933).

Lazarev, N. V., E. I. Liublina, and R. Ya. Madorskaya, Biological action of xenon, *Fiziol. Zh. SSSR*, **34**(1), 131–134 (1948).

Lazarev, N. V., E. I. Liublina, and M. A. Rozin, The state of nonspecifically enhanced resistivity, *Patol. Fiziol. Eksp. Ter.*, **4**, 16–21 (1959).

Lehmann, K. B., *Kurzes Lehrbuch der Arbeits- und Gewerbehygiene*, Verlag von S. Hirzel, Leipzig, 1919.

Lester, D., and L. A. Greenberg, The inhalation of ethyl alcohol by man, *Quart. J. Stud. Alcohol.*, **12**, 167–173 (1951).

Letavet, A. A., Establishment of MACs for toxic agents: principles and practices, in A. A. Letavet and A. A. Kanarevskaya, Eds., *Promyshlennaya Toksikologiya i Klinika Professionalnykh Zabolevaniy Khimicheskoi Etiologii*, pp. 3–5, Medgiz, Moscow, 1962.

Levina, E. N., Relationship between the irritant action of nonelectrolytes and their physicochemical properties, in *Referaty Rabot LenNII Gigiyeny Truda i Profzabolevanii za 1951 G.*, pp. 102–108, Institut Gigiyeny Truda i Profzabolevaniy, Leningrad, 1952.

Levina, E. N., *Obshchaya Toksikologiya Metallov* [*General Toxicology of Metals*], Meditsina, Leningrad, 1972.

Levy, G., Relationship between rate of elimination of tubocurarine and rate of decline of its pharmacological activity, *Br. J. Anaesth.*, **36**, 694–695 (1964).

Levy, G., and E. Nelson, Theoretical relationship between dose, elimination rate, and duration of pharmacologic effect of drugs, *J. Pharm. Sci.*, 54, 812 (1965).

Lim, K. S., K. G. Rink, K. G. Glass, and E. Soaje-Echague, A method for the evaluation of cumulation and tolerance by the determination of acute and subchronic median effective doses, *Arch. Intern. Pharm. Ther.*, **130**, 336–352 (1961).

Lindenberg, A. B., Isotoxicité des hydrocarbures aromatiques, *C. R. Acad. Sci.*, **241**, 2011–2013 (1955).

Lindenberg, A. B., Densité d'énergie cohesive et activité thermodynamique des composés aliphatiques et aromatiques au seuil de leur action toxiques reversible, *C. R. Acad. Sci.*, **242**, 2880–2883, (1956).

Lindenberg, B. A., and C. Gary-Bobo, Concentration thermodynamique narcotisante des alcohols, *C. R. Acad. Sci.*, **233**, 212–214 (1951).

Lindenberg, B. A., and C. Gary-Bobo, La narcose alcoholique chez les poissons, *Arch. Sci. Physiol.*, **6**, 3–24 (1952).

Lindenberg, A. B., M. Massin, and G. Gauchat, La cytolyse de la levure causée par les narcotiques en tant que phénomène physique indifférent, *C. S. Soc. Biol.*, **151**, 1369–1372 (1957).

Liniucheva, L. A., and L. A. Tiunov, Effect of phenylethylhydrazine on liver monoamine oxidase activity in man and in animals, in *Materialy Tretiei Konferentsii po Toksikologii i Gigiyene Vysokomolekuliarnykh Soyeninenii i Khimicheskogo Syriya, Ispolzuyemogo dlya ikh Sinteza*, pp. 18–19, Khimiya, Leningrad, 1966.

Liniucheva, L. A., L. A. Tiunov, and T. S. Kolosova, Effect of acetone on the blood and urine levels of ketone bodies in experimental animals of various species, *Farmakol. Toksikol.*, **21**(4), 465–467 (1969).

Liozner, L. D., Z. A. Riabinina, and V. F. Sidorova, Some patterns of mitosis in the liver during its reparative regeneration, *Biull. Eksp. Biol. Med.*, **47**(5), 96–99 (1959).

Liublina, E. I., Measurement of characteristics of the flexor reflex, *Issledovaniya v Oblasti Promyshlennoi Toksikologii*, Vol. 12, No. 5, pp. 51–66, Institut Gigiyeny Truda i Profzabolevaniy, Leningrad, 1948.

Liublina, E. I., Effect of some pharmacological agents on the duration of narcosis induced by various narcotics, *Farmakol. Toksikol.*, **17**(6), 6–12 (1954).

Liublina, E. I., "Issledovaniye Deistviya Malykh Kontsentratsii Narkotikov na Tsentralnuyu Nervnuyu Sistemu" ["A Study into the Effects of Low Concentrations of Narcotics on the Central Nervous System"], unpublished doctoral dissertation, Leningrad, 1955.

Liublina, E. I., *Dva Tipa Deistviya Primeniayemykh v Promyshlennosti Organicheskikh Rastvoritelei (Narkotikov) na Nervnuyu Sistemu [Two Types of Action on the Nervous System of Industrially Used Organic Solvents (Narcotics)]*, Institut Gigiyeny Truda i Profzabolevaniy, Leningrad, 1956.

Liublina, E. I., Parabiosis and nonelectrolytes, *Ucheniye Zapiski Leningradskogo Gosudarstvennogo Universiteta*, No. 222, Issue No. 43: Seriya Biologicheskikh Nauk, pp. 142–159, 1957

Liublina, E. I., Establishment by calculation of tentative values for MACs, in *Trudy Nauchnoi Sessii, Posviashchennoi Itogam Ratoty za 1958 God*, pp. 218–223, Institut Gigiyeny Truda i Profzabolevaniy, Leningrad, 1959.

Liublina, E. I., Establishing tentative values of MACs for organic substances by calculation, *Gig. Sanit.*, **12**, 20–25 (1960).

Liublina, E. I., On unnecessary experimental studies conducted for the purpose of establishing maximum allowable concentrations of vapors and gases in the air of working areas, in A. A. Letavet and A. A. Kanarevskaya, Eds., *Promyshlennaya Toksikologiya i Klinika Professionalnykh Zabolevaniy Khimicheskoi Etiologii*, pp. 55–57, Medgiz, Moscow, 1962.

Liublina, E. I., Relationships between physicochemical properties and toxicities of organic compounds using different modes of expressing their effective concentrations, in N. V. Lazarev, Ed., *Voprosy Obshchei Promyshlennoi Toksikologii*, pp. 48–55, Institut Gigiyeny Truda i Profzabolevaniy, Leningrad, 1963a.

Liublina, E. I., Analysis of correlations between physicochemical properties, toxicities, and MACs, in *Materialy Nauchnoi Sessii po Itogam Rabotyza 1961–1962 Gody*, pp. 114–117, Institut Gigiyeny Truda i Profzabolevaniy, Leningrad, 1963b.

Liublina, E. I., On the possibility of calculating concentrations of nonelectrolytes in the blood of rabbits depending on exposure conditions, in P. V. Terentiev, Ed., *Primeneniye Matematicheskikh Metodov v Biologii*, Vol. 3, pp. 155–158, Leningradskiy Universitet, Leningrad, 1964.

Liublina, E. I., Relationships between toxicity and physicochemical properties of metals, in I. D. Gadaskina, A. A. Golubev, and E. T. Lykhina, Eds., *Voprosy Obshchei i*

Chastnoi Promyshlennoi Toksikologii, pp. 26–36, Institut Gigiyeny Truda i Profzabolevaniy, Leningrad, 1965.

Liublina, E. I., The toxicity of some substances as related to the periodic table, *Gig. Tr. Prof. Zabol.*, **12**, 9–13 (1967).

Liublina, E. I., Relations of physicochemical properties of hydrocarbons to their toxicity, *Gig. Sanit.*, **7**, 20–25 (1969).

Liublina, E. I., Parabiosis and the physicochemical properties of nonelectrolytes, in N. V. Lazarev, A. A. Golubev, and E. T. Lykhina, Eds., *Aktualniye Voprosy Promyshlennoi Toksikologii*, pp. 59–72, Institut Gigiyeny Truda i Profzabolevaniy, Leningrad, 1970.

Liublina, E. I., Habituation under various conditions of exposure to industrial poisons, in E. I. Liublina and N. A. Minkina, Eds., *Problema Adaptatsii v Gigiyene Truda*, pp. 14–19, Moskovskiy Institut Gigiyeny, Moscow and Leningrad, 1973a.

Liublina, E. I., Correlations between molecular weight and MAC in some classes of organic compounds in relation to the state of aggregation of the compound, *Gig. Tr. Prof. Zabol.*, **4**, 37–40 (1973b).

Liublina, E. I., and V. A. Filov, Physicochemical properties of organic substances and their toxicity indices, in I. D. Gadaskina, A. A. Golubev, and E. T. Lykhina, Eds., *Voprosy Obshchei i Chastnoi Promyshlennoi Toksikologii*, pp. 7–16, Institut Gigiyeny Truda i Profzabolevaniy, Leningrad, 1965.

Liublina, E. I., and A. A. Golubev, Application of the method of correlational pleiads to detect correlations between properties and toxicities of substances, in P. V. Terentiev, Ed., *Primeneniye Matematicheskikh Metodov v Biologii*, Vol. 2, pp. 90–93, Leningradskiy Universitet, Leningrad, 1963.

Liublina, E. I., and A. A. Golubev, *Instruktsiya po Ustanovleniyu Rastchetnym Sposobom Orientirovochnykh Predelno Dopustimykh Kontsentratsii Promyshlennykh Yadov v Vozdukhe Rabochikh Pomeshchenii* [*Instructions for Establishing by Calculation of Approximate Maximum Allowable Concentrations in the Air of Work Areas*], 2nd ed., Institut Gigiyeny Truda i Profzabolevaniy, Leningrad, 1967.

Liublina, E. I., and N. A. Minkina, Exposure conditions promoting or hindering habituation to poisons, *Gigiyena Primeneniya, Toksikologiya Pestitsidov i Klinika Otravleniy*, No. 7, pp. 182–188, Institut Gigiyeny i Toksikologii Pestitsidov, Polimernykh i Plasticheskikh Mass, Kiev, 1969.

Liublina, E. I., and L. V. Rabotnikova, Possibility of predicting the toxicity of volatile organic compounds from their physical constants, *Gig. Sanit.*, **8**, 33–37 (1971).

Liublina, E. I., N. A. Minkina, and M. L. Rylova, The problem of habituation to industrial poisons, in L. I. Medved, Ed., *Gigiyena i Toksikologiya Pestitsidov i Klinika Otravleniy*, pp. 113–120, Zdoroviye, Kiev, 1965.

Liublina, E. I., A. A. Golubev, and V. A. Filov, Determination by computing methods of approximate values of toxicity indices for chemical agents, in G. A. Stepansky, Ed., *Farmakologiya. Toksikologiya, Problemy Toksikologii*, pp. 11–44, VINITI, Moscow, 1967.

Liublina, E. I., N. A. Minkina, and M. L. Rylova, *Adaptatsiya k Promyshlennym*

Vrednym Veshchestvam kak Faza Intoksikatsii [*The Adaptation to Harmful Industrial Substances as a Phase of Intoxication*], Meditsina, Leningrad, 1971.

Livshits, P. Z., A note on the calculation of the median lethal dose, *Farmakol. Toksikol.*, **29**(1), 113–118 (1966).

Loewe, S., Die quantitatiwen Probleme der Pharmakologie, *Ergen. Physiol.*, **27**, 47–187 (1928).

Lohs, K., *Synthetische Gifte*, Verlag des Ministeriums für nationale Verteidigung, Berlin, 1958.

Loit, A. O., *Rekomendatsii dlya Predvaritelnoi Otsenki Toksichnosti Letuchikh Organicheskikh Veshchestv Skorostnym Metodom* [*Recommendations for the Rapid Preliminary Assessment of the Toxicity of Volatile Organic Substances*], Medgiz, Leningrad, 1964.

Lukomsky, Ya. I., *Teoriya Korreliatsii i eye Primeneniye k Analizu Proizvodstva* [*Correlation Theory and Its Application in Industrial Analyses*], Gosstatizdat, Moscow, 1958.

Marchenko, E. N., and I. F. Zapalkevich, Air pollution by a combination of industrial poisons, *Gig. Truda Prof. Zabol.*, **8**, 3–9 (1965).

Martin, B. K., Drug urinary excretion data—some aspects concerning the interpretation, *Br. J. Pharmacol. Chemother.*, **29**, 181–183 (1967a).

Martin, B. K., Treatment of data from drug urinary excretion, *Nature*, **214**, 247–249 (1967b).

Matthews, A. P., *Am. J. Physiol.*, **10**, p. 280 (1904), cited in J. R. E. Jones, *J. Exp. Biol.*, **16**, 425–437 (1939).

Mayer, S., R. P. Maickel, and B. B. Brodie, Kinetics of penetration of drugs and other foreign compounds into cerebrospinal fluid and brain, *J. Pharmacol. Exp. Ther.*, **127**, 205–211 (1959).

McGowan, J. C., The physical toxicity of chemicals. I. Vapours, *J. Appl. Chem.*, **1**, Suppl. 2, S120–S126 (1951a).

McGowan, J. C., Physical toxicity in aqueous solutions, *Proc. Biochem. Soc.*, **50**, VII (1951b).

McGowan, J. C., Factors affecting physical toxicity in aqueous solutions, *J. Appl. Chem.*, **2**, 323–328 (1952a).

McGowan, J. C., Systematic treatment of physical toxicity in aqueous solutions, *J. Appl. Chem.*, **2**, 651–658 (1952b).

McGowan, J. C., Solubilities, partition coefficients and physical toxicities, *J. Appl. Chem.*, **4**, 41–47 (1954).

McGowan, J. C., Physically toxic chemicals and industrial hygiene, *Arch. Ind. Health*, **11**, 315–323 (1955).

McGowan, J. C., Partition coefficients and biological activities, *Nature*, **200**, 1317 (1963).

Medved, L. I., Yu. S. Kagan, and E. N. Spynu, Pesticides and problems of health, *Zh. Vses. Khim. O-va Mendeleeva*, **13**(3), 263–271 (1968).

Milne, M. D., Potentiation of excretion of drugs, *Proc. Roy. Soc. Med.*, **57**, 809–811 (1964).

Mironos, E. S., "Voprosy Deponirovaniya Benzola i Serougleroda v Zhirovoi Tkani" ["Deposition of Benzene and Carbon Disulfide in Fatty Tissues"], unpublished candidate's dissertation, Leningrad, 1970.

Molinengo, L., Sulla applicabililita del principio di Ferguson e della "sieve theory" a composti ad azione inotropa negativa, *Arch. Int. Pharmacodyn. Ther.*, **143**, 90–107 (1963).

Morris, L. E., E. L. Frederickson, and O. S. Orth, Differences in the concentration of chloroform in the blood of man and dog during anesthesia, *J. Pharmacol. Exp. Ther.*, **101**, 56–62 (1951).

Moshkovsky, Sh. D., Basic principles of the quantitative study of chemotherapeutic agents, *Med. Parazitol.*, **5**, 713–724 (1936).

Moshkovsky, Sh. D., Functional curves and types of experiment in quantitative chemotherapy, *Med. Parazitol.*, **10**, 204–216 (1941).

Moshkovsky, Sh. D., Methodological considerations concerning the quantitative evaluation of the combined effect produced by physiologically active substances, *Med. Parazitol.*, **3**, 30–42 (1943).

Mullins, L. J., Some physical mechanisms in narcosis, *Chem. Rev.*, **54**, 289–323 (1954).

Navrotsky, V. K., Industrial dust, in Z. I. Izraelson and Z. B. Smeliansky, Eds., *Rukovodstvo po Gigiyene Truda*, Vol. 2, pp. 15–33, Medgiz, Moscow, 1963.

Nelson, E., Kinetics of drug absorption, distribution, metabolism, and excretion, in *Proceedings, 3rd International Congress on Chemotherapy, Stuttgart, 1963*, Vol. 2, pp. 1657–1666, Georg Thieme Verlag, Stuttgart, 1964.

Nofre, C., H. Dufour, and A. Cier, Toxicité générale comparée des anions mineraux chez la souris, *C. R. Acad. Sci.*, **257**, 791–794 (1963).

Onchi, Y., and Y. Asao, Absorption, distribution and elimination of diethyl ether in man, *Br. J. Anaesth.*, **33**, 544–548 (1961).

Ostrenga, J. A., Correlation of biological activity with chemical structure. Use of molar attraction constants, *J. Med. Chem.*, **12**, 349–352 (1969).

Pakhomychev, A. I., T. A. Kozlova, and A. I. Korenevskaya, Observations on the combined effect of poisons and high ambient temperature, in V. M. Zhdanov, Ed., *Trudy XIII Vsesoyuznogo Siezda Gigiyenistov, Epidemiologov, Mikrobiologov i Infektsionistov*, Vol. 1, pp. 337–339, Medgiz, Moscow, 1959.

Paribok, V. P., The toxicity of poisonous nonelectrolytes and some anthelmintics to nematodes, *Farmakol. Toksikol.*, **20**(4), 74–75 (1957).

Paribok, V. P., and F. A. Ivanova, Toxicity of nitrogen oxides to animals with continuous and discontinuous exposure, *Farmakol. Toksikol.*, **28**(4), 484–488 (1965a).

Paribok, V. P., and F. A. Ivanova, Effect of ambient temperature on the toxic action of nitrogen oxides, *Gig. Tr. Prof. Zabol.*, **7**, 22–26 (1965b).

Paton, W. D. M., and R. N. Speden, Uptake of anaesthetics and their action on the central nervous system, *Br. Med. Bull.*, **21**, 44–48 (1965).

Pattison, F. L. M., *Toxic Aliphatic Fluorine Compounds*, Elsevier, Amsterdam, 1959.

Pelikan, E. V., *Opyt Prilozheniya Sovremennykh Fiziko-Khimicheskikh Issledovanii k Ucheniyu o Yadakh* [*Experience with the Application of Modern Physicochemical Concepts to the Study of Poisons*], St. Petersburg, 1854.

Pelikan, E. V., *Toksikologiya Tsianistykh Metallov* [*The Toxicology of Cyanides of Metals*], St. Petersburg, 1855.

Piotrowski, J., Zlozone wydalanie jednorazowey dawki substancji obcej, *Med. Pr.*, **14**, 61–73 (1963).

Piotrowski, J., Wydalanie cial obcych w przypadkach ciaglego lub periodycznego wchlaniania, *Med. Pr.*, **16**, 150–165 (1965).

Piotrowski, J., Chemiczne zagadnienia przemyslowej toksykologii nitrobenzenu, *Med. Pr.*, **17**, 519–534 (1966).

Piotrowski, J., *The Application of Metabolic Excretion Kinetics to Problems of Industrial Toxicology*, U.S. Department of Health, Education and Welfare, Government Printing Office, Washington, D.C., 1971.

Plokhinsky, N. A., *Algoritmy v Biometrii* [*Algorithms in Biometrics*], Moskovskiy Universitet, Moscow, 1967.

Pokrovsky, V. A., "Kombinirovannoye Deistviye Vysokoi Temperatury i Nekotorykh Yadov na Zhivotnyi Organizm" ["Combined Action of High Temperature and Some Poisons on the Animal Organism"], unpublished candidate's dissertation, Voronezh, 1946.

Pokrovsky, V. A., Effect of some organic poisons on the female organism, *Gig. Tr. Prof. Zabol.*, **2**, 17–30 (1967).

Pomorsky, Yu. L., *Metody Biometricheskikh Issledovanii* [*Methods in Biometric Research*], Leningradskoye Oblastnoye Izdatelstvo, Leningrad, 1935.

Posternak, J., Théories de la nacrose et propriétés cellulaires, *Rev. Med. Suisse Rom.*, **73**, 550–555 (1953).

Posternak, J., and M. G. Larrabee, Action de narcotiques sur les synapses et sur les axones dans un ganglion sympathique, in *CNRS, 26, Méchanisme de la Narcose*, pp. 41–45, Paris, 1951.

Pozzani, U. C., C. S. Weil, and C. P. Carpenter, The toxicological basis of threshold limit values. 5. The experimental inhalation of vapor mixtures by rats, with notes upon the relationship between single dose inhalation and single dose oral data, *Am. Ind. Hyg. Assoc. J.*, **20**(5), 364–369 (1959).

Pravdin, N. S., *Metodika Maloi Toksikologii Promyshlennykh Yadov* [*Methods for the Toxicology of Low Concentrations of Industrial Poisons*], Medgiz, Moscow, 1947.

Pravdin, N. S., Ed., *Voprosy Promyshlennoi Toksikologii* [*Aspects of Industrial Toxicology*], Institut Gigiyeny Truda i Profzabolevaniy, Moscow, 1960.

Prozorovsky, V. B., Selecting the criterion of tolerance in toxicological studies, *Farmakol. Toksikol.*, **30**(2), 240–243 (1967).

Quick, A. J., The relationship between chemical structure and physiological response, *J. Biol. Chem.*, **96**, 83–101 (1932).

Rabotnikova, L. V., The toxicity of metal oxides in relation to the physicochemical properties and normal body levels of the metal, in I. D. Gadaskina, A. A. Golubev, and E. T. Lykhina, Eds., *Voprosy Obshchei i Chastnoi Promyshlennoi Toksikologii*, pp. 52–55, Institut Gigiyeny Truda i Profzabolevaniy, Leningrad, 1965.

Rabotnikova, L. V., "Materialy k Uskorennym Metodam Opredeleniya Toksichnosti Okislov Metallov" ["Rapid Methods for Determining the Toxicity of Metal Oxides"], unpublished candidate's dissertation, Leningrad, 1966.

Rabotnikova, L. V., Assessing the relative importance of the routes of administration of poisons, in N. V. Lazarev, A. A. Golubev, and E. T. Lykhina, Eds., *Aktualniye Voprosy Promyshlennoi Toksikologii*, pp. 180–185, Institut Gigiyeny Truda i Profzabolevaniy, Leningrad, 1970.

Rapoport, I. A., Toxicogenetika [Toxicogenetics], in E. M. Vermel and G. A. Stepansky, Eds., *Farmakologiya. Toksikologiya*, pp. 3–46, VINITI, Moscow, 1966.

Rashevsky, N., *Mathematical Principles in Biology and Their Applications*, Charles C. Thomas, Springfield, Ill., 1961.

Rashevsky, N., *Some Medical Aspects of Mathematical Biology*, Charles C. Thomas, Springfield, Ill., 1964.

Rentz, F., Zur Systematik und Nomenklatur der Kombinationswirkungen, *Arch. Int. Pharmacodyn. Ther.*, **43**, 337–362 (1932).

Renzetti, N. A., Atmospheric sampling for aldehydes and eye irritants in Los Angeles smog, *J. Air Pollut. Control Assoc.*, **11**, 421–427 (1961).

Rythmic Functions in the Living System, *Ann. N. Y. Acad. Sci.*, **98**(4), 753–1326 (1962).

Rich, S., and J. G. Horsfall, The relations between fungitoxicity, permeation and lipid solubility, *Phytopathology*, **43**, 457–460 (1952).

Richardson, B. W., Physiological research on alcohols, *Med. Times Gaz.* **2**, 703 (1869).

Richardson, C. H., Comparative toxicity of the vapors of several chlorinated methane and ethane derivatives to the rice weevil, *Iowa State Coll. J. Sci.*, **26**, 357–369 (1952).

Riegelman, S., J. Loo, and M. Rowland, Concept of a volume of distribution and possible errors in evaluation of this parameter, *J. Pharm. Sci.*, **57**, 128–133 (1968).

Ross, R. G., and R. A. Ludwig, A comparative study of fungitoxicity in an homologous series of N-n-alkylethylene-thioureas, *Can. J. Bot.*, **35**, 65–95 (1957).

Rybak, E. I., Yu. I. Lisunkin, and O. M. Kalinin, Finding the 50% and other doses by the method of stochastic approximation, *Farmakol. Toksikol.*, **29**(3), 368–370 (1966).

Ryzhik, L. A., Hygienic measures to be observed when using fireproof liquids for regulators of steam turbines, *Gig. Tr. Prof. Zabol.*, **3**, 41–43 (1967).

Saccardo, P., Rappresentaz periòdica e tossicològica degli elementi, *Chimica*, **31**, 411–414 (1955).

Sacher, G. A., The dimensionality of the life span, in B. L. Strehler, Ed., *The Biology of Aging*, pp. 251–252, American Institute of Biological Sciences, Washington, D.C., 1960.

Samedov, I. G., "Ob Osobennostiakh Deistviya na Organizm Malykh Kontsentratsiy Uglevodorodov Nefti" ["Effect on the Body of Low Concentrations of Hydrocarbons Contained in Petroleum"], unpublished doctoral dissertation, Baku, 1967.

Samsonov, G. V., Role of stable electron configurations in the establishment of properties of chemical elements and compounds, *Poroshk. Metal.*, **10**, 49–60 (1966).

Sanotsky, I. V., Calculation of the safety factor in establishing MACs for industrial poisons in experiment, in A. A. Letavet and A. A. Kanarevskaya, Eds., *Promyshlennaya Toksikologiya i Klinika Professionalnykh Zabolevanii Khimicheskoi Etiologii*, pp. 35–37, Medgiz, Moscow, 1962.

Sanotsky, I. V., On rational forms of toxicological information presentation, *Farmakol. Toksikol.*, **27**(5), 620–627 (1964).

Sanotsky, I. V., Current status of research into the combined action of gases, vapors, and aerosols, *Toksikologiya Novykh Promyshlennykh Khimicheskikh Veshchestv*, No. 11, pp. 6–13, Meditsina, Moscow, 1969.

Sarkisov, D. S., Recent developments in the study of regeneration and some problems of clinical medicine, *Klin. Med.*, **48**(11), 14–20 (1970).

Sarkisov, D. S., and B. V. Vtiurin, *Elektronnomikroskopicheskii Analiz Povysheniya Vynoslivosti Serdtsa [Electron Microscopic Analysis of Enhanced Endurance of the Heart]*, Meditsina, Moscow, 1969.

Sarkisov, D. S., L. D. Krymsky, and K. V. Botsmanov, Relationship between the cellular and intracellular forms of reparative regeneration in the liver, *Biull. Eksp. Biol. Med.*, **3**, 103–105 (1969a).

Sarkisov, D. S., L. D. Krymsky, K. V. Botsmanov, B. V. Vtiurin, and K. I. Dzarakhokhov, An autoradiographic study of relationships between the frequency of exposure to a stimulus and the rate of reparative regeneration, *Arkh. Patol. Anat. Patol. Fiziol.*, **3**, 22–26 (1969b).

Sarkisov, D. S., L. D. Krymsky, K. I. Dzarakhokhov, and L. S. Rubetskoi, On the paradoxical effect from carbon tetrachloride administered at varying time intervals, *Biull. Eksp. Biol. Med.*, **7**, 115–117 (1969c).

Saunders, B. Ch., *Some Aspects of the Chemistry and Toxic Action of Organic Compounds Containing Phosphorus and Fluorine*, Cambridge University Press, London, 1957.

Savchenkov, M. F., "Vliyaniye Nekotorykh Promyshlennykh Yadov na Zhivotnykh Raznogo Vozrasta" ["Effect of Some Industrial Poisons on Animals of Various Ages"], unpublished candidate's dissertation, Leningrad, 1969.

Savitsky, I. V., Effect of high ambient temperature on the course of intoxication by thiolic poisons, *Gig. Tr. Prof. Zabol.*, **10**, 30–35 (1967).

Schatz, A., E. B. Schalscha, and V. Schatz, The occurrence and importance of paradoxical concentration effects in biological systems, *Compost Sci.*, **5**(1), 26–31 (1964).

Sechzer, P. H., H. W. Linde, R. D. Dripps, and H. L. Price, Uptake of halothane by the human body, *Anesthesiology*, **24**, 779–783 (1963).

Sexton, W. A., *Chemical Constitution and Biological Activity*, Spon, London, 1949; 3rd ed., 1963.

Shadursky, K. S., *Lektsii po Obshchei Farmakologii [Lectures in General Pharmacology]*, Ministerstvo Vysshego i Srednego Spetsialnogo Obrazovaniya Byelorusskoi SSR, Minsk, 1961.

Shakhparonov, M. I., *Vvedeniye v Molekuliarnuyu Teoriyu Rastvorov [Introduction to the Molecular Theory of Solutions]*, Gosudarstvennoye Izdatelstvo Tekhniko-Teoreticheskoi Literatury, Moscow, 1956.

Shaw, W. H. R., Cation toxicity and the stability of transition-metal complexes, *Nature*, **192**, 754–755 (1961)

Shekhtman, B. A., On the mechanism of action of two types of industrial narcotics, in *Materialy Nauchnoi Konferentsii, Posviashchennoi Voprosam Gigiyeny Truda, Promyshlennoi Toksikologii i Professionalnoi Patologii v Neftianoi i Neftekhimicheskoi Promyshlennosti*, pp. 18–19, Institut Gigiyeny Truda i Profzabolevaniy, Baku, 1966.

Shekhtman, B. A. "Usloviya Truda pri Pererabotke Malosernistykh Neftei i ikh Vliyaniye na Organizm" ["Working Conditions during Processing of Low-Sulfur Oils and Their Effect on the Organism"], unpublished doctoral dissertation, Baku, 1969.

Sheppard, C. W., and A. S. Householder, The mathematical basis of the interpretation of tracer experiments in closed steady-state systems, *J. Appl. Phys.*, **22**, 510–520 (1951).

Shirk, U. G., R. R. Corey, and P. L. Poelma, The influence of chemical structure on fungal activity, *Arch. Biochem. Biophys.*, **32**, 392–396 (1951).

Shtabsky, B. M., Hygienic evaluation of cumulative properties of harmful substances, in D. N. Koliuzhniy, Ed., *Gigiyena Naselennykh Mest*, pp. 41–42, Institut Obshchei i Kommunalnoi Gigiyeny, Kiev, 1969.

Shtabsky, B. M., Relationship between material and functional cumulation, in *Primeneniye Matematicheskikh Metodov dlya Otsenki i Prognozirovaniya Realnoi Opasnosti Nakopleniya Pestitsidov vo Vneshnei Srede i Organizme. Materialy Pervogo Simpoziuma*, pp. 43–46, Institut Gigiyeny i Toksikologii Pestitsidov, Polimernykh i Plasticheskikh Mass i Institut Kibernetiki Akad. Nauk Ukr. SSR, Kiev, 1971.

Shugayev, B. B., L. A. Timofievskaya, and G. N. Zayeva, Forecasting the carcinogenic effects of industrial products, in *Otdalenniye Posledstviya Vliyaniya na Cheloveka Khimicheskikh Veshchestv, Primeniayemykh v Promyshlennosti i Selskom Khoziaystve. Nauchniy Obzor*, pp. 101–122, Vsesoyuzniy Institut Meditsinskoi i Mediko-Tekhnicheskoi Informatsii, Moscow, 1969.

Sidorenko, G. I., and M. A. Pinigin, A contribution to the study of intermittent exposure to atmospheric pollutants, *Gig. Sanit.*, **10**, 94–97 (1969).

Sidorov, K. K., Some methods for quantitative evaluation of the cumulative effect, *Toksikologiya Novykh Promyshlennykh Khimicheskikh Veshchestv*, No. 9, pp. 19–27, Meditsina, Moscow, 1967.

Sidorov, K. K., Calculation of the safety factor in establishing MACs for harmful substances in the air of work areas, *Gig. Tr. Prof. Zabol.*, **6**, 54–56 (1971).

Snedecor, G. W., and W. G. Cochran, *Statistical Methods*, 6th ed., Iowa State University Press, Ames, Ia., 1968.

Sochava, E. A., "Materialy k Toksikologii Nekotorykh Kislorodsoderzhashchikh Geterotsiklicheskikh Soyedinenii (Proizvodnykh Pirana)" ["Toxicology of Some Oxygen-Containing Heterocyclic Compounds (Pyran Derivatives)"], unpublished candidate's dissertation, Leningrad, 1969.

Sollberger, A., *Biological Rhythm Research*, Elsevier, Amsterdam, 1963.

Spector, W. S., Ed., *Handbook of Toxicology. Vol. I: Acute Toxicities*, W. B. Saunders, Philadelphia and London, 1956.

Speransky, S. V., Modification of methods for measuring muscle strength in white mice, in A. A. Letavet and A. A. Kanarevskaya, Eds., *Promyshlennaya Toksikologiya i Klinika Professionalnykh Zabolevanii Khimicheskoi Etiologii*, pp. 63–64, Medgiz, Moscow, 1962.

Speransky, S. V., Advantages of using incremental current in studying the capacity of white mice to summate subthreshold impulses, *Farmakol. Toksikol.*, **28**(1), 123–124 (1965).

Stasenkova, K. P., and T. A. Kochetkova, Comparative toxicity of furan compounds, *Toksikologiya Novykh Promyshlennykh Khimicheskikh Veshchestv*, No. 10, pp. 35–44, Meditsina, Moscow, 1968.

Suvorov, S. V., Relation of the toxicity of inorganic substances to the electronic structure of their atoms, *Gig. Sanit.*, **11**, 98–101 (1968).

Swintosky, J. V., Excretion equations and interpretation for digitoxin, *Nature*, **179**, 98–99 (1957).

Terentiev, P. V., Further development of the method of correlational pleiads, in *Primeneniye Matematicheskikh Metodov v Biologii*, pp. 27–36, Leningradskiy Universitet, Leningrad, 1960.

Ter Haar, D., and H. Wergeland, *Elements of Thermodynamics*, Addison-Wesley, Reading, Mass., 1966.

Timofeev-Resovsky, N. V., V. I. Ivanov, and V. I. Korogodin, *Primeneniye Printsipa Popadanii v Radiobiologii* [*Application of the Hit Theory in Radiobiology*], Atomizdat, Moscow, 1968.

Tiunov, L. A., Approaches to the determination of species differences in sensitivity of experimental animals for toxicological studies, in *Obshchiye Voprosy Promyshlennoi Toksikologii*, pp. 55–59, Institut Gigiyeny Truda i Profzabolevaniy, Moscow, 1967.

Tiunov, L. A., and S. A. Keizer, On procedures for validating the selection of experimental animals for toxicological studies, in *Toksikologiya i Gigiyena Vysokomolekuliarnykh Soyedineniy i Khimicheskogo Syriya, Ispolzuemogo dlya ikh Sinteza*, pp. 16–18, Khimiya, Moscow and Leningrad, 1966.

Tiunov, L. A., and V. V. Kustov, *Toksikologiya Okisi Ugleroda* [*The Toxicology of Carbon Monoxide*], Meditsina, Leningrad, 1969.

Tiunov, L. A., T. I. Sokolova, and A. L. Bandman, Benzene transformations in the liver of experimental animals, *Farmakol. Toksikol.*, **32**(2), 185–188 (1969).

Tiunov, L. A., G. A. Vasilyev, and L. V. Ivanova, Patterns of the toxic action of furfural administered at different rhythms, *Biull. Eksp. Biol. Med.*, **9**, 29–30 (1970).

Tolokontsev, N. A., Mathematical expression of relationships governing the absorption of harmful gaseous substances, in *Tesizy Dokladov Vtorogo Soveshchaniya po Primeneniyu Matematicheskikh Metodov v Biologii*, pp. 50–52, Leningradskiy Universitet, Leningrad, 1959.

Tolokontsev, N. A., "Toksicheskii Effekt Neelektrolitov pri ikh Nepreryvnom i Intermittiruyushchem Vozdeistvii" ["Toxic Effects of Nonelectrolytes with Continuous and Intermittent Exposure''], unpublished candidate's dissertation, Leningrad, 1960a.

Tolokontsev, N. A., A comparative study of continuous and intermittent exposure to volatile toxic nonelectrolytes, *Gig. Sanit.*, **3**, 29–35 (1960b).

Tolokontsev, N. A., Mathematical expression of relationships governing the absorption of toxic gaseous nonelectrolytes, in *Primeneniye Matematicheskikh Metodov v Biologii*, pp. 186–191, Leningradskiy Universitet, Leningrad, 1960c.

Tolokontsev, N. A., Some general aspects of quantitative toxicology, in N. V. Lazarev, Ed., *Voprosy Obshchei Promyshlennoi Toksikologii*, pp. 85–93, Institut Gigiyeny Truda i Profzabolevaniy, Leningrad, 1963.

Tolokontsev, N. A., Some methods for quantitative evaluation of toxicity of chemicals, in P. V. Terentiev, Ed., *Primeneniye Matematicheskikh Metodov v Biologii*, No. 3, pp. 135–154, Leningradskiy Universitet, Leningrad, 1964.

Tolokontsev, N. A., Prospects for the application of mathematical methods in toxicology, in *Obshchiye Voprosy Promyshlennoi Toksikologii*, pp. 96–100, Institut Gigiyeny Truda i Profzabolevaniy, Moscow, 1967.

Trakhtenberg, I. M., I. V. Savitsky, and R. Ya. Shterengarts, Effect of mercury in low concentrations, *Gig. Tr. Prof. Zabol.*, **12**, 7–12 (1965).

Trčka, V., and A. Dlabač, Vliv alifatických substituentů na biologickou účinnost. III, *Česk. Fisiol.*, **11**, 533 (1962).

Ulanova, I. P., Establishment of hygiene standards for mixtures of gases and vapors, *Toksikologiya Novykh Promyshlennykh Khimicheskikh Veschestv*, No. 11, pp. 33–39, Meditsina, Moscow, 1969.

Ulanova, I. P., Degree of hazard, species sensitivity, and margin of safety as factors to be considered in establishing MACs for industrial substances, in A. A. Letavet and I. V. Sanotsky, Eds., *Printsipy i Metody Ustanovleniya Predelno Dopustimykh Kontsentratsii Vrednykh Veshchestv v Vozdukhe Proizvodstvennykh Pomeshchenii*, pp. 65–76, Meditsina, Moscow, 1970.

Ulanova, I. P., K. K. Sidorov, and A. I. Khalepo, Determination of cumulative properties of occupational poisons, in A. A. Letavet and I. V. Sanotsky, Eds., *Printsipy i Metody Ustanovleniya Predelno Dopustimykh Kontsentratsii Vrednykh Veshchestv v Vozdukhe Proizvodstvennykh Pomeshchenii*, pp. 101–108, Meditsina, Moscow, 1970.

Van der Waerden, B. L., *Matematische Statistik*, Springer-Verlag, Berlin, Göttingen, and Heidelberg, 1957.

Vogel, A. J., W. T. Cresswell, G. H. Jeffrey, and J. Leicester, Physical properties and chemical constitution, *J. Chem. Soc.*, pp. 514–549, February 1952.

Volkova, Z. A., Validation of maximum allowable concentrations for toxic substances in the air of working areas by studying working conditions in relation to the health status of workers, *Gig. Tr. Prof. Zabol.*, **8**, 19–24 (1965).

Volkova, Z. A., N. P. Kokorev, I. F. Zapalkevich, A. P. Martynova, E. N. Marchenko, and B. V. Shafranov, Combined action of industrial poisons: some hygienic aspects, *Toksikologiya Novykh Promyshlennykh Khimicheskikh Veshchestv*, No. 11, pp. 14–22, Meditsina, Moscow, 1969.

Wagner, J. G., Method for estimating rate constants for absorption, metabolism, and elimination from urinary excretion data, *J. Pharm. Sci.*, **56**, 489–494 (1967).

Wagner, J. G., and E. Nelson, Kinetic analysis of blood levels and urinary excretion in the absorptive phase after single doses of drug, *J. Pharm. Sci.*, **53**, 1392–1403 (1964).

Wang Weng-Yang, A contribution to the toxicology of fatty aldehydes, in N. V. Lazarev and I. D. Gadaskina, Eds., *Materialy po Toksikologii Veshchestv, Primeniayemykh v Proizvodstve Plasticheskikh Mass i Sinteticheskikh Kauchukov*, pp. 42–60, Institut Gigiyeny Truda i Profzabolevaniy, Leningrad, 1957.

Weber, E., *Grundriss der biologischen Statistik. Anwendungen der matematischen Statistik in Naturwissenschaft und Technik*, 7th ed., Fischer, Jena, 1972.

Weil, C. S., M. D. Woodside, J. B. Bernard, and C. P. Carpenter, Relationship between single peroral, one-week, and ninety-day rat feeding studies, *Toxicol. Appl. Pharmacol.*, **14**, 426–431 (1969).

Wiegand, R. C., and P. G. Sanders, Calculation of kinetic constants from blood levels of drugs, *J. Pharmacol. Exp. Ther.*, **146**, 271–275 (1964).

Wilbrandt, W., Die biologische Halbwertzeit von Medikamenten, ihre Ermittlung und Bedeutung, *Schweiz. Med. Wschr.*, **94**, 737–745 (1964).

Wilder, J., *Stimulus and Response. The Law of Initial Value*, John Wright, Bristol, 1967.

Williams, R. J., *Biochemical Individuality*, John Wiley, New York, 1956.

Williams, R. T., *Detoxication Mechanisms*, 2nd ed., Chapman and Hall, London, 1959.

Worthing, A. G., and J. Geffner, *Treatment of Experimental Data*, Chapman and Hall, London, 1946.

Yakovlev, K. P., *Matematicheskaya Obrabotka Rezultatov Izmerenii* [*Mathematical Treatment of Measurement Data*], Gostekhizdat, Moscow, 1953.

Zahradnik, R., Influence of the structure of alphatic substituents on the magnitude of the biological effect of substances, *Arch. Int. Pharmacodyn. Ther.*, **135**, 311–329 (1962a).

Zahradnik, R., Correlation of the biological activity of organic compounds by means of the linear free energy relationships, *Experientia*, **18**, 534–541 (1962b).

Zahradnik, R., M. Chvapil, J. Vostál, and J. Teisinger, The toxicity of alcohols and potassium salts of alkylxanthic acids, *Farmakol. Toksikol.*, **25**(5), 618–622 (1962).

Zahradnik, R., F. Boček, and J. Kopecký, Empirical equations for correlating biological efficiency of organic compounds, in *Proceedings, 3rd International Pharmacological Meeting, São Paulo, 1966*, Vol. 7, pp. 127–139, Pergamon, New York, 1968.

Zalesov, V. S., V. E. Kolla, L. M. Filatova, and G. A. Yuzhakova, Relationship between the chemical structure and toxicity of organoboron compounds, *Nauchniye Trudy Permskogo Farmatsevticheskogo Instituta*, No. 2, pp. 27–36, 1967.

Zayeva, G. N., On the application of computing methods, *Toksikologiya Novykh Promyshlennykh Khimicheskikh Veshchestv*, No. 6, pp. 150–164, Medgiz, Moscow, 1964.

Zayeva, G. N., Establishing MACs for occupational poisons, in *Metody Opredeleniya Toksichnosti i Opasnosti Khimicheskikh Veshchestv*, pp. 37–46, Meditsina, Moscow, 1970.

Zayeva, G. N., L. A. Timofievskaya, L. A. Bazerova, and N. V. Migukina, Comparative toxicities of cyclic imino compounds, *Tokcikologiya Novykh Promyshlennykh Khimicheskikh Veshchestv*, No. 10, pp. 25–35, Meditsina, Moscow, 1968.

Zhdanov, Yu. A., Correlation equations in biochemistry, *Usp. Sovrem. Biol.*, **61**(2), 187–197 (1966).

Zilber, Yu. D., Establishing hygienic standards for tricresyl phosphate, in *Materialy Respublikanskoi Itogovoi Nauchnoi Konferentsii po Gigiene*, pp. 71–72, Ministerstvo Zdravookhraneniya RSFSR, Leningrad, 1963.

Zilber, Yu. D., and E. T. Lykhina, Guidelines for the replacement of toxic chemicals in industry, in Yu. A. Osipov, Ed., *Materialy k Nauchnoi Sessii, Posviashchennoi 40-letiyu Instituta Gigiyeny Truda i Profzabolevaniy*, pp. 51–54, Institut Gigiyeny Truda i Profzabolevaniy, Leningrad, 1964.

Zimmer, K. G., *Studies on Quantitative Radiation Biology*, Oliver and Boyd, Edinburgh and London, 1961.

INDEX

Absolute lethal dose, 26
Absolute temperature, 58, 73, 91
Absorption, via gastrointestinal tract, 99-
    100
    via respiratory tract, of gases and vapors,
        94-98
        of particulate matter, 98-99
    route of and toxic effect, 10-11
    via skin, 99
        calculation of LD_{50} from data on, 404-
        405
    see also Absorption kinetics; Sorption
Absorption kinetics, 110-112 (Fig. 17)
    of gaseous substances inhaled periodically,
        125-129 (Fig. 23, 125)
    of heavy radioactive elements, 218-220
        (Fig. A19 and A20)
    of inert gases, 122-124 (Fig. 22)
    of known dose, 135-136 (Fig. 25)
    of metabolizable substances, 130-135
        (Fig. 24, 132)
    models for, see Kinetic model(s), for
        absorption
    nonlinear, 178-180 (Fig. A5)
    rate constant for, see Kinetic (rate) con-
        stant(s)
    relation to partition coefficient, 214-215
    of substances entering tissues from blood
        plasma, 139-140 (Fig. 27)
Acute action zone, 35
Adaptation (to poisons), 254, 257-258, 263,
    264
    defined, 258

mathematical model for, 269
    relation to cumulation, 258
Additivity, 272, 273, 279, 283, 285, 287,
    288
    formulas for, 285, 306, 307
    see also Combined effects; Combined
        exposure
Aerosols, estimation of toxicity indices for,
    381, 390, 397, 398 (Fig. A1), 414
    retention of in respiratory tract, 98
    role of in toxic mixtures, 296, 297, 298-
        299 (Table A5)
Affinity, for receptor sites, 244
    for tissues, 95, 100, 213, 218
Age, relation to kinetic parameters, 186-187
    sensitivity to poisons and, 5
Air humidity, influence on toxicity, 302
Alcohols, equation(s) for calculating LC_{50}
    of, 374
    plot of, 379 (Fig. 49)
    MAC for, 382, 387
        plots of, 387 (Fig. 51), 388 (Fig. 52)
    oil/water partition coefficient for, 394
        plots of, 395 (Fig. 54)
    water solubility of, 394
        plots of, 396 (Fig. 55)
Aldehydes
    equation(s) for calculating LC_{50} of, 379
    MAC for, 387, 412
        plot of, 387 (Fig. 51)
    oil/water partition coefficient for, 394
        plots of, 395 (Fig. 54)
All-or-none responses, see Quantal responses

Amines
  equation(s) for calculating LC_{50} of, 374, 381
    plots of, 379 (Fig. 49), 380 (Fig. 50)
  LD_{50} of, 381
  MAC for, 382, 387
    plots of, 387 (Fig. 51), 388 (Fig. 52)
  oil/water partition coefficient for, 394
    plots of, 395 (Fig. 54)
  threshold concentration of, 380
  water solubility of, 394
    plots of, 396 (Fig. 55)
Amount of effect (response), methods of measurement, 25
  of poison, units of, 24
Anilines, equation for calculating threshold concentration of, 380
Antagonism, 271, 272
Atomic charges, correlation with biological activity, 347
  relation to toxic properties of metal ions, 354
Atomic numbers of elements, relationship to toxicity, 341-344 (Fig. 44; Table 30)

Bactericidal activity, in homologous series, 317, 320
Balance equations, 234-237, 240
Barometric pressure, and toxicity, 14-15, 303
Basimetry, 10
Benzene, concentration-time curves for, 49
Benzene derivatives, disubstituted, structure-activity relationships among, 325
Binding of xenobiotics, 29, 102, 221
  to complexones, 354
  to plasma proteins, 167, 168, 169
  to tissue structures, 233
Biochemical individuality, 6, 26, 43, 98
Biochemical status, 191
Biochemistry, 323
Biological action zone, use of to assess cumulation, 256
Biological clock, 6
Biological variability, 6, 26, 29, 117, 146.
    See also (Inter)individual differences
Biopharmaceutics, 201
Biophases, 54

accumulation of substances in, 55-56, 69
Biorhythms, 6-10, 419
  circadian, see Circadian rhythms
  importance of for toxicology, 8, 10
  seasonal, 7
Biosphere, pollution of, xi-xii, 227
Biotransformation, 96, 101-102
  of benzidine, interspecies differences in, 16 (Table A1)
  general scheme of, 102
  kinetic aspects of, 130-133, 154-156, 166, 173-175, 225
  of rapidly metabolizable substances, 96, 97 (Fig. 12), 98
  types of reactions involved, 102
  see also Metabolism
Blastomogenic activity, 256
Body weight, correlation with species-related variables, 3
  with toxicity parameters, 18-20
  "determining principle" of, 18
  and kinetic parameters, 185, 191, 214 (Table A13)
  relation to volume of distribution, 118, 214-215
Boiling point, correlation with MAC, 333, 357, 367-368, 371, 412, 413
  with saturated vapor pressure, 374, 392
  with toxicity indices, 333, 336, 345, 369, 371, 374, 375, 379, 380, 397, 398
  relation to other constants (diagrams), 375, 393
Bologram, 274, 280-281 (Fig. 38-41), 283
Bromohydrocarbons, equation for calculating LC_{50} of, 374
Bromsulphalein test, 197, 261

C_{min}, see Threshold concentration
Carbon monoxide, equation for calculating MAC for, 42
Carcinogenic activity, 25
  of biotransformation products, 100
  of jointly acting substances, 291, 292 (Table A1)
  relation to chemical structure, 318-319, 347
Cephalization, index of, 3, 18
Charge-transfer constant, 346
Charge-transferring capacity, 346

Chemical potential, 56, 58, 59, 91, 92
  formula for, 57
  physical meaning of, 57
Chlorohydrocarbons
  equation(s) for calculating LC_{50} of, 374
    plot of, 379 (Fig. 49)
  MAC for, 387
    plot of, 387 (Fig. 51)
  oil/water partition coefficient for, 394
    plots of, 395 (Fig. 54)
Chromatographic parameters, correlation
    with lipophilicity, 350
Chromatography, 171, 172, 237, 241, 350
Chronic action zone, 35
Circadian rhythms, 8, 9 (Table 3)
  effect of on kinetic parameters, 196
Clearance, of endogenous creatinine, 198,
    199 (Table A14)
  plasma, formula for, 119
  of xenobiotics from the body, 167
  factors affecting rate of, 168
Combined effects, additive, 273, 274, 275,
    279, 285, 287, 288, 289, 290-291,
    307
  less than additive, 289-290, 291, 293,
    294, 307
  more than additive, 276, 289, 291, 292,
    307
  nomenclature for, 271-273 (Tables 22-24)
  of vapor-gas-aerosol mixtures, 294-300
  see also Combined exposure; Joint action
    studies
Combined exposure, 48, 51
  acute, 287-290
  to chemical and physical agents, 300-305
  chronic, 290-294
  and complex exposure, 306-307
Compartmental analysis, 171, 172
  in environmental toxicokinetics, 228, 232
  see also Compartments; Kinetic model(s)
Compartment(s), 106-108 (Figs. 14-16)
  central, 108
  deep, 168, 170, 244
  peripheral, 108, 179 (Fig. A3)
  shallow, 170
Competition among xenobiotics, 169, 208
Complex exposure, 48, 51, 305-308
  and combined exposure, 306-307
    formula for, 306
  defined, 306

effects from, 307-308
  formula for, 306
  and MAC, 306
Complexone(s), 356
  efficiency of, 211 (Fig. A17)
  model for action by, 209-212 (Fig. A16,
    210)
Complexone therapy, 209
  model for, 212
Computers, use of in QSAR studies, 349
  in toxicokinetics, 105, 166-167, 180, 197,
    240
  analogue, 105-106, 124, 171, 172, 232
Concentration, units of, 24, 362, 370
Concentration-time curves, 49, 94. See also
    Dose (concentration)-time relation-
    ships
Congeneric compounds, 213
  calculation of biological activity of, 322-
    328
Conjugation, 102
Correction factors, 39, 285
  to MAC, 368 (Table 32), 409, 413
  see also Safety factors
Correlation analysis, 369, 370, 379
  use of in structure-activity studies, 322
Critical dose, use of in study of cumulation,
    253, 263, 265
Crystal lattice, relation to MAC, 354-355
  to toxicity, 355
Cumulation, 25, 47, 252ff., 388, 409, 413
  and adaptation, 258
  classification of by degree, 253-254, 255,
    256 (Table 21), 399 (Table A1)
  coefficient of, see Cumulation coefficient
  evaluation of, 419
    at lethal level, 252-257
    methods, 253-255, 256, 257, 260-261,
    268
    at threshold level, 257-266
    choice of tests and doses, 264
  and habituation, 258, 259, 263
  importance of, in toxicology, 252, 257
  index of, 268
  kinetic approach to study of, 243
  prediction of, 234, 267-268
  relation to receptors, 267
  types of, 252, 267
Cumulation coefficient, 252 ff., 389, 390,
    400, 419

formulas for, 253, 254, 268
measurement of at lethal level, 253-255
   at threshold level, 257, 260-264
   difficulties of, 259-260
   relation to MAC, 256, 265
   standardization of, 268-269
   and toxicokinetics, 244
Cutoff (in toxicity), 62, 321
   prediction of, 75

D_{min}, see Threshold dose
DDT, cumulative action of, 47
   effect of in mixtures, 290, 291, 293
   on half-lives of drugs, 203
Density, correlation with MAC, 333, 367, 368, 371
   with toxicity indices, 333, 339, 369, 371
Design of new compounds, factors to be considered in, 213
Desorption, 238-239
Detoxication, 100
   mechanisms of, 102, 182, 191
Dissociation constants, for benzoic acid derivatives, 322
Distribution, 100-101
   equilibrium, see Equilibrium distribution law of, 88, 91-92
Distribution coefficient, see Partition coefficient
Dose(s) for chronic tests, equations for calculation of, 412 (Table A6), 413
   units of, 24, 362
Dose(concentration)-time relationships, 24, 42-43, 48-51
   approximation of, 30, 48
   uses of, 48, 51
      to classify substances by hazard, 50 (Table A1)
Dose-response curves, 28 (Fig. 1), 38
   approximation of, 29
   reasons for sigmoid shape of, 29
Dose-response lines, 36 (Fig. 2), 37, 42 (Fig. 3)
Dose-response relationships, 24, 25
   and mechanism of substance action, 29
   multimodal, 43-44
Dose-time-response relationships, 274
   representation of, 24
   and target and hit theories, 30
Dummy variables, 349, 352

Dynamics of uptake of xenobiotics into tissues, elements of a theory, 232-243

Ecosystem, definition of, 230
Effective doses (concentrations), median (ED_{50}), 33, 34, 35, 36, 37, 39, 41, 42
   zone of, 26
Electrolytic dissociation, 206
Electronegativity, relation to toxicity of metal oxides, 356-357
Electronic stability, relation to toxicity, 343, 354
Electronic structure, relation to biological activity, 319, 343-344
Elements, relation of toxicity to body content of, 339-340
   to electronic stability of, 343-344
   to position of in periodic table, 340-343, 354
   structures of most and least toxic, 343, 344 (Table 30)
Elimination, 102-104
   relation to decline in biological activity, 162-164
   types of, 198-199 (Fig. A14)
   see also Elimination kinetics
Elimination kinetics, 112-114 (Fig. 19), 210-211
   complex, 144-147 (Figs. 28, 145)
   determinants of, 167-169
   and interaction between xenobiotics, 203-204
   of heavy radioactive elements, 218-221 (Figs. A19 and A21)
   of mercury, 222-225 (Fig. A22, 222)
   of metabolite(s), 150-153 (Figs. 30 and 31)
   models for, see Kinetic model(s), for elimination
   by more than one route, 142-143, 176-177, 207
   nonlinear, 176-177
   rate constant for, see Kinetic (rate) constant(s)
   of substance undergoing distribution, 147-150
   of unchanged substance and metabolite(s), 154, 155-156, 158-160
   for urinary excretion, 141-142

see also Metabolites, kinetics of
Environmental factors, relation to pharma-
    cokinetics, 202-203
    to toxicity, 13-15, 301-305
Enzyme induction, 102, 202, 205, 208,
    230, 258
Enzyme kinetics, 174-175
Equieffective concentration
    as criterion of toxicity, 56
    use of to judge mode of substance action,
        66
    values of for lethal action, 61 (Table 5)
        for narcotic action, 69-71 (Table 8)
        for threshold action, 72-73 (Table 9)
Equilibrium constants, 322, 323
Equilibrium distribution (of nonelectro-
    lytes), 54 ff., 100, 419
    condition for, 57
    determination of, 68
    time taken to attain, 69
Ethers, equations for calculating LC_{50} of,
    374, 379 (Fig. 49), 380 (Fig. 50)
Exercise, relation to toxicokinetics, 195
    (Table A6)
Exposure, continuous, 12, 13
    intermittent, 12-13
    to variable concentrations, 12-13
Exposure regimen, general considerations,
    10-13
    and kinetic parameters, 202
    in study of cumulation, choice of, 264
    importance of, 255
Extrapolation of animal data to man, 1, 15,
    16, 17, 18, 51, 99, 243, 320, 419.
    See also Interspecies scaling
Extrathermodynamic approaches to QSAR
    problems, 347-353
    Hammett-Taft's 322-323, 347-348
    Hansch's, 325-328, 348-350
    and Free and Wilson's method, 328,
        350-352
    and Kubinyi's bilinear model, 352

Ferguson's principle, 56 ff., 321
    essence of, 56-57, 60
    role of in study of interaction between
        xenobiotics and organism, 92-93
    use of to evaluate mechanism of substance
        action, 68
    to judge type of activity, 65

in studies on mammals, 68-76
Food intake, effect on toxicokinetics, 194-
    195
Foreign substances, nonspecifically (non-
    electrolytically) acting, 54-56
    specifically acting, 54-56
    see also Xenobiotics
Free and Wilson's method, 328, 348
    compared with Hansch's, 328, 350-352
    mathematical expression of, 350, 351
Freundlich's adsorption isotherm, 29
Fugacity, 58-59
Fungicides, 28, 294

Gas constant, 58, 73
Genetic factors in pharmacokinetics, 185,
    186 (Fig. A8)
Graded responses, 25, 32, 34, 277
    estimation of in study of cumulation, 265
    measurement of, 25

Haber's formula, 11
    applicability of, 11-12
Habituation, 13, 47, 258, 261-263
    coefficient of, 265
    defined, 258
    importance of in study of cumulation, 261
    mechanisms of, 258-259
Half-life, 115-117
    defined, 115
    dependence of on exposure level, 182
        (Table A2)
    determination of, 113 (Fig. 18), 114 (Fig.
        19), 163-164
    effect of disease on, 196 (Table A7), 200
        (Tables A9 and A10)
    of interaction between xenobiotics on,
        203-204 (Table A12)
    formula for, 116
    interindividual differences in, 184 (Fig.
        A7), 185
    interspecies differences in, 190 (Table A5)
    relation to body weight, 194 (Fig. A12)
        to creatinine clearance, 199
Hammett's constant, 322, 326, 348
    equation, 322
Hansch's constant, 326, 349, 350, 351
    method, 325-328, 348-350
    compared with Free and Wilson's, 328,
        350-352

parabolic equation, 213, 325, 349
  physical essence of, 326
  uses of, 326-327 (Table 25)
Hazards, real, from volatile substances, 76-
    84
  compared, 82, 84
  scales of, 80-81 (Table 10), 82 (Table 11),
    83 (Table 12)
Hemodynamic factors, relation to toxico-
    kinetics, 195
Hemolytic activity, in homologous series,
    317, 320
Henry's law, 59
Heterocyclic compounds
  equation for calculating LC_{50} of, 374
  MAC of, 387
Homologous series
  calculation of toxicity indices in, graphic
    method, 321, 362-365
  Zayeva's method, 321-322, 365-366
  structure-activity relationships in, 320-
    322
  values of Zahradnik's constant for, 363
    (Table 31), 364 (Fig. 45)
  variation of properties in, 90, 91 (Fig. 8),
    92
  of thermodynamic activity in, 60 ff.
Hoorweg-Weiss' strength-duration curves,
    30
  equation, 42
Hydrocarbons, combined effects of, 287-
    288
  equation(s) for calculating LC_{50} of, 374
    plots of, 379 (Fig. 49), 380 (Fig. 50)
  MAC for, 387
    plot of, 387 (Fig. 51)
  oil/water partition coefficient for, 394
    plots of, 395 (Fig. 54)
  threshold concentration of, 380
  water solubility of, 394
    plots of, 396 (Fig. 55)
  estimation of constants and LC_{50} of,
    373-374, 376-377
  diagram, 375
  halogen-containing, comparison of LC_{50}
    values of, 377-378 (Fig. 48)
Hydrodynamics, physicochemical, 240
Hydrogen bonds, 55
Hygienic standards, for toxic substances,
    principles of establishment, 407-408

  see also Maximum allowable concentration;
    Tentative safe exposure level
Hypoxia, effect on toxicity, 303

Ideal-gas laws, 58, 73
Individual differences, see (Inter)individual
    differences
Inert gases, 54, 101
  absorption kinetics of, 122-124, 216-217
    (Fig. A18)
Inhibitory action of chemicals on mitochon-
    dria, correlation with toxicity, 401-
    404
Initial and boundary conditions, formulation
    of, 241-242
Inorganic substances, calculation of toxicity
    indices and MAC for, 382-383, 384
    (Table 37), 390
  structure-activity relationships among,
    337-344, 353-357
Insecticides, 29
  effect of solvent on toxicity of, 89
Interaction between xenobiotics, toxicoki-
    netic aspects of, 203-212
(Inter)individual differences, in kinetic para-
    meters, 183-186
  in sensitivity to poisons, 6, 27, 29, 30, 277
Interrelationship of chemical structure,
    chemical activity, physicochemical
    properties, and biological activity
    (scheme), 313
(Inter)species differences, in biotransforma-
    tion, 16 (Table A1), 188, (Table A3),
    189, 190 (Table A5)
  in kinetic parameters, 188-193
  in physiological parameters, 123
  in sensitivity to poisons, 1-3, 15-22, (Table
    A2, 17; Table A3, 18; Fig. A1, 19),
    256, 399-400 (Table A2)
  and metabolism, 2, 17
Interspecies scaling, 20-21, 191-193. See
    also Extrapolation of animal data to
    man
Ionizing radiation, and toxicity, 305
Irritant activity, in homologous series, 317-
    318, 320
Irritant gases, effect of mixtures of, 288,
    297
  equations for calculating MAC for, 386
  safe levels (TSEL) for, 401

Isobol, 274, 278-279 (Fig. 37)
Isodynamic diagram, 279, 285

Joint action of poisons, 270 ff, types of, 272
  see also Combined effects; Combined exposure
Joint action studies, analytic methods, 283-284
  graphic methods, 274-283
    deviation from additivity method, 274-278
    Loewe's method, 278-283
  nomenclature for, 271-273 (Tables 22-24)

Ketones
  equation for calculating LC_{50} of, 374
    plot of, 379 (Fig. 49)
    MAC for, 412
    threshold concentration of, 380
Kidney disease, effect of on kinetic parameters, 197-200
Kinetic (rate) constant(s)
  for absorption, calculation of, 134-135, 164-166
    formulas for, 111, 214
  for degradation, 130-131
    interindividual differences in, 183 (Fig. A6)
    role of in accumulation of xenobiotics, 214-215
    values of in different species, 188 (Table A3)
  for elimination, calculation of, 162, 163-164, 164-166
    formulas for, 113, 205
    relation to clearance of endogenous creatinine, 198, 199 (Fig. A14)
    to volume of distribution, 167
    examples of calculation, 116, 119-121
  see also Half-life
Kinetic model(s)
  for absorption into cerebrospinal fluid from blood plasma, 139
  of a known dose, 135-138
  of metabolizable substances, 130-131
  for occupational exposure to gaseous substance, 125-128
  simplest, 110-112
  taking account of physiological

parameters, 123-124
  for complexone action, 209-212
  construction of, 106, 108
  for elimination, bi- and multiexponential, 144-145
    of mercury from the body, 222-224
    of metabolite(s), 150-152, 156-160, 161
    by more than one route, 142-143, 176-178, 207-208
  for elimination, simplest, 112-114
    of substance undergoing distribution, 147-150
    of unchanged substance along with metabolite, 154, 155-156, 158-161
    by urinary excretion, 141-142
  kinds of, 104-106
  for mercury in soil and atmosphere, 228-229
  of pesticide behavior in ecosystems, 230-232
  for uptake of xenobiotics into tissues, 234-242
  uses of, 108, 109, 129

Langmuir's adsorption isotherm, 29
Lazarev's system of nonelectrolytes, 287, 376, 391, 393, 397, 404
  described, 329
LC_{50}, see Median lethal concentration
LD_{50}, see Median lethal dose
Lead, distribution of in the body, 101
  elimination of, 145, 218-219 (Fig. A19)
Lethal concentrations, 26-31, median, see Median lethal concentration
  See also Lethal doses
Lethal doses, 26-31
  median, see Median lethal dose
  quantities used for characterization of, 26-29
  zone of, 26, 27, 32
Lethal synthesis, 100
Life span, correlation with species-related variables, 2-3, 18
Lipophilicity, 329, 352
  and chromatographic parameters, 350
  parabolic relationship with absorption, 213
    with biological activity, 349
Liver disease, effect of on kinetic parameters, 196-197

MAC, see Maximum allowable concentration
MAC-time relationships, 42-43
Mass action, law of, 206
Mass transport phenomena, in living systems, 233
Mathematical models, see Kinetic model(s)
Maximum allowable concentration (MAC), 39-43
  calculation of, in homologous series, 365-366
    from inhibitory concentration, 404, (Table A4)
    for inorganic substances, 384 (Table 37), 390
    from narcotic concentration, 346
    for nonvolatile organic substances, from molecular weight, 382 (Table 36)
    from toxicity indices, 389, 390
    from saturation concentration, 414
    for volatile organic substances, from properties, 367, 372, 382 (Table 36), 384 (Table 37)
      from toxicity indices, 385, 386 (Tables 38 and 39), 387 (Table 40)
  correlation of with LD$_{50}$ of metal oxides, 356
    with properties of metal oxides, 357 (Table A4)
  correlation with properties, of organic compounds, 330, 333-334 (Table 27), 335, 336 (Fig. 43), 337, 346, 371 (Fig. 46)
    with threshold limit values, 412 (Table A6), 413
    with type of crystal lattice, 354-355
  between various kinds of, 408-409, 410-411 (Table A5), 412 (Table A6), 415, 421
  kinds of, 407
  for mixtures, 300
  plots of regression equations for, 387 (Fig. 51), 388 (Fig. 52)
  relation to cumulation, 252, 256, 265
    to inhibitory concentrations, 402-403 (Table A3)
  for residential areas and for water, calculation of, 410-411 (Table A5), 412 (Table A6), 413
    principles of establishment, 407-408

rule of setting of for multiple contaminants, 284
Maximum permissible doses (concentrations), 39-43. See also Maximum allowable concentration
Maximum permissible level, 244, 285, 308, 419. See also Maximum allowable concentration
Median lethal concentration (LC$_{50}$), calculation of from inhibitory concentration, 404 (Table A4)
  from other toxicity indices, 383, 386, (Table 38)
  from physicochemical properties, 369 (Table 33), 372, 374 (Table 34), 379, 384 (Table 37), 386 (Table 38)
  correlation of with MAC, 386 (Table 38), 387 (Table 40), 410-411 (Table A5)
  correlation of, with properties of organic substances, 330, 333-334 (Table 27), 335, 336 (Fig. 43), 371 (Fig. 46)
  diagram for estimation of for hydrocarbons, 375
  plots of regression equations for, 379 (Fig. 49), 380 (Fig. 50), 387 (Fig. 51)
  relation to inhibitory concentrations, 402-403 (Table A3)
  variation of with boiling and melting points, 398
  see also Median lethal dose
Median lethal dose (LD$_{50}$), 27-29
  calculation of for absorption via skin, 404-405
    according to Boček, 325, 366
    from inhibitory concentration, 404 (Table A4)
    from molecular weight, 381-382
    for one route of entry from value for another route, 406
  correlation of with dose for chronic tests, 412 (Table A6), 413
    with Hammett-Taft's constants, 347-348
    with MAC, 386 (Table 38), 387 (Table 40), 388 (Fig. 52) 410-411 (Table A5), 412 (Table A6)
    with normal body levels of metals, 339
    with properties of metal oxides, 356
    of metals, 339
    of metal salts, 355 (Table A3)

of organic compounds, 330, 333-334 (Table 27), 335, 337, 346, 347-348

with stabilities of metal complexes, 355-356

with threshold dose, 356

with TSEL, 400

relation to inhibitory concentrations, 402-403 (Table A3)

to route of administration, 405-406

statement in terms of probability, 27-28, 36

utility of, 28

variation of with atomic numbers of elements, 341-343 (Fig. 44)

with boiling and melting points, 397-398

in relation to route of entry, 365

Median narcotic concentration (NC_{50}), calculation of from physicochemical properties, 369 (Table 33)

correlation with properties of organic compounds, 330, 333-334 (Table 27), 335, 336 (Fig. 43), 337, 346, 371 (Fig. 46)

Melting point, correlation with MAC, 333, 357, 367-368, 371, 412

with toxicity indices, 333, 336, 369, 371, 397, 398

Mercury, toxicokinetics of, 220-225, 228-230 (Fig. A23, 229)

Metabolic rate, correlation with body weight, 3

with life span, 3

Metabolism, effect of chemical structure on, 315

of interaction between xenobiotics on, 207-208

and thermodynamic activity, 89

see also Biotransformation

Metabolites, kinetics of, 150-153, 155, 156-158, 158-160, 161, 162, 225-227

toxicity of, 100, 102

Metals, compounds of, reasons for differences in biological activity, 353-354

ions of, correlation between toxicity and properties of, 338-339 (Table 29)

periodicity of toxic properties of, 354

oxides of, correlation between toxicity and properties of, 356-357 (Table A4)

Methotrexate, clearance of from plasma in different species, 191-193 (Figs. A10 A11), 194 (Fig. A12)

Michaelis constant, 175

Michaelis-Menten's equation, 175

Model(s) for adaptation to poisons, 269

kinetic, see Kinetic model(s)

of structure-activity relationships, 323 ff., 348 ff.

Modeling, 53, 266. See also Model(s)

of toxicokinetic processes, 146-147, 171, 232, 233

scope and purposes, 104-110

Molar attraction constant, 328

Molar polarization, correlation with MAC, 346

with narcotic concentration, 346

Molar refraction, calculation of, 391

correlation of with Hansch's constant, 350

with other properties, 391, 394-397

relation to other constants (diagram), 393

with toxicity indices, 333, 369, 371, 372

Molar volume, correlation with MAC, 333, 371, 372

with other properties, 394, 395, 396

Molecular weight, correlation with dose, 330

with MAC, 333, 367-368, 371, 380, 382

with other properties, 394, 395

with toxicity indices, 333, 369, 371, 374, 375, 379, 381, 382

relation to other constants (diagram), 375

Multiple contaminants of work environment, hygienic standards for, 284-286, 295

Mutagenic activity, 256

relationship to chemical structure, 319

Narcotic concentration, 134

median, see Median narcotic concentration

relation to lethal, 84

Narcotics, combined effects of, 288

types of, 376

described, 317

Navier-Stokes equation, 240

NC_{50}, see Median narcotic concentration

Neutron activation analysis, 171, 184

Nitriles and cyanides, equation for calculating LC_{50} of, 374
Nitro compounds, equation(s) for calculating LC_{50} of, 374
    plot of, 380 (Fig. 50)
    MAC for, 382, 387, 412
    plots of, 387 (Fig. 51), 388 (Fig. 52)
    water solubility of, 394
    plots of, 396 (Fig. 55)
No-effect doses (concentrations), 41, 51
Noise, and toxicity, 303
Nonelectrolytes, distribution of in the body, 100
    equilibrium distribution of, 56 ff.
    Lazarev's system of, see Lazarev's system of nonelectrolytes
    narcotic effects of, 316-317
Nonelectrolytic action (activity), 54, 316, 362
    degree of, 56
    features of, 54-56
    of potent poisons, 55
    and thermodynamic activity, 59, 63-65, 79
Nonlinear effects, 172-182
    causes of, 173-176
    quantitation of, 174-177
    transition to as characteristic of toxicity, 181-182
Nonparametric statistics, 418
    use of to assess threshold actions, 33, 41
Nonspecific action (activity), see Nonelectrolytic action (activity)
Nonspecifically (nonelectrolytically) acting substances, definition, 284
Nonvolatile organic substances, calculation of toxicity indices and MAC for, 381-382, 389-390, 412
    relation of toxicity of to boiling and melting points of, 397-398
Normality, limits of, 31

Olfactory thresholds, correlation with physical properties of benzene derivatives, 345 (Table A1)
Oligodynamic substances, 43
Organic solvents, habituation to, 259
Organic substances, nonvolatile, see Nonvolatile organic substances
    structure-activity relationships among,

320-337, 345-353
    volatile, see Volatile organic substances
Organoboron compounds, 315
Organochlorine compounds, cumulative action of, 255, 261, 262, 263
    equation for calculating MAC for, 389
    toxicokinetics of, 230-232
Organofluoric compounds, 295
    structure-activity relationships among, 315
Organophosphorus compounds, cumulative action of, 255, 258, 261, 262 (Fig. 33), 263
    equation(s) for calculating LD_{50} of, 381
    MAC for, 389
    safe levels (SEL) for, 400
    joint action of, 288, 289
    and chlorinated hydrocarbons, 290
    structure-activity relationships among, 315, 316, 347
Organosilicon compounds, 300
    structure-activity relationships among, 315
Overton-Mayer's equation, 326
Oxygen tension, effect of on half-life of antipyrine, 195-196

Parabiosis, 259
Parachor, use of to calculate toxicity, 326, 328
Paradoxical effects, 43-47, (Fig. 4, 44)
    defined, 43
    importance of, 44, 47
    mechanisms of, 45-47
    and statistics, 44-45
Partial vapor pressure, 58
Partition coefficient, 110ff.
    between biophases, 57
    blood/air, 10, 11, 123, 133, 361
    calculation of, 119, 121
    definition of, 239
    formula for, 91
    octanol/water, 326, 348, 352
    oil/water, calculation of, 391, 394, 395
        correlation with toxicity indices and MAC, 333, 371
    relation to absorption, 214-215, 216-217 (Fig. A18)
    tissue/blood, 100, 101
    water/air, 133
        formula for, 392
        relation to other properties (diagram), 393

Pathologic conditions, effect of on toxicokinetic parameters, 196-201
Pattern recognition methods, use of in
QSAR studies, 352-353
Periodic table, and MAC, 343
use of to evaluate biological activity, 340-
344 (Fig. 44, 342; Table 30, 344)
Permeability, 68
of cell membranes, 206
of cuticles, 89
of skin, 99
Permeability constant, 139
Pesticides, 227, 347
cumulation of, 255, 256, 257
effect from consecutive exposure to, 294
of at high altitude, 303
of under high temperature, 302
equation(s) for calculating LD_{50} of, 381
MAC for, 389
safe levels (TSEL) for, 400
model for toxicokinetics of, 230-232
routes of absorption, 305
Pharmacokinetics, linear and nonlinear, 173
relation to toxicokinetics, 170
see also Toxicokinetics
Pharmacology, 34, 201, 203, 213, 270
Phenols, equation for calculating LD_{50} of,
382
Physical toxicity, 63, 316
Physicochemical constants, see Physicochemical properties
Physicochemical properties, of inorganic
substances, correlation with toxicity
indices and MAC, 337 ff., 353 ff.,
382-383, 384
of organic substances, classification of,
335-337
correlation with each other, 391ff.
with toxicity indices and MAC, 330
ff., 345 ff., 361-362, 367 ff., 397-
398, 412
diagram for estimation of for hydrocarbons, 375
values of, 331-332
relation to kinetic parameters, 213
variation of in homologous series, 90, 91,
92
see also Boiling point; Density; Melting
point; Molar refraction; Molar volume; Molecular weight; Parachor;

Partition coefficient; Refractive index; Saturated vapor pressure; Solubility; Surface tension
Physiologic variables, model for absorption
taking account of, 123-124
modifying effects of on toxicokinetics,
194-196
Polyarthritis, effect of on pharmacokinetics,
201
Position isomerism, 314
Potentiation, 271, 273
Probit analysis, use of to describe dose-
response relationships, 37-38
in study of cumulation, 264, 265
of joint action of poisons, 277 (Fig. 36),
278

Quantal responses, 25, 32, 34, 277
estimation of in study of cumulation, 264,
265
measurement of, 25
Quantitative structure-activity relationships,
see Structure-activity relationships,
role of
Quantum-chemical concepts, 338, 347

Radiant energy, relation to toxicity, 304
Radioactive elements, 171, 172, 210
heavy, toxicokinetics of, 218-220 (Fig.
A19 and A20), 221 (Fig. A21)
Range, of biological activity as defined in
terms of thermodynamic activity,
85, 86 (Table 13), 87
therapeutic, see Therapeutic range
Rank(-order) tests, 33, 34
Refractive index, correlation with LC_{50},
333, 369, 371
with MAC, 333, 367-368
"Rate" method, of treating excretion data,
158-160
"Rate versus amount" method, of treating
excretion data, 162
Regression coefficients, comparison of for
equations relating MAC and LC_{50}
to boiling point, 413-414
Relative lethal toxicity, 339-340
Relative toxicity assays, 30, 36, 38
Retention (of xenobiotics) in respiratory
tract, 96, 97 (Figs. 11 and 12), 98
interindividual differences in, 98

Rhythmometry, 10
Richardson's rule, 62

Safe doses (concentrations), 41, 42 (Fig. 3)
Safety factors, 51, 215, 388, 389
  calculation of, 390, 399
  and permissible doses, 39-40
  relation to cumulation coefficient, 256
Saturated vapor pressure, calculation of from boiling point, 374, 392
  correlation with toxicity indices and MAC, 333, 367, 371
  relation to other properties, 375
    to volatility, 78
Sensitivity to poisons, factors contributing to, 2
  individual differences in, 6, 27, 29, 30, 277
  life span and, 2
  relation to age, 5
  seasonal variations in, 7
  sex differences in, 3-4 (Table 1)
  species differences in, see (Inter)species differences, in sensitivity to poisons
Sensitization, 256
Sex differences, in retention of xenobiotics, 187-188
  in sensitivity to poisons, 3-4 (Table 1)
"Sigma-minus" method (of treating excretion data), 160-161
Sign test, 33
Solubility, absorption via skin and, 99
  biotransformation and, 99, 103
  calculation of from other properties, 394, 396
  correlation with toxicity indices and MAC, 333, 371
  of metal compounds, relation to toxicity of, 339, 353
  relation to other properties (diagrams), 375, 393
    to permeability, 89
    to range of substance action, 88
    to thermodynamic activity, 88, 90 (Table 14)
  retention of xenobiotics in respiratory tract and, 94, 96, 98-99
Solubility coefficient, water/air, 110

Sorption (of xenobiotics into tissues), defined, 233
  equations for kinetics of, 238, 239
    for statics of, 239
  relative, 237
Species differences, see (Inter)species differences
Specific action (activity), features of, 54-56
  relation to thermodynamic activity, 64, 79
Specifically acting substances, definition, 284
Spectrometry, mass, 172
Spectrophotometry, 171
Stability constant(s), 209, 210, 356
Standard potential of metals, relation to toxicity of, 338, 339, 356, 357
Steric effects of substituents, 323, 349
Structure-activity relationships, among inorganic substances, 337-344, 353-357
  among organic substances, 320-337, 345-353
  in homologous series, 320-322
  outside groups of congeners, 329-337
  in various groups of congeners, 322-328
Structure-activity studies, role of, 313, 315-316, 420
Structural nonspecificity, 316
Summated threshold index, use of in study of cumulation, 260-262, 264, 266
Summation, 271. See also Additivity
Susceptibility to poisons, see Sensitivity to poisons
Surface tension, correlation with LC_{50}, 333, 369
  with MAC, 333, 336, 367-368
  with threshold concentration, 333, 336, 369
Synergism, 271, 272

Taft's equation, 323
Temperature, effect on toxicity, 13-14, 203, 301-302, 304
  relation to MAC, 302
    to pharmacokinetics, 202-203
Tentative safe exposure level (TSEL), calculation of by stepwise method, 399-400
  equations for, 400, 401
Teratogenic activity, 25
  relationship to chemical structure, 319-320

Therapeutic range, definitions of, 34-35,
    85
  quantitative uncertainty of, 35
  relation to toxicity zone, 38
Thermal trauma, effect of on calcium elim-
    ination, 201
Thermodynamic activity, 58 ff., 202, 371
  bactericidal, values of, 62 (Table 6)
  as criterion of type of substance action,
    63-64, 92
  determination of by inter- or extrapola-
    tion, 75
  in solution, 59
  empiric use of by Fühner, 60
  equieffective, values of for lethal action,
    61 (Table 5)
    for narcotic action, 69-71 (Table 8)
    for threshold action, 72-73 (Table 9)
    variation of in homologous series, 60˙
      ff., 68, 74 ff., 88, 92
  fictitious, 79, 88
  formulas for, 58, 59
  and metabolism, 89, 93
  physical meaning of, 58
  range of, 60, 63-64, 74, 75, 85, 88
  relation to insecticidal potency, 88
    to solubility, 88, 90 (Table 14)
  rule of equal activity for equal effect,
    66-68
  use of to classify substances by type of
    action, 69-71, (Table 8), 74-75
    by hazard, 79, 80-81 (Table 10), 82
      (Table 11), 83 (Table 12), 84
Thermodynamic capacity, 88, 202
Thermodynamic concentration, 58
Thermodynamic equilibrium, 54, 56 ff.
Threshold concentration (C_{min}), 7, 31-34,
    85, 86
  calculation of from other toxicity indices,
    383, 385, 386 (Table 38)
    from properties, 369 (Table 33), 372,
      380 (Table 35)
  correlation of with properties of organic
    substances, 330, 333-334 (Table
    27), 335, 336 (Fig. 43), 371 (Fig.
    46)
  irritant, correlation with MAC, 386
    (Table 39)
    with TSEL, 401
  see also Threshold dose (D_{min})

Threshold dose (D_{min}), 31-34
  correlation with LD_{50}, 356
    with properties of metal oxides, 356-
      357
  definition of, 31
  determination of, 32-34
  importance of, 31
  statement of in terms of probability, 34,
    41
  uncertainty of, 31-32
Threshold limit values, 412, 413
Thyroid dysfunction, effect of on half-lives
    of substances, 200-201
Time-response curves, reasons for sigmoid
    shape of, 30
Time-response relationships, 24, 30
Tolerance, 255. See also Habituation
Total body burden, 48, 51
  maximum permissible, formula for, 307
Toxic action zone, see Toxicity zone
Toxicity, absolute (theoretical), 77
  chemical, 64
  cutoff in, 62, 75, 321
  importance of quantitative assessment of,
    23, 25-26
  physical, 63
  time-dependent and time-independent, 11
  two-phase, 77
    defines, 77-78
    relation to thermodynamic activity, 79
    uses of, 78, 79
    variation of in homologous series, 78
  variation of with atomic numbers of ele-
    ments, 341-344 (Figs. 44, 342; Table
    30, 344)
    with valency, 341
Toxicity criteria
  importance of, 23
  kinds of, 25
  see also Toxicity indices
Toxicity indices, correlation with each other,
    383 ff., 399 ff., 408 ff.
  with physicochemical properties, 330 ff.,
    345-347, 353 ff., 361 ff., 409, 412,
    413
  determination of by calculation, 361 ff.,
    397 ff.
  prospects for, 420-421
  quantitative uncertainty of, 28, 31, 35-36,
    42

statement in terms of probability, 28, 33-
   34, 38, 41, 418
see also Maximum allowable concentration; Median lethal concentration;
   Medial lethal dose (LD$_{50}$); Median
   narcotic concentration (NC$_{50}$);
   Tentative safe exposure level
   (TSEL); Threshold concentration;
   Threshold dose
Toxicity parameters, correlation with body
   weight, 18-19
rational assessment of, 244
and route of absorption, 11
see also Toxicity indices
Toxicity zone, 34-39
characterization of, 36-38
definitions of, 35
and mechanism of substance action, 36
quantitative uncertainty of, 35
relation to permissible doses and concentrations, 39, 40
to therapeutic range, 38
Toxicokinetics, 104, 106
chemical structure, physicochemical properties, and, 212-215
defined, 170
ecological (environmental), 227-232
defined, 227
of mercury, 228-230
of organochlorine pesticides, 230-232
of heavy radioactive elements, 218-220
linear, 110 ff.
mechanisms of toxic action and, 243
methods used in, 171-172
modifying factors, 182 ff.
   exposure regimen, 201-202
   route of absorption, 202
nonlinear, 172-182. See also Nonlinear
   effects
   compared with linear, 175
and pollution control, 244
prospects for, 244-245
relation to pharmacokinetics, 170
Toxicological experiments, kinds of, 24,
   25
Transfer of animal data to man, see Extrapolation of animal data to man;
   Interspecies scaling
Transition metals, 355
correlation between toxicity and

properties of, 338-339
Transport-distribution relationships, 69,
   213, 315
Trichloroethylene and its metabolites, tox-
   icokinetics of, 225-227 (Table A15)
TSEL, see Tentative safe exposure level

Ultrasound, and toxicity, 303-304

Valency, relation to toxicity, 341
Van der Waals forces, 55
Vapor-gas-aerosol mixtures, 294-300
approaches to setting hygienic standards
   for, 286, 295-296, 300
classification of, 295
mechanism of action, 296-297
role of aerosols in, 296 (Table A4), 297,
   298-299 (Table A5)
of gaseous components of, 297, 300
Vibration, effect on toxicity, 303
Vinyl esters, narcotic action of, 55
paradoxical effect of, 46
relationship between narcotic and lethal
   concentrations of, 84
transformation in the body, 74-75, 89,
   318
Volatile organic substances, calculation of
   toxicity indices and MAC for, 367-
   372, 383, 385-389, 412, 413
for individual classes of, 372-381, 382
   (Table 36), 387 (Table 40; Fig. 51),
   388 (Fig. 52), 412 (Table A6), 413
correlations between physicochemical
   properties of, 392-397
between toxicity indices and properties
   of, 330-337 (Table 27, 333-334; Fig.
   43, 336), 361-362, 367-372 (Fig. 46,
   371), 372-381
see also Volatile substances
Volatile substances, absorption of, 94-98,
   122-129
elimination of, 102-103
evaluation of cumulative properties of,
   259
habituation to, 259
organic, see Volatile organic substances
real hazards from, 76-84
Volatility, 77, 78, 363, 381
Volume of distribution, 117-121
characterization of, 168

definition of, 117
methods of determination, 117-118
relation to half-life, 119, 199
Weber-Fechner's law, 29
Wilcoxon's test, 34
Wilder's law of initial value, 8, 10

Xenobiotics, general scheme of passage
    through the body, 103 (Fig. 13),
    104

see also Foreign substances

Zahradnik's constants, 323, 326, 362-365
    diagram, 364 (Fig. 45)
    equations, 323, 324
    applicability of, 324-325
Zayeva's method of calculating toxicity in-
    dices and MAC, 321-322, 365-366
Zero-order processes, 154, 163,
    174